NUTRITION AND DIET RESEARCH PROGRESS

DIETARY FIBER

SOURCES, PROPERTIES AND THEIR RELATIONSHIP TO HEALTH

NUTRITION AND DIET RESEARCH PROGRESS

Additional books in this series can be found on Nova's website
under the Series tab.

Additional e-books in this series can be found on Nova's website
under the e-book tab.

NUTRITION AND DIET RESEARCH PROGRESS

DIETARY FIBER

SOURCES, PROPERTIES AND THEIR RELATIONSHIP TO HEALTH

DAVID BETANCUR-ANCONA, M.D.
LUIS CHEL-GUERRERO, M.D.
AND
MAIRA RUBI SEGURA-CAMPOS, M.D.
EDITORS

New York

For permission to use material from this book please contact us:
Telephone 631-231-7269; Fax 631-231-8175
Web Site: http://www.novapublishers.com

Library of Congress Cataloging-in-Publication Data

Library of Congress Control Number: 2013947629

ISBN: 978-1-62808-931-8

Published by Nova Science Publishers, Inc. † New York

Contents

Preface

Dietary fiber is the edible portion of plants or analogous carbohydrates that are resistant to digestion and adsorption in the human small intestine with complete or partial fermentation in the large intestine. Dietary fiber includes polysaccharides, oligosaccharides, and associated plant substances. According to solubility, dietary fiber may be classified as soluble dietary fiber or insoluble dietary fiber, and both types are associated with particular metabolic and physiological effects in human. High dietary fiber diets are associated with the prevention, reduction and treatment of some diseases. Dietary fiber intake provides many health benefits. A generous intake of dietary fiber reduces risk for developing the diseases as coronary heart disease, stroke, hypertension, diabetes, obesity, and certain gastrointestinal disorders. Furthermore, increased consumption of dietary fiber improves serum lipid concentrations, lowers blood pressure, improves blood glucose control in diabetes, promotes regularity, aids in weight loss, and appears to improve immune function. The physiological effects are related to the physicochemical and functional properties of dietary fiber. It is widely known that dietary fibers obtained by different methods and from different sources, performs differently during their transit through gastrointestinal tract, depending on their chemical composition and physicochemical characteristics and on the processing that food undergo. The interest in food rich in fiber increased in the recent decades, and the importance of this food constituent has led to the development of a large market for fiber-rich products and ingredients. Current recommendations for dietary fiber intake are related to age, gender, and energy intake, and the general recommendation for adequate intake is 14 g/1000 kcal. This adequate intake includes non-starch polysaccharides, analogous carbohydrates (e.g., resistant starches), lignin, and associated substances. Using the energy guideline of 2000 kcal/day for women and 2600 kcal/day for men, the recommended daily dietary fiber intake is 28 g/day for adult women and 36 g/day for adult men. The role of dietary fiber in health and nutrition has stimulated a wide range of research activities.

For the above mentioned the purpose of this book is to analyze the sources, properties and the relationship from dietary fiber with the health. The book has eleven chapters: (1) Dietary fiber from the food industry byproducts, (2) Pectins: source, properties and their relationship to health, (3) Dietary fiber as ingredient for the meat industry, (4) Dietary fiber in meat products: functional and bioactive ingredient, (5) Antioxidant dietary fiber: sources and applications, (6) Antioxidant dietary fiber from tropical fruits, (7) Pomegranate. A potential source of antioxidant dietary fiber, (8) Characterization and functionality of by-products from chia (*Salvia hispanica* L.) seeds of Argentina, (9) Effect of drying treatment on primary nutrients and antioxidant activities of *Stevia rebaudiana* Bertoni stems, (10) fibrous fraction of hard-to-cook bean (*Phaseolus vulgaris*) as potential additive in food industry and (11) dietary fiber: from concept to realization.

We are grateful to all internationally expertize and renowned authors for their state-of-the-art compilation of recent rapid developments in this field, which made possible the publication of this book. We believe that this book deserves a broad readership in the disciplines of nutrition, food science, pharmaceuticals, and biochemistry and nutraceutical/functional foods. This book could also be useful as a comprehensive reference book by senior undergraduate and graduate students, as well as by nutraceutic and pharmaceutical industries. We thank members of the production team at NOVA for their time, effort, advice and expertise.

Maira Rubi Segura Campos,
Luis Chel Guerrero,
David Betancur Ancona,
Universidad Autónoma de Yucatán

In: Dietary Fiber
Editors: D. Betancur-Ancona, L. Chel-Guerrero et al.
ISBN: 978-1-62808-931-8

Chapter 1

Dietary Fiber from the Food Industry by-Products

Inmaculada Mateos-Aparicio*[*], *Araceli Redondo-Cuenca* and *M. José Villanueva

Departamento de Nutrición y Bromatología II, Bromatología,
Facultad de Farmacia, Universidad Complutense de Madrid, Madrid, Spain

Abstract

The production of processed food is on the rise and the food industries are producing large amounts of by-products, such as those generated by the juice industry or when processing vegetables and legumes for the frozen and canned food industries. By-products are generated during the processing of plant food in large quantities and pose economic and environmental problems due to their high volumes and disposal costs. They are abundant and represent an inexpensive material that has been undervalued until now, being only used as fuel or fertilizer. However, there is an increasing interest in recovering these waste materials because of their technological or nutritional properties. Today they are considered as a possible source of functional compounds, such as dietary fiber, which can be used to develop dietary supplements such as additives for low-in-fiber food products and in the design of new functional foods.

Consumers are becoming increasingly aware of the importance of diet and health, but a large proportion of the population lacks of an adequate intake of fruits and/or vegetables. Dietary supplements and food fortification could be an alternative route to the consumption of plant components that may provide health benefits. Dietary fiber has all the characteristics to be considered an important ingredient in the formulation of functional foods, playing an important role in many physiological processes and in the prevention of diseases of different origins.

[*] E-mail: inmateos@ucm.es.

1. Introduction

The food industry is increasingly taking steps to reduce the environmental impact of organic waste, including the recovery and utilization of by-products for use as livestock feed, composting, or for the production of electrical or thermal energy. These by-products can also be used as a source of functional ingredients, since they contain a large quantity of high-value compounds such as fiber, proteins, antioxidants, etc.

Dietary fiber has all the characteristics to be considered an important ingredient in the formulation of functional foods, playing an important role in many physiological processes and in the prevention of diseases of different origins. The recommended intake of dietary fiber is not the same in all countries; while the UK proposes 18 g/day of dietary fiber expressed as non-starch polysaccharides (NSP), this amount increases to 30 g/d in Germany, and the United States recommends 38 g/d for men and 26 g/d for women. A Mediterranean diet, typical in Spain, Italy and Greece, provides a significant amount of dietary fiber as it is rich in vegetables, cereals, fruits and legumes; the recommended intake in these countries being 20 g/d for men and 15.7 g/d for women (Rodríguez et al. 2006). Considering that actual western fiber intake falls far short of these amounts, the search for appropriate sources to enrich low-fiber foods becomes more necessary. The study of the different by-products, especially those with a high yield and a good insoluble dietary fiber (IDF) / soluble dietary fiber (SDF) ratio, is thus required to maintain good health and prevent food-related diseases (Mateos-Aparicio, 2012).

The role of plant components and their potential effects on human health has been thoroughly studied in recent years. Epidemiological studies have found that eating fruits, vegetables and legumes provides health benefits, such as reducing the risk of both coronary heart disease and certain kinds of cancer. A minimum of five servings a day of vegetables and fruits is suggested (Heimendinger and Chapelsky, 1996). Consumers are becoming aware of the importance of diet in relation to health problems, but a large proportion of the population lacks of an adequate intake of fruits, vegetables and/or legumes. Thus, dietary supplements and food fortification may be an alternative route to the consumption of plant components that have health benefits. Since consumers tend to refuse synthetic additives, functional ingredients should preferably be from natural sources.

Globally, around one-third of the edible parts of food produced for human consumption gets lost or wasted. This amounts to about 1.3 billion tn/year and reflects not only food processing wastes, but also food losses (Gustavsson et al. 1996; Galanakis, 2012). Food wastes and by-products are residues with a high organic load, which are usually produced during raw materials processing of foodstuffs and can be liquid or solid. The fact that these substances are separated during the production process as undesirable materials defines them as wastes in most European legislations (Galanakis, 2012; EEC, 1975 and 1991). In contrast, the term *food by-products* is increasingly used by scientists in the field to indicate that these substrates have functional compounds and they should be taken into account when developing new products with a market value. In low-income countries, food wastes are primary generated during agricultural production and secondarily during postharvest handling or storage. Food losses in industrialized countries occur in both the agricultural and consumption stages (Gustavsson et al. 1996; Galanakis, 2012). Scientists focus mainly on the recovery of functional compounds derived from agricultural and food processing by-products. These sources are abundant, are located in relatively few locations and are less susceptible to deterioration compared to the waste produced at the end of the food supply chain (Galanakis, 2012).

The wastes generated by various branches of the food industry can be divided into two main groups, plant or animal origin. Although, there are many examples of valorisation of animal wastes such as using the whey from cheese processing as a source of lactose and proteins (Madureira et al. 2010), or protein hydrolyzates from fish by-products (Kristinsson and Rasco, 2000), currently there is considerable emphasis on the recovery of vegetable wastes (Elleuch et al. 2011). Schieber et al. 2001 described plant by-products as those substances generated during the processing of plant food in large quantities that pose economic and environmental problems due to their high volumes and disposal costs. Therefore, the components that remain after isolating the main constituent are abundant and represent an inexpensive material that has been undervalued until now, being only used as fuel or fertilizer. The problem of disposing by-products is made even more difficult due to legal limitations. Today, they are considered a promising source of functional compounds.

As a result, the exploitation of agro-food wastes may help resolve economic and environmental problems and would open the possibility of reusing them to obtain different functional ingredients such as dietary fiber. The importance of these substances has led to the development of a large and potential market for products and ingredients, and there is currently a trend to find new sources.

2. Dietary Fiber as Functional Ingredient

To appreciate the importance of functional foods it helps to understand how nutrition research has changed in the last century. For the first half of the twentieth century nutrition science focused on establishing minimum requirements for essential nutrients to avoid deficiency diseases. At present, the centre of attention in developed countries is on the concept of balanced nutrition based on a well-rounded diet to promote health and decrease the risks of diet-related diseases (Mateos-Aparicio, 2012).

The use of functional food in optimum nutrition is aimed at improving individual physiological functions to ensure greater well-being and health throughout life. At the beginning of 1980, the Japanese government funded research into the analysis, development and design of functional foods. In 1991, as part of a national effort to reduce the increasing costs of medical care, a category of potentially beneficial foods called Foods for Specific Health Use (FOSHU) was established. More recently, many new terms have appeared related to FOSHU such as nutraceuticals, designed food, enriched food or functional food. In Europe, the most significant effort in the scientific approach to functional foods can be found in the task force from the International Life Science Institute-ILSI Europe, sponsored by the European Commission under the project entitled Functional Food Science in Europe (FUFOSE). This project established that "a food product can be considered as functional if it has satisfactorily been proved that it produces a beneficial effect on one or more physiological functions, besides its conventional nutritional effects, this being relevant for improving human health". It is important to note that functional foods, in the amounts normally ingested in our diet, must keep their nutritional role together with their capacity for producing beneficial effects on specific physiological functions (Roberfroid, 2000; Ashwell, 2002; Howlet, 2008; FECYT, 2005). Different compounds can be considered functional ingredients, and the health properties of dietary fiber, which is the focus of this chapter, are well-known and have been extensively tested.

The concept of dietary fiber has changed considerably in recent years. It is now recognized that dietary fiber encompasses a much broader range of substances than was acknowledged previously and that it has greater physiological significance than previously thought. The most accepted definitions are from American Association of Cereal Chemists (2001), ILSI and Codex Alimentarius (Gray, 2006). In Europe, EFSA (2010) recently issued a document that describes dietary fiber as the "non-digestible carbohydrates plus lignin, including non-starch polysaccharides (NSP) – celluloses, hemicelluloses, pectins, hydrocolloids (i.e., gums, mucilages, β-glucans), resistant oligosaccharides – fructo-oligosaccharides (FOS), galacto-oligosaccharides (GOS), other resistant oligosaccharides, resistant starches – consisting of physically enclosed starch, some types of raw starch granules, retrograded amylose, chemically and/or physically modified starches, and lignin". The characteristics of dietary fiber make it an important ingredient in formulating diverse functional foods due to its beneficial effects (AACC, 2001; Gray, 2006; Rodríguez et al. 2006; EFSA, 2010) (Table 1).

Table 1. Health improvement characteristics of dietary fiber

Satiety
Decreased intestinal transit time
Greater excretion of fat and protein
Delayed glucose absorption
Decreased glycemic index
Maintenance of intestinal microbiota
Metabolites production
Energy production
Prebiotic effect
Prevention of colon cancer
Immune system enhancement
Hypocholesterolemic effect
Prevention of cardiovascular diseases

Dietary fiber is frequently divided into soluble and insoluble fiber, and the solubility appears to confer a range of health benefits. Thus, soluble dietary fiber (SDF) is generally associated with potential prebiotic characteristics due to the fermentation process, which produces short-chain fatty acids, principally acetate, propionate and butyrate. Butyrate has been found to act as a protective agent against experimental tumorigenesis, and propionate could have hypocholesterolemic effects (Martínez-Villaluenga et al. 2005; Gray, 2006). Furthermore, SDF is usually considered a significant factor in the prevention of cardiovascular disease due to its role in reducing cholesterol levels; it also appears to improve glucose tolerance in diabetic patients, has anti-inflammatory and anti-carcinogenic effects on the digestive system, and shows a positive effect on diarrhoea, constipation and irritable bowel (Chandalia et al., 2000; Bosaeus, 2004; Gray, 2006). Insoluble dietary fiber (IDF), on the other hand, is frequently related to an increase in faecal bulk and a reduction in gastrointestinal transit time (Gray, 2006).

3. Recovery of Dietary Fiber from by-Products and Applications

3.1. Fruit and Vegetables By-Products

Fruits and vegetables produce large amounts of waste in the different stages of food processing such as seeds, skins, peels, stones, pips and whole fruits that do not meet quality standards. These discards are usually reused as animal or supplement feeds, fertilizers or to generate energy (Schieber et al. 2001). However, they present different high-added value compounds including the fiber fraction, which contains both soluble and insoluble fiber compounds, and minor components such as polyphenols or vitamins that can be used for designing new functional foods.

The most widely investigated by-products with potential health benefits are fruits such as orange (*Citrus sinensis*), apple (*Malus domestica*), grape (*Vitis vinifera* L.), pineapple (*Ananas comosus*), mango (*Mangifera indica*) or stones from fruit such as the peach (*Prunus persica*). Other research has been carried out on vegetable by-products such as the tomato (*Lycopersicon esculentum*), onion (*Allium cepa* L.), asparagus (*Asparagus officinalis*), potato (*Solanum tuberosum* L.) or artichoke (*Cynara scolymus*). During their industrial processing, high percentages of solid wastes are produced, eg. citrus (up to 50%), apple (40%), pineapple (50%), peach (25%), tomato (15%), asparagus (40-50%), onions (50%), and artichoke (65-70%) (Goñi and Hervert-Hernámdez, 2011; Pérez-Cózar, 2011; Ros et al. 2012).

In recent decades the literature has reported that plant by-products contain high levels of fiber with a great potential as a functional ingredient. Total dietary fiber (TDF) content from orange peel, cv Valencia, was 54% DM and from cv Liucheng 51.5% DM (Chau and Huang, 2003; Figuerola et al. 2005). Orange by-products are particularly rich in pectins, especially in the albedo tissue. Pectic polysaccharides (about 55%) are made up of homogalacturonan (HG), rhamnogalacturonan I (RGI), rhamnogalacturonan II (RGII) with arabinogalactan Type- I and arabinan. They also contain cellulose (22%) and other non-cellulosic polysaccharides (14 %), including xyloglucans (10%), heteromannans (2%) and heteroxylans (2%) (Prasabari et al. 2011). Apple pomace is the by-product obtained after the elaboration of cider (a low alcohol content beverage) and contains the remains of pressed apples (skins, deeds, pulp). TDF values of this by-product range from 42.5 to 65.6% DM (Sudha et al. 2007; Pérez-Cózar, 2011; Ktenioudaki et al. 2013). Apple pomace fiber polysaccharides are represented mainly by glucose and uronic acids. Arabinose and galactose have an important contribution that suggests the presence of pectic substances made up of homogalacturonans and arabinans, arabinogalactans and galactans that may come from the side chains (Mateos-Aparicio et al. 2011; Pérez-Cózar, 2011). Benítez et al. (2011) reported TDF results for onion bagasse of between 36.1 and 45.3% DM depending on cultivar. The monosaccharide composition of dietary fiber is mainly made up of glucose, uronic acids and galactose; whereas xylose, mannose, and arabinose occurred in small amounts. This fact could indicate that the cellulosic matrix was closely related to hemicelluloses (probably xyloglucans) and pectic polysaccharides, mainly homogalacturonans, whereas arabinans and galactans had a smaller role in this matrix. These authors indicated that onion waste is unfortunately not ideal for the usual outlets for vegetable wastes. Its aromatic characteristics are too pungent for animal feed and it cannot be used as a fertilizer due to its phytopathogenic effects. Therefore, the authors propose applying sterilization to stabilize onion by-products and to improve their composition and physico-chemical fiber properties in order to use them as a potential ingredient in functional foods. The TDF content of industrial white asparagus by-product ranged from 62% to 77% DM. Fuentes-Alventosa et al. (2009) showed that cellulose was the main polymer in this fiber (up to 3 fold higher) and suggest the presence of arabinoxylans and xyloglucans as the main hemicelluloses since xylose accounted for more than 50% of the monomeric composition. The by-products from Artichoke (outer bracts, stems, leaves and apical zone) are rich in dietary fiber (61-66 % DM) (Lutz et al. 2011; Pérez-Cózar, 2011). The monomeric composition of the polysaccharide fiber from artichokes includes high amounts of glucose, arabinose, xylose and uronic acid and minor proportions of rhamnose, mannose and galactose, which evidence the presence of cellulose, pectic substances (rhamnogalacturonans) and hemicelluloses such as arabinoxylans (Pérez-Cózar, 2011). Li et al. (2010) reported that the Jerusalem artichoke stalk contained cellulose (43.7% DM), hemicelluloses (25.6% DM), and lignin (14.1% DM), thus 70% of the weight of the stem is made up of cellulose and hemicelluloses. Tomato-processing by-product, also known as tomato pomace, contains the peel and seeds and represents around 4% of the fruit weight and 59% of the fiber on a dry weight basis (Del Valle et al. 2006). Navarro-Gonzalez et al. (2011) showed that tomato peels contain 86.1% of the TDF and that the most representative fraction was the IDF (71.82%). The main hemicellulosic polysaccharides are xyloglucomannans and there is also a small amount of xylan-pectic complex (Seymour et al. 1990). Side chain pectic polysaccharides from tomato are composed mainly of β-(1-4)-linked galactopyranosyl and α-(1-5)-linked arabinofuranosyl residues (Chandra et al. 2009).

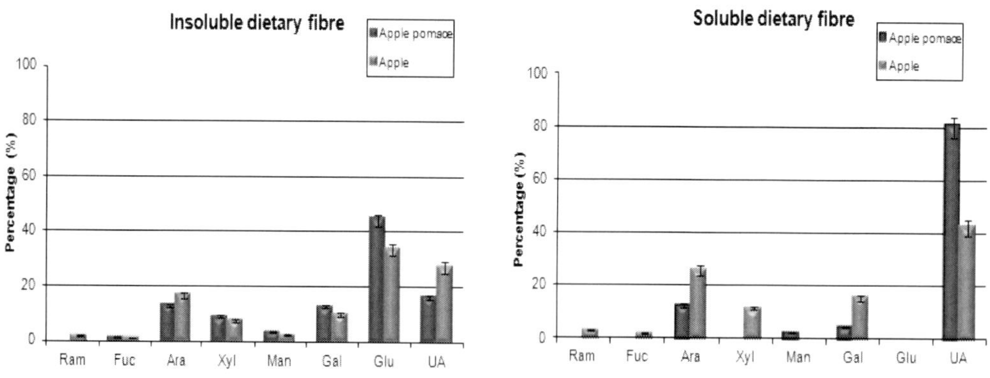

Figure 1. Comparison of the monosaccharide composition in apple and apple pomace (% DM).

Apple pomace has an IDF/SDF ratio of 2.5 to 5.5 (Sudha et al. 2007; Pérez-Cózar, 2011; Ktenioudaki et al. 2013). Onion by-products range from 3.1 to 9.0 due to the different IDF content that depends on the cultivar (Benítez et al. 2011). The IDF/SDF proportion varied from 7.2 to 4.6 in asparagus by-product depending on the applied treatment (Fuentes-Alventosa et al. 2013), so the observed decrease in this ratio is due to a reduction in the percentage of IDF in the gently extracted asparagus. The IDF/SDF relation is lower (2.9) in the artichoke by-product (Pérez-Cózar, 2011) and therefore more balanced.

It has now been reported that the by-products from the fruits and vegetable processing industry could be a rich source of dietary fiber and bioactive compounds (phenolic compounds such as flavonoids, phenolic acids, or catechins etc., essentials oil, lycopene or other carotenoids). Marín et al. (2007) reported by-products from different citrus processes as a source of functional fibers and also flavonoids. Navarro-Gonzalez et al. (2011) revealed that tomato peel may be considered a source of insoluble hemicelluloses and antioxidant bioactive compounds (lycopene, rutin or chlorogenic acid). Some polyphenols bound to dietary fiber are not hydrolysable by digestive enzymes in the upper area of the intestine as they are entrapped by dietary fiber. The non-fermentable and non-absorbable polyphenols present in the large intestine that remain in the colonic lumen may contribute to a healthy antioxidant environment by scavenging the free radicals and counteracting the effects of dietary pro-oxidants (Goñi and Serrano, 2005). Thus, polyphenols bound to dietary fiber exert beneficial effects by creating an antioxidant environment in the large intestine.

In vivo experiments are important to evaluate the properties that are attributed to fiber and to better understand the underlying mechanisms of each physiological effect. A hypercholesterolemic diet supplemented with 20% of apple pomace increased ($p \leq 0.001$) faecal bulk and lowered lipid parameters in Wistar rat serum, but without significant differences. Significant increases of lipids ($p \leq 0.001$) and bile acids ($p \leq 0.01$) in the faeces were also observed, meaning a potential reduction of fat by faecal excretion. Colonic fermentation in the caecum of rats produced a significant decrease in the pH of caecal content ($p \leq 0.001$) and a significant increase in short chain fatty acids ($p \leq 0.001$) (Pérez-Cózar, 2011). A positive effect for the risk of atherosclerosis was observed in Wistar rats fed with a high-fat diet supplemented with onion by-product. This effect could be due to the pectin and quercetin derivatives present in the onion by-product (Hamauzu et al. 2011). In Syrian golden hamsters fed a high-fat diet with 20% artichoke by-product there was an increase ($p \leq 0.001$) of stool bulk and a decrease ($p \leq 0.01$) of LDL cholesterol and triglyceride levels in serum as well as total cholesterol ($p \leq 0.01$) in the liver. The triglyceride, bile acid and protein content of the faecal excretion increased ($p \leq 0.01$) (Pérez-Cózar, 2011). Shao et al. (2013) observed lower plasma total cholesterol and LDL cholesterol, reduced hepatic cholesterol and an increase in the excretion of bile acids, triglycerides and total cholesterol in hamsters fed with high-fat diets supplemented with tomato pomace (42%) or defatted tomato seeds (18%). Chau and Huang (2003) demonstrated that hamsters fed a diet which included 5.38% orange by-product could significantly ($p \leq 0.05$) decrease the levels of serum triglycerides, serum total cholesterol, liver total lipids and liver cholesterol, and moreover significantly ($p \leq 0.05$) increase the levels of faecal total lipids, faecal cholesterol, and faecal bile acids, as well as the faecal bulk and moisture. The pronounced hypocholesterolemic and hypolipidemic effects of by-products could be attributed to their ability to enhance cholesterol and bile acid excretion.

The production of functional foods could include healthy ingredients such as dietary fiber or other bioactive compounds from fruit and vegetable by products generated in agro-food processing. The substitution of wheat flour with an apple by-product in different proportions (15%, 25% and 35%) provided good compositional/nutritional properties, but the changes in the rheological characteristics could affect its baking quality (Ktenioudaki et al. 2013). Cakes prepared from blends of wheat flour containing 0–30% apple pomace affected the rheological properties but they were a good source of dietary fiber (Suhda et al. 2007). Takeuchi and Nagashima (2011) prepared dried chips from artichoke tubers and studied their properties (sensory evaluation, visual acceptability, physicochemical properties) and showed that it could partially replace potato starch in industrial uses where viscosity is not required, such as in the production of snacks and frozen foods. Sáyago-Ayerdi et al. (2009) suggested that grape antioxidant fiber introduced as an ingredient in chicken hamburgers is a very effective inhibitor of lipid oxidation and has potential as a natural antioxidant.

Dietary fibers are not only desirable for their nutritional and functional effect but also for their technological properties. Citrus fruits are particularly rich in pectin, especially in the albedo tissue and the large quantities of citrus (lemon, lime, orange and grapefruit) wastes generated by the fruit juice industry have become the most important raw material for the production of commercial pectin. Pectins obtained from either lemon or lime are reported to predominantly contain homogalacturonan (HG) (with varying degrees of methyl/acetyl esterification) and smaller quantities of rhamnogalacturonan (RG) I and RG II. They are highly modified as a consequence of the harsh acidic extraction procedures that strip away the side chains, particularly RG I and arabinose containing polymers (Yapo et al. 2007; Prabasari et al. 2011). Rezzadori et al. (2007) reviewed the technological use of orange by-product for pectin production. Its extraction with water has been studied at different sample-to-solvent ratios, different pHs and with different extraction methods. The combination of hand-pressure and microwave on pectin yield was 12% better than hand-pressure alone, which was also better than microwave extraction alone (Liu et al. 2006).

The traditional problems by-products pose are the seasonality of supply and their high water content. This makes storage difficult and, therefore, they must be used quickly to prevent microbiological contamination and fermentation. Consequently, it is necessary to improve the management of these wastes by developing processes to achieve an adequate recovery of high added-value compounds. Fuentes-Alventosa et al. (2013) have proposed very recently a hydrothermal process for the valorisation of asparagus by-product. Moreover, Galanakis (2012) have lately reviewed the extraction, fractionation and isolation of these compounds from agro-food wastes applying conventional and emerging technologies to maximize the yield of the target compounds, extracting the high added-value ingredients from impurities and toxic compounds or avoiding deterioration and loss of functionality during processing.

3.2. Pulse Food By-Products

Legumes are considered to be good for health due to their compatibility with cereals and their properties in disease prevention. The most common legumes for human consumption are bean, lentil, pea, chickpea, broad bean and soybean (Guillon and Champ, 2002). Most legume beans are consumed after a simple industrial process in which the pod is removed or more complex processes to obtain different final products. The by-products generated in the processing of these legumes should be studied to understand their potential use as sources of functional ingredients.

There are many studies that focus on by-products from cereals, vegetables and fruits; however research on legume by-products is limited. Pea pods, broad beans pods and okara have been studied previously to assess their potential as sources of functional by-products (Redondo et al. 2008; Mateos-Aparicio et al. 2010a,b,c,d).

Most legumes are consumed after a simple industrial process, in which the pod is removed and the legume itself is frozen, tinned or sold fresh. Peas (*Pisum sativum L)* and broad beans (*Vicia faba* L) are widely consumed, and are grown all over the world. Large quantities of pods are produced and are underutilized, and using them to obtain functional ingredients such as dietary fiber has not been sufficiently considered. Soybean (*Glycine max.* L) processing also leads to a large amount of by-products. Soybeans are commonly processed to obtain protein isolates and other end products such as soymilk and tofu. During this process a fiber-rich residue called okara is removed in large quantities. Discarding okara as waste is a potential environmental problem because it is highly susceptible to putrefaction. Okara's high moisture content (≈80%) makes it difficult to handle and too expensive to dry by conventional means (Charalampopoulos and Rastall, 2012). In China about 20,000,000 tons of moist okara are produced annually from the soybean production industry. However, until now it has been consumed only as feed, or even incinerated as factory waste, and the reuse of okara, especially in food applications, is very difficult (Jinhong et al. 2012).

Pea and broad bean by-products, basically pods and okara residue from the process of making soy beverages and tofu from soybeans, have a great amount of dietary fiber, with pea pods having the most (pea pod: 58.6 g/100 g; okara: 54.3 g/ 100 g; broad bean pod: 40.1 g/100 g) (Mateos-Aparicio et al. 2010a). The importance of dietary fiber has led to the development of a large and potential market for fiber-rich products and ingredients and nowadays there is a trend to find new sources, such as agronomic by-products that have traditionally been undervalued (Jones et al. 2006). Dietary fiber plays an important role in many physiological processes and in the prevention of diseases of different aetiology. Thus, the study of the content, type and the main monomers (Redondo et al. 2008; Mateos-Aparicio et al. 2010a,d), the characterization of cell wall polysaccharides (Mateos-Aparicio et al. 2010b,c), the *in vitro* physicochemical properties (swelling, and water and oil retention capacity) (Mateos-Aparicio et al. 2010b) and the *in vitro* and animal studies of health properties (Préstamo et al. 2007; Jiménez-Escrig et al. 2008; Villanueva et al. 2011) can predict the potential physiological effects *in vivo* of dietary fiber of these aforementioned bean by-products.

The monosaccharide composition of the total dietary fiber in these legume by-products is quite different with glucose and galactose being the main monomers in okara, uronic acids and glucose in broad bean pods and glucose and xylose in pea pods (Mateos-Aparicio et al. 2009) (Table 2). These legume by-products have a greater amount of IDF than SDF. IDF represents 93% of the TDF in the case of pea pods, 77% in broad bean pods and 92% in okara (Mateos-Aparicio et al. 2010a). Broad bean pods have the most balanced fiber because the IDF/SDF relationship is close to 3, while in okara it is near 11 and in pea pods it is 13. The proportion calculated in broad bean pods is lower than the IDF/SDF in soybean seeds (Redondo et al. 2008), chickpeas and lentils (Martín-Cabrejas et al. 2006) or in other non-conventional legumes such as cowpesa, jack beans, dolichos and mucunas (Martín Cabrejas et al. 2008) but greater than in raw or germinated peas (Martín-Cabrejas et al. 2003).

Table 2. Percentage of each monomer in the total dietary fiber from okara, broad bean and pea pods (% DM)

% DM	OKARA	BROAD BEAN POD	PEA POD
Rhamnose	1.37	1.39	1.29
Fucose	1.20	0.52	-
Arabinose	13.92	13.63	3.22
Xylose	9.42	5.26	35.07
Mannose	3.77	1.61	1.10
Galactose	24.95	12.11	6.28
Glucose	34.25	28.54	36.17
Uronic Acids	10.77	36.97	16.75

Mateos-Aparicio et al. (2010b,c) have studied the isolation of cell wall polysaccharides (CWP) from okara and Mateos-Aparicio et al. (2010b) reported also the composition of CWP from pea pods and broad bean pods. Pea pods, broad bean pods and okara display different polymeric structures with cellulose as the main polymer. The high amount of xylose in pea pods may be due to the presence of xylans and xyloglucans, the most widespread neutral hemicelluloses. Okara and broad bean pods are made up of slightly methylated rhamnogalacturonan regions very substituted with arabinans, galactans and/or arabinogalactans. Pectic acids from the primary cell wall appear, due to the highly ramified non-solubilised pectic material, in association with other polymers, mostly cellulose. Xylogalacturonan regions appear in okara, and are probably replaced with short oligomeric side-chains of xylose in pea pods. These xylogalacturonan regions have been described previously in pea pods (Mateos-Aparicio et al. 2010b), pea hulls (Weightman et al. 1994; Renard et al. 1997; LeGoff et al. 2001), apples (Schols et al.1995), melons and cotton (Yu and Mort, 1996), soybean meal (Huisman et al. 1996, 1998, 1999) and okara (Mateos-Aparicio et al. 2010b,c). Glucuronic and galacturonic acids are the main components of broad bean pods because this by-product is very rich in soluble fiber (Mateos-Aparicio et al. 2010b). Mateos-Aparicio et al. (2010c) observed a strong link between structural proteins, cellulose-xyloglucans and pectin networks in okara by-products. The antioxidant activity of the soluble fractions from okara would confirm the strong role of pectins in the reduction power and free radical scavenging activity of the cell-wall polysaccharides from edible plants found by other authors.

The functional prebiotic α-galactosides (stachyose and raffinose) are in greater concentration in okara than in broad bean pods and inulin is presented in okara (Mateos-Aparicio et al. 2010a). Oligosaccharides, such as fructo-oligosaccharides or α-galactosides have a very important role in human health, particularly, in the positive balance of the intestinal microbiota, since they can control pathogenic bacteria (Martínez-Villaluenga et al. 2005).

As previously mentioned, few studies have been conducted on legume by-products, with okara, broad bean and pea pods receiving the most attention. However the only *in vivo* animal studies have been conducted with okara. Préstamo et al. (2007), Jiménez-Escrig et al. (2008) have studied the health effects of dietary fiber from okara in Wistar rats and Villanueva et al. (2011) in Syrian hamsters. Préstamo et al. (2007) showed that *in vivo* colonic fermentation of okara resulted in a lower pH and higher total short chain fatty acid production. Jimenez-

Escrig et al. (2008) observed that dietary fiber from okara protects the gut environment in terms of antioxidant status and prebiotic effect. Villanueva et al. (2011) suggested that the main components of okara, dietary fiber and protein, could be related with the total lipids and cholesterol decrease in plasma and the liver, as well as with the faecal output increase in hamsters fed a high-fat diet. Thus, okara might play an interesting role in the prevention of hyperlipidemia and could be used as a natural ingredient or supplement for functional food preparation. On the other hand, the swelling and water retention capacity of okara (Figure 2), and also of broad bean and pea pods, indicates their potential application as a texturing additive (Mateos-Aparicio et al. 2010b).

In spite of its high amount of total fiber, okara is not particularly rich in the soluble fraction. Mateos-Aparicio et al. (2010d) studied the effect of a treatment combining hydration, mild temperatures and high hydrostatic pressure to improve the SDF content, IDF/SDF ratio and its associated physicochemical properties *in vitro* of okara (Figure 2). On the other hand, Villanueva et al. (2013) studied okara that was subject to an enzymatic treatment with Ultraflo L® to produce a product (okara^{ET}) which has a higher content of soluble dietary fiber, an enhanced IDF/SDF ratio and better physicochemical properties (Figure 2). Moreover, the fermentation of okara^{ET} using a pure culture of *Bifidobacterium bifidus* showed short chain fatty acid production, a pH decrease and substrate consumption, which indicated the potential bifidogenic capacity of okara^{ET}.

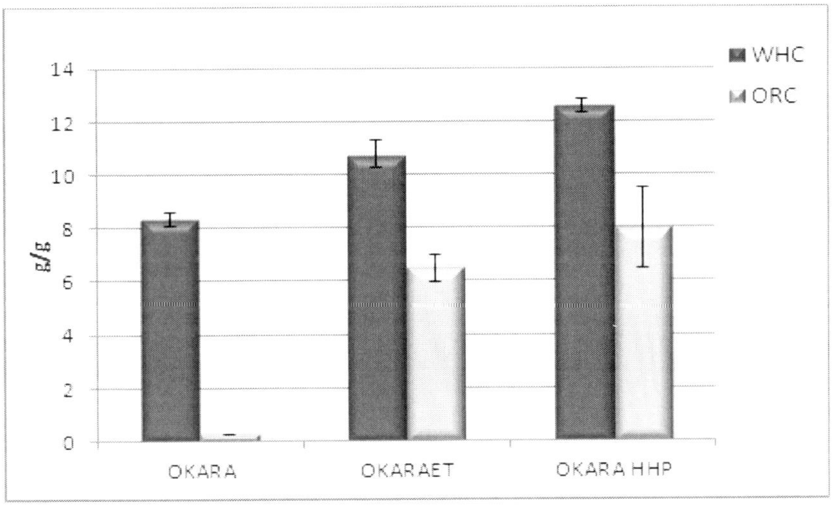

Figure 2. The water holding capacity (WHC) and oil retention capacity (ORC) (g/g) of okara, high hydrostatic pressure-treated okara (okara^{HHP}) and enzymatically treated okara (okara^{ET}).

The use of legume by-products as sources of dietary fiber for the production of functional foods is very limited. However, they should be considered as functional ingredients, especially in the case of okara, due to the presence of high quality fat and proteins, as well as the absence of colour and taste. There are very few studies into the potential use of okara, so Silva et al. (2009) added okara flour to the wheat flour to study its effect on the technological properties and behaviour during storage of bread. They concluded that the addition of 10% okara flour to bread yielded acceptable technological and sensory characteristics and recommended this percentage. Bedani et al. (2013) researched the effect of okara flour on

Lactobacillus acidophilus La-5 and *Bifidobacterium animalis* Bb12 viability in a fermented soy product and on probiotic survival under *in vitro* simulated gastrointestinal conditions. The fermented soy product matrix improved Bb-12 survival on day 1 of storage and may be considered a good vehicle for Bb-12. It could also play an important role in probiotic protection against gastrointestinal juices.

Since the production of legume-based foods (beverages, oils, snacks, etc.) generates millions of tons of legume by-products, such as pods or other waste, studies are needed to find their potential use as sources for functional ingredients. Bean by-products might be regarded as functional ingredients for the fiber fortification of common foods, which has the advantage of requiring the fewest dietary changes in our current lifestyle to increase the consumption of functional ingredients.

3.3. Cereals By-Products

Generally, fruit and vegetable processing wastes are the most widely investigated substrates for extracting several types of antioxidants and dietary fibers. This is because the corresponding by-products are made up of soft tissues rich in both ingredients (Galanakis, 2012). However, cereals are a rich source of fermentable carbohydrates including dietary fiber, resistant starch and non-digestible oligosaccharides. The dietary fiber is concentrated in the outer layers of the grain, with the highest dietary fiber found in the cereal by-products (after the refinement process). One issue to consider is the presence of phytic acid in the insoluble fiber from cereals. It is considered an antinutrient, mainly due to its ability to bind with essential minerals and also to interact non-specifically with protein and starch and consequently reduce their uptake in the human intestine (Khattab and Arntfield, 2009). On the other hand, phytic acid may play a role in reducing the risk of cancer, possibly because of its antioxidant effects (Kumar et al. 2010).

Wheat is the dominant crop in Western countries, and rice is more prevalent in Asia (Gustavsson et al. 2011). Wheat grinding generates by-products such as bran or straw, which are rich in highly nutritional proteins Prakash, 1996), dietary fibers and particularly glucuronoarabinoxylans (Sun and Tomkinson, 2002; Hollmann and Lindhauer, 2005). Wheat bran fiber contributes to the modulation of intestinal transit and increases stool volume (Regulation (EU) N° 432/2012). Rice bran is a by-product obtained from the outer layers of rice and is a good source of protein, minerals, fatty acids and dietary fiber content (Mccaskill and Zhang, 1999; Guohua et al. 2009), plus it is used for the enrichment of some foods, due to its high dietary fiber content. Rice bran hemicellulose B (RBHB) and rice bran insoluble dietary fiber (RBDF) have been reported to have a high water-binding and fat-binding capacity, swelling capacity and many other biological activities including the potential to decrease blood cholesterol and reduce the incidence of colon cancer (Guhua et al. 2009).

Oat mill waste, a by-product of rolled oat grain, has been suggested for the extraction of β-glucan with gelling properties (Patsiouraa et al. 2011). Barley and oats have the highest concentrations of β-glucan of all cereals. The β-glucan content can range from 1% in wheat grains, to 3-7% in oats, and 5-11% in barley (Sullivan et al. 2013). Nutritional studies into β-glucan have shown a link between its regular consumption and a number of health benefits, including a decrease in the risk of chronic heart disease by lowering blood cholesterol (Onning, 2007) and an increased insulin response in diabetics (Poutanen et al. 2007). The food industry is therefore faced with the challenge of producing novel barley-based foods that are healthy but also that will satisfy the consumer's needs. In recent years, the potential use of β-glucan from barley and other sources as a functional food ingredient has gained attention (Malkki, 2004; Trepel, 2004). β-glucan can be described as a functional food as it provides some of the quality attributes desired in a food such as texture, but also has the ability to confer specific health benefits to the consumer. Barley bran has received some attention, particularly because it has been shown to contain high levels of fiber. It is often assumed that like wheat bran, barley bran consists of the pericarp, germ, aleurone, and the subaleurone layers; however its composition may differ depending on the degree of pearling implemented prior to milling, and needs to be better defined (Izydorczyk and Dexter, 2004). Barley bran is high in both insoluble and soluble fiber, and as a result has the ability to accelerate gastrointestinal transit time when incorporated into a food (Regulation (EU) Nº 432/2012) and also has a hypocholesterolemic effect (Lupton et al. 1993). Barley husks constitute 10–13 wt% of the whole crop and are today mainly regarded as a low profit product (Bhatty and Rossnagel, 1998). More than one third of these husks is made up of hemicelluloses, with arabinoxylan being the most abundant (MacGregor and Fincher, 1993).

The first commercialized dietary fibers were those from cereals. Wheat bran is the most classic form of fiber-rich concentrate and contains around 44% fiber, most of it insoluble (Hollmann and Lindhauer, 2005). As an alternative, oat bran that has lower amount of total dietary fiber but the proportion of soluble fiber is higher than in the wheat bran. The nutritional value of regular consumption of wheat bran in terms of its protective effect against colon cancer is still a matter of debate. Although several laboratory animal model studies have shown results which were interpreted as indicating protective effects (Harris and Ferguson, 1999), several large epidemiological studies (Sengupta et al. 2001) have not provided conclusive evidence that the risk of colon cancer is reduced.

Intestinal anaerobic fermentation of wheat bran produces butyrate that inhibits proliferation, induces differentiation and enhances apoptosis in colon cancer cells and acts as a growth factor for a healthy colon epithelium. Wheat bran sustains butyrate levels throughout the entire lumen of the colon in contrast to most fiber sources. It is hypothesized that the protective effects of wheat bran against colon cancer may be associated with increased colonic butyrate. The arabinoxylans of wheat bran (25–28% dm) are a major source of fermentable and butyrate producing polysaccharides. Bacterial fermentation of arabinoxylans from wheat and sorghum has been studied *in vitro* (Van Laere et al. 2000).

Another agricultural residue, although less used, is wheat straw, which has a hemicellulose content of 35-38%. These hemicelluloses have interesting applications. The highly branched heteroxylans from corn hulls, a by-product of starch production, is being used as a new food gum. Xylans from cereals are part of the insoluble fiber and contribute to raising the volume of faecal bulk, decreasing intestinal transit time and trapping substances that can be dangerous for the human organism (mutagenic and carcinogenic agents) (Sun and Tomkinsom, 2002).

3.4. Other Sources

Chitin is the second most abundant natural biopolymer after cellulose. The chemical structure of chitin is similar to that of cellulose with 2-acetamido-2-deoxy-β-D-glucose

(NAG) monomers linked by β(1-4) linkages. Chitin is abundantly found in crustacean shells and other sources such as fungus and yeasts. Chitosan is the deacetylated (to varying degrees) form of chitin, which, unlike chitin, is soluble in acidic solutions. Chitin and its deacetylated form, chitosan, have been of interest in the past few decades due to their potential broad range of industrial applications. However, only limited attention has been paid to using these versatile biopolymers in the food industry. Conversion of by-products and wastes into valuable ingredients has been identified as a challenge for food research and development. These biopolymers offer a wide range of applications including food packaging films, preservation of foods from microbial deterioration or the purification of water and clarification and deacidification of fruit juices. They can also be used as hypocholesterolemic agents because of their ability to bind fat, or as thickeners, gelling agents and emulsifiers (Sahidi et al. 1999; Aranaz et al. 2009; Mengíbar et al. 2011,2012). Their application in the encapsulation of antioxidants has also been discussed in the literature (Harris et al. 2009).

The utilization of the brewer's yeast cells from the beer industry for the production of food-grade yeast extract is promising. Brewer's yeast has three groups of polysaccharides: mannoprotein, ß-D-glucans and chitin. The ß-D-glucans from yeast can be divided into two subtypes: ß-1,3-D-glucose and ß-1,6-D-glucose (Klis et al. 2002). These products are used to obtain ß-D-glucans since they have important effects on health including: better cardiovascular health through a decrease in LDL cholesterol (Bell et al. 1999) improved glycemic response (Jenkins et al. 2002), and anti-inflammatory (Li et al. 2004) and antitumor (Cheung et al. 2002) effects. Moreover, β-glucan obtained from brewer's yeast can be used in food products as a thickening, water-holding, or oil-binding agent and emulsifying stabilizer (Thammakiti et al. 2004). Saccharomyces yeast biomass is the second major by-product from the brewing industry. It can be of value as a raw material with different uses; however it is still underutilized (Ferreira et al. 2010).

Conclusion

The exploitation of large quantities of plant by-products as a source of functional compounds and their application in the food industry is a promising field, which requires interdisciplinary research by food technologists, food chemists, nutritionists and toxicologists. Indeed, functional foods represent an important, innovative and rapidly growing part of the whole food market. Dietary fibers have all the characteristics needed to be an important ingredient in the formulation of functional foods. Increased dietary fiber intake can be achieved by changing dietary habits, increasing the consumption of high-fiber foods, and moreover, consuming fortified foods and supplements. Since consumers tend to reject synthetic additives, functional ingredients should preferably be from natural sources.

The food industries generate millions of tons of by-products that produce economic and environmental problems. Research is required to evaluate their potential reuse as sources of functional ingredients, such as dietary fiber, which can be used for the production of dietary supplements, to improve the technological properties and/or the fortification of common foods.

References

AACC (American Association of Cereal Chemist) (2001). The Definition of Dietary Fiber. *Cereal Foods World, 46,* 112-126.

Aranaz, I.; Mengibar, M.; Harris, R.; Panos, I.; Miralles, B.; Acosta, N.; Galed, G. & Heras, A. (2009). Functional characterization of chitin and chitosan. *Current Chemical Biology, 3,* 202-230.

Ashwell, M. (2002). *Concepts about functional food.* Brussels, Belgium: ILSI Europe Concise Monograph Series.

Bedani, R.; Rossi, E.A. & Isay Saad, S.M. (2013). Impact of inulin and okara on Lactobacillus acidophilus La-5 and Bifidobacterium animalis Bb-12 viability in a fermented soy product and probiotic survival under in vitro simulated gastrointestinal conditions. *Food Microbiology, 34,* 382-389.

Bell, S.; Goldman, V.M.; Bistrian, B.R.; Arnold, A.H.; Ostroff, G. &Forse, R.A. (1999). Effects of β-Glucan from oats and yeaston serum lipids. *Critical Reviews in Food Science and Nutrition, 39,* 189-202.

Benítez, V.; Mollá, E.; Martín-Cabrejas, M.A.; Aguilera, Y.; López-Andréu, F.J. & Esteban, R.M. (2011). Effect of sterilisation on dietary fiber and physicochemical properties of onion by-products. *Food Chemistry, 127,* 501–507.

Bhatty, R.S. & Rossnagel, B.G. (1998). Comparison of pearled and unpearled Canadian and Japanese barleys. *Cereal Chemistry, 75,* 5-21.

Bosaeus, I. (2004). Fiber effects on intestinal functions (diarrhoea, constipation and irritable bowel syndrome). *Clinical Nutrition Supplements, 1,* 33-38.

Chandalia, M.; Garg, A.; Lutjohann, D.; von Bergmann, K.; Grundy, S.M. & Brinkley, L.J. (2000). Beneficial effects of high dietary fiber intake in patients with type 2 diabetes mellitus. *New England Journal of Medicine, 342,* 1392–1398.

Chandra, K.; Ghosh, K.; Ojha, A.K. & Islam, S.S. (2009). Chemical analysis of a polysaccharide of unripe (green) tomato (*Lycopersicon esculentum*). *Carbohydrate Research, 344,* 2188–2194.

Charalampopoulos, D. & Rastall, R.A. (2012). Prebiotics in foods. *Current Opinion in Biotechnology, 23,* 187-191.

Chau, C.F. & Huang, Y.L. (2003). Comparison of the chemical composition and physicochemical properties of different fibers prepared from the peel of *Citrus sinensis* L.Cv. Liucheng. *Journal of Agricultural and Food Chemistry, 51,* 2615–2618.

Cheung, N.K.; Modak, S.; Vickers, A. & Knuckles, B. (2002). Orally administered beta-glucan enhance anti-timor effects of monoclonal antibodies. *Cancer Inmunology, Immunotherapy, 51,*55-564.

Del Valle, M.; Cámara, M. &Torija, M.-E. (2006). Chemical characterization of tomato pomace. *Journal of the Science and Food and Agriculture, 86,* 1232-1236.

EEC Commission Regulation 442 (1975). Waste. *Official Journal of European Community, L194,* 39-41.

EEC Commission Regulation 689 (1991). Hazardous waste. *Official Journal of European Community, L377,* 20-27.

EFSA (European Food Safety Authority) (2010). Scientific Opinion on Dietary Reference Values for carbohydrates and dietary fiber. *EFSA Journal, 8 (3),* 1462.

Elleuch, M.; Bedigian, D.; Roiseux, O.; Besbes, S.; Blecker, C. & Attia, H. (2011). Dietary fiber and fiber-rich by-products of food processing: Characterisation, technological functionality and commercial applications: A review. *Food Chemistry, 124,* 411–421.

FECYT (Fundación Española para la Ciencia y la Tecnología) (2005). *Alimentos funcionales.* Madrid, Spain: FECYT.

Ferreira, I.M.P.L.V.O.; Pinho, O.; Vieira, E. & Tavarela, J.G. (2010). Brewer's Saccharomyces yeast biomass: characteristics and potential applications. *Trends in Food Science & Technology, 21*, 77-84.

Figuerola, F.; Hurtado, M.L.; Estévez, A.M.; Chiffelle, I. & Asenjo, F. (2005). Fiber concentrates from apple pomace and citrus peel as potential fiber sources for food enrichment. *Food Chemistry, 91,* 395–401.

Fuentes-Alventosa, J.M.; Jaramillo-Carmona, S.; Rodríguez-Gutiérrez, G.; Guillén-Bejarano, R.; Jiménez-Araujo, A.; Fernández-Bolaños, J. & Rodríguez-Arcos, R. (2013). Preparation of bioactive extracts from asparagus by-product. *Food and Bioproducts Processing, 91,* 74–82.

Fuentes-Alventosa, J.M.; Rodríguez-Gutiérrez, G.; Jaramillo-Carmona, S.; Espejo-Calvo J.A.; Rodríguez-Arcos, R.; Fernández-Bolaños, J.; Guillén-Bejarano, R. & Jiménez-Araujo, A. (2009). Effect of extraction method on chemical composition and functional characteristics of high dietary fiber powders obtained from asparagus by-products. *Food Chemistry, 113,* 665–671.

Galanakis C.M. (2012). Recovery of high added-value components from food wastes: Conventional, emerging technologies and commercialized applications. *Trends in Food Science & Technology, 26,* 68-87.

Goñi, I. & Hervert-Hernández D. (2011). By-Products from Plant Foods are Sources of Dietary Fiber and Antioxidants. In I. Rasooli (Ed). *Phytochemicals - Bioactivities and Impact on Health.* Rijeka, Croatia: InTech.

Goñi, I. & Serrano, J. (2005). The intake of dietary fiber from grape seeds modifies the antioxidant status in rat cecum. *Journal Science Food Agricultural*, 85, 1877–81.

Gray, J. (2006). *Dietary fiber. Definition, analysis, physiology and health*, Brussels, Belgium: ILSI Europe Concise Monograph Series.

Guillon, F. & Champ, M.M.J. (2002). Carbohydrate fractions of legumes: uses in human nutrition and potential for health. *British Journal of Nutrition, 88*, 293-306.

Guohua Hu; Shaohua Huang; Shuwen Cao & Zhengzhi Ma (2009). Effect of enrichment with hemicellulose from rice bran on chemical and functional properties of bread. *Food Chemistry, 115,* 839-842.

Gustavsson, J.; Cederberg, C.; Sonesson, U.; van Otterdijk, R. & Meybeck, A. (2011). Global food losses and food waste. Extend, causes and prevention. Rome: Food and Agriculture Organization of the United Nations. http://www.fao.org/fileadmin/user_upload/ags/publications/GFL_web.pdf

Hamauzu, A.; Nosaka, T.; Ito, I.; Suzuki, T.; Torisu, S.; Hashida, M.; Fukuzawa A.; Ohguchi, M. & Yamanaka, S. (2011). Physicochemical characteristics of rapidly dried onion powder and its anti-atherogenic effect on rats fed high-fat diet. *Food Chemistry, 129,* 810–815.

Harris, P.J. & Ferguson, L.R. (1999). Dietary fibers may protect or enhance carcinogenesis. *Mutation Research, 443,* 95–110

Harris, R.; Lecumberri, E.; Mateos-Aparicio, I.; Mengíbar, M.; Heras, A. (2009). Chitosan nanoparticles and microspheres for the encapsulation of natural antioxidants extracted from *Ilex paraguariensis*. *Carbohydrate Polymers, 84,* 803-806.

Heimendinger, J. & Chapelsky, D. (1996). The national 5 a day for better health program. *Advances in Experimental Medicine and Biology, 401,* 199-206.

Hollmann, J. & Lindhauer, M. G. (2005). Pilot-scale isolation of glucuronoarabinoxylans from wheat bran. *Carbohydrate Polymers, 59,* 225-230.

Howlet, J. (2008). *Functional Foods from Science to Health and Claims*. Brussels, Belgium: ILSI Europe Concise Monograph Series.

Huisman, M.M.H.; Schols, H.A. & Voragen, A.G.J. (1996). Isolation and sequential extraction of cell wall polysaccharides from soy meal. *Carbohydrate Polymers*, *37*, 87–95.

Huisman, M.M.H.; Schols, H.A. & Voragen, A.G.J. (1998). Cell wall polysaccharides from soybean (*Glycine max*) meal. Isolation and characterisation. *Carbohydrate Polymers*, *37*, 87-95.

Huisman, M.M.H.; Schols, H.A.; Voragen, A.G.J. (1999). Enzymatic degradation of cell wall polysaccharides from soybean meal. *Carbohydrate Polymers*, *38,* 299-307.

Izydorczyk, M.S. & Dexter, J.E. (2004). Barley: milling and processing. *Encyclopaedia of Grain science*, Oxford, UK: Elsevier.

Jenkins, A.L.; Jenkins, D.J.; Zdravkovic, U.; Wursch, P. & Vuksan, V.(2002). Depression of the glycemic index by high levels of beta-glucan fiber in two functional foods tested in type 2 diabetes. *European Journal of Clinical Nutrition*, *56*, 622-628

Jiménez-Escrig, A.; Tenorio, M.D.; Espinosa-Martos, I. & Rupérez, P. (2008). Health-promoting effects of a dietary fiber concentrate from the soybean by-product okara in rats. *Journal of Agriculture and Food Chemistry, 56,* 7495-7501.

Jinhong Wu, Y.W.; Chunmei Y. & Zhengwu W. (2012). Enzymatic Preparation and Characterization of Soybean Oligosaccharides from Okara. *Procedia Engineering*, *37,* 186 – 191.

Jones, J.; Lineback, D. & Levine, M. (2006). Dietary reference intakes: implications for fiber labelling and consumption. *Nutrition Reviews*, *64*, 31-38.

Khattab, R.Y. & Arntfield, S.D. (2009). Nutritional quality of legume seeds as affected by some physical treatments. 2. Antinutritional factors. *LWT-Food science and Technology*, *42*, 1113-1118

Klis, F.M.; Mol, P.; Hellingwerf, K. & Brul, S. (2002). Dynamics of cell wall structure in *Saccharomyces cerevisiae*. *FEMS Microbiology Reviews*, *26*, 239-256.

Kristinsson, H.G. & Rasco, B.A. (2000). Fish protein hydrolysates: production, biochemical, and functional properties. *Critical Reviews in Food Science and Nutrition*, *40*, 43-81

Ktenioudaki, A.; O'Shea, N. & Gallagher, E. (2013). Rheological properties of wheat dough supplemented with functional by-products of food processing: Brewer's spent grain and apple pomace. *Journal of Food Engineering*, *116*, 362–368.

Kumar, V.; Sinha, A.K.; Makkar, H.P.S. & Becker, K. (2010). Dietary roles of phytate and phytase in human nutrition: A review. *Food Chemistry*, *120*, 945-959

Le Goff, A.; Renard, C.M.G.C.; Bonnin, E. & Thibault, J.-F. (2001). Extraction, purification and chemical characterisation of xylogalacturonans from pea hulls. *Carbohydrate Polymers*, *45*, 325-334.

Li, C.; Ha, T.; Kelley, J.; Gao, X.; Qiu, Y. & Kao, R.L. (2004). Modulating Toll-like receptor mediated signalling by (1-3)-beta-D-glucan rapidly induces cardioprotection. *Cardiovascular Research, 61*, 538-547.

Li, D.; Dai, J.Y. & Xiu, Z.L. (2010). A novel strategy for integrated utilization of Jerusalem artichoke stalk and tuber for production of 2,3-butanediol by Klebsiella pneumoniae. *Bioresource Technology, 101,* 8342-8347.

Liu, Y.; Shi, J. & Langrish T.A.G. (2006).Water-based extraction of pectin from flavedo and albedo of orange peels. *Chemical Engineering Journal*, 120 203–209.

Lupton, J.R.; Morin, J.L. & Robinson, M.C. (1993). Barley bran flour accelerates gastrointestinal transit time. *Journal of the American Dietetic Association*, 93, 881-885.

Lutz, M.; Henríquez, C. & Escobar, M. (2011). Chemical composition and antioxidant properties of mature and baby artichokes (*Cynara scolymus* L.), raw and cooked. *Journal of Food Composition and Analysis, 24*, 49-54.

MacGregor, A.W. & Fincher, G.B. (1993). Carbohydrates of the barley grain. In A.W. MacGregor and R.S. Bhatty (Eds), *Barley: Chemistry and technology*. St Paul, USA: American Association of Cereal Chemistry.

Madureira, A.R.; Tavares, T.; Gomes, A.M.P.; Pintado, M.E. & Malcata, F.X. (2010). Invited review: physiological properties of bioactive peptides obtained from whey proteins. *Journal of Dairy Science, 93*, 437-455.

Malkki, Y. (2004). Trends in dietary fiber research and development. *Acta Alimentaria, 33*, 39-62.

Marín, F.R.; Soler-Rivas, C.; Benavente-García, O.; Castillo, J. & Pérez-Álvarez, J.A. (2007). By-products from different citrus processes as a source of customized functional fibres. *Food Chemistry, 100*, 736–741.

Martín-Cabrejas, M.A.; Aguilera, Y.; Benítez, V.; Mollá, E.; López Andréu, F.J. & Esteban, R.M. (2006). Effect of Industrial Dehydratation on the Soluble Carbohydrate and Dietary Fiber Fractions in Legumes. *Journal of Agriculture and Food Chemistry, 54*, 7652-7657.

Martín-Cabrejas, M.A.; Ariza, N.; Esteban, R.M.; Mollá, E.; Waldron, K. & López-Andreu, F.J. (2003). Effect of Germination on the Carbohydrate Composition of the Dietary Fiber of Peas (*Pisum sativum* L.). *Journal of Agriculture and Food Chemistry, 51*, 1254-1259.

Martín-Cabrejas, M.A.; Díaz, M.F.; Aguilera, Y.; Benítez, V.; Mollá, E. & Esteban, R.M. (2008). Influence of germination on the soluble carbohydrates and dietary fiber fractions in non-conventional legumes. *Food Chemistry, 107*, 1045-1052.

Martínez-Villaluenga, C.; Frías, J. & Vidal-Valverde, C. (2005). Raffinose family oligosaccharides and sucrose contents in 13 Spanish lupin cultivars. *Food Chemistry, 91*, 645-649.

Mateos-Aparicio, I. (2009). Aprovechamiento de subproductos de leguminosas para la obtención de ingredientes funcionales. Comparación de metodologías para la caracterización de fibra alimentaria. PhD Thesis. Madrid, Spain: *Colección Digital de Tesis de la UCM* (http://eprints.ucm.es/)

Mateos-Aparicio, I. (2012). Beans by-products, potential sources for functional ingredients. In: E. Popescu and I. Golubev (Eds). *Beans: Nutrition, Consumption and Health*. New York, USA: Nova Science Publishers.

Mateos-Aparicio, I.; Pérez-Cózar, M.L.; Villanueva, M.J.; Redondo, A. & Tenorio, M.D. (2011). Potential prebiotic effect of apple pomace fiber. *In vivo* assay. Ponencia Sesión

Nutrición e Inmunología. III Workshop Probióticos, Prebióticos y Salud: Evidencia Científica. Barcelona, Spain.

Mateos-Aparicio, I.; Redondo-Cuenca, A.; Villanueva-Suárez, M.J.; Zapata-Revilla, M.A. &Tenorio-Sanz, M.D. (2010). Okara, broad bean pod and pea pod, potential sources of functional compounds. *LWT- Food Science and Technology*, *43*, 1467-1470.

Mateos-Aparicio, I.; Redondo-Cuenca, A. &Villanueva-Suárez, M.J. (2010). Isolation and characterization of cell wall polysaccharides from legume by-products: okara, pea pod and broad bean pod. *Food Chemistry*, *122*, 339-345.

Mateos-Aparicio, I.; Mateos-Peinado, C.; Jiménez-Escrig, A. & Rupérez, P. (2010). Multifunctional antioxidant activity of polysaccharide fractions from the soybean by-product okara. *Carbohydrate Polymers*, *82*, 245-250.

Mateos-Aparicio, I.; Mateos-Peinado, C. & Rupérez, P. (2010). High hydrostatic pressure treatment modifies the content and physicochemical properties of dietary fiber in okara by-product from soybean. *Innovative Food Science and Emerging Technologies*,*11*, 445-450.

Mccaskill, D. & Zhang, F. (1999). Use of rice bran oil in foods. *Food Technology*, *53*, 50–51.

Mengíbar, M.; Ganan, M.; Miralles, B.; Carrascosa, A.V.; Martínez-Rodríguez, A.J.; Peter, M.G. & Heras, A. (2011). Antibacterial activity of products of depolymerization of chitosans with lysozyme and chitosanase against *Campylobacter jejuni*. *Carbohydrate Polymers*, *84*, 844-848.

Mengíbar, M. (2012). Obtención y caracterización de quitosanos modificados: ingredientes funcionales con aplicaciones tecnológicas y biológicas en la industria alimentaria. PhD Thesis. Madrid, Spain: *Colección Digital de Tesis de la UCM* (http://eprints.ucm.es/)

Navarro-González, I.; García-Valverde, V.; García-Alonso, J. & Periago, M.J. (2011). Chemical profile, functional and antioxidant properties of tomato peel fiber. *Food Research International*, *44*, 1528–1535.

Onning, G. (2007). Carbohydrates and the risk of cardiovascular disease. In C.G. Biliaderis & M.S. Izydorczyk (Eds), *Functional food carbohydrates*. Boca Raton, USA: CRC Press, Taylor and Francis Group.

Patsiouraa, A.; Galanakis, C.M. & Gekas, V. (2011). Ultrafiltration optimization for the recovery of β-glucan from oat mill waste. *Journal of Membrane Science, 373*, 53-63.

Pérez Cózar, M.L. (2011). Fibra alimentaria procedente de subproductos vegetales, preparación, caracterización y efectos funcionales. PhD Thesis. Madrid, Spain: *Colección Digital de Tesis de la UCM* (http://eprints.ucm.es/)

Poutanen, K.; Laaksonen, D.; Autio, K.; Mykkanene, H. & Niskanen, L. (2007). The role of carbohydrates in the prevention of and Management of type 2 diabetes. In C.G. Biliaderis & M.S. Izydorczyk (Eds), Functional food carbohydrates. Boca Raton, USA: CRC Press, Taylor and Francis Group.

Prabasari, I.; Pettolino, F.; Liao, M.-L. & Bacic, A. (2011). Pectic polysaccharides from mature orange (*Citrus sinensis*) fruit albedo cell walls: Sequential extraction and chemical characterization. *Carbohydrate Polymers*, *84*, 484-494.

Prakash, J. (1996). Rice bran proteins: properties and food uses. *Critical Reviews in Food Science and Nutrition, 36*, 537-552

Préstamo, G.; Rupérez, P.; Espinosa-Martos, I.; Villanueva, M.J. & Rupérez, P. (2007). The effects of okara on rat growth, cecal fermentation and serum lipids. *European Food Research and Technology,225*, 925-928.

Redondo-Cuenca, A.; Villanueva-Suárez, M.J. & Mateos-Aparicio, I. (2008). Soybean seeds and its by-products okara as sources of dietary fiber. Measurement by AOAC and Englyst method. *Food Chemistry, 108,* 1099-1105.

Regulation (EU) Nº 432/2012 European Comission (2012). Lista de declaraciones autorizadas de propiedades saludables de los alimentos distintas de las relativas a la reducción del riesgo de enfermedad y al desarrollo y la salud de los niños. *Diario Oficial de la Unión Europea, L136/1.*

Renard, C.M.G.C.; Weightman, R.M. & Thibault, J.-F. (1997). The xylose-rich pectins from pea hulls. *International Journal of Biological Macromolecules, 21,* 155-162.

Rezzadori, K.; Benedetti, S. & Amante, E.R. (2007). Proposals for the residues recovery: Orange waste as raw material for new products. *Food Chemistry*, 100, 736–741.

Roberfroid, M.B. (2000). Defining Functional Foods. In: G. Gibson & C. Williams (Eds). *Functional Foods.* Cambridge, UK: Woodhead Publishing Ltd.

Rodríguez, R.; Jiménez, A.; Fernández-Bolaños, J.; Guillén, R. & Heredia, A. (2006). Dietary fiber from vegetable products as source of functional ingredients. *Trends in Food Science & Technology, 17,* 3-15.

Ros, M.; Pascual J.A.; Ayuso M.; Morales, A.B.; Miralles, J.R. & Solera, C (2012). Salidas valorizables de los residuos y subproductos orgánicos de la industria de los transformados de frutas y hortalizas. Murcia, Spain: CEBAS-CSIC.

Sáyago-Ayerdi, S.G.; Brenes, A.; Goñi, I. (2009). Effect of grape antioxidant dietary fiber on the lipid oxidation of raw and cooked chicken hamburgers. *LWT - Food Science and Technology, 42,* 971-976.

Schieber, A.; Stintzing, F.C. & Carle, R. (2001). By-products of plant food processing as a source of functional compounds recent developments. *Trends in Food Science and Technology, 12,* 401–413.

Schols, H.A.; Vierhuis, E.; Baks, E.J. & Voragen, A.G.J. (1995). Different populations of pectic hairy regions occur in apple cell walls. *Carbohydrate Research, 275,* 343-360.

Sengupta, S.; Tjandra, J.J. & Gibson, P.R. (2001). Dietary-fiber and colorectal neoplasia. *Diseases of Colon and Rectum, 44,* 1016–1033.

Seymour, G.B.; Colquhoun, I.J.; Dupont, M.S.; Parsley, K.R. & Selvendran, R.R. (1990). Composition and structural features of cell wall polysaccharides from tomato fruits. *Phytochemistry, 29,* 725-573.

Shahidi, F.; Arachchi, J.K.V. & Jeon, Y.-J. (1999). Food applications of chitin and chitosans. *Trends in Food Science & Technology, 10,* 37-51.

Shao, D.; Bartley, G.E.; Yokoyama,W.; Pan, Z.; Zhang, H. & Zhang, A. (2013). Plasma and hepatic cholesterol-lowering effects of tomato pomace, tomato seed oil and defatted tomato seed in hamsters fed with high-fat diets. *Food Chemistry, 139,* 589–596.

Silva, L.H.; Paucar-Menacho, L.M.; Vicente, C.A.; Salles, A.S.; Steel, C.J. & Chang YoonKil (2009). Development of loaf bread with the addition of okara flour. *Brazilian Journal of Food Technology, 12,* 315-322.

Sudha, M.L.; Baskaran, V. & Leelavathi, K. (2007). Apple pomace as a source of dietary fiber and polyphenols and its effect on the rheological characteristics and cake making. *Food Chemistry, 104,* 686-692.

Sullivan, P.; Arendt, E. & Gallagher, E. (2013). The increasing use of barley and barley by-products in the production of healthier baked goods. *Trends in Food Science & Technology, 29,* 124-134.

Sun, R. C., & Tomkinson, J. (2002). Characterization of hemicelluloses obtained by classical and ultrasonically assisted extractions from wheat straw. *Carbohydrate Polymers, 50,* 263-271.

Takeuchi, J. & Nagashima, T. (2011). Preparation of dried chips from Jerusalem artichoke (*Helianthus tuberosus*) tubers and analysis of their functional properties. *Food Chemistry, 126,* 922–926.

Thammakiti, S.; Suphantharika, M.; Phaesuwan, T. & Verduyn, C. (2004). Preparation of spent brewer's yeast β-glucans for potential applications in the food industry. *International Journal of Food Science & Technology, 39,* 21-29.

Trepel, F. (2004). Dietary fiber: more than a matter of dietetica. I. Compounds, properties, physiological effects. *Wiener klinische Wochenschrift, 116,* 465-476.

Van Laere, K.M.J.; Hartemink, R.; Bosveld, M.; Schols, H.A.; Voragen, A.G.J. (2000). Fermentation of plant cell wall derived polysaccharides and their corresponding oligosaccharides by intestinal bacteria. *Journal of Agricultural and Food Chemistry, 48,* 1644–1652.

Villanueva, M.J.; Yokoyama, W.H.; Hong, Y.J.; Barttley, G.E. & Rupérez, P. (2011). Effect of high-fat diets supplemented with okara soybean by-product on lipid profiles of plasma, liver and faeces in Syrian hamsters. *Food Chemistry, 124,* 72–79.

Villanueva-Suárez, M.J.; Pérez-Cózar; M.L. & Redondo-Cuenca, A. (2013). Sequential extraction of polysaccharides from enzymatically hydrolyzed okara by-product: physicochemical properties and in vitro fermentability. *Food Chemistry* http://dx.doi.org/10.1016/j.foodchem.2013.03.066.

Weightman, R.M.; Renard, C.M.G.C. & Thibault, J.-F. (1994). Structure and properties of the polysaccharides from pea hull. Part 1: Chemical extraction and fractionation of the polysaccharides. *Carbohydrate Polymers, 24,* 139-148.

Yapo, B.M.; Lerouge, P.; Thibault, J.-F. & Ralet, M.C. (2007). Pectins from citrus peel cell walls contain homogalacturonans homogenous with respect to molar mass, rhamnogalacturonan I and rhamnogalacturonan II. *Carbohydrate Polymers, 69,* 426–435.

Yu, L. & Mort, A.J. (1996). Pectins and Pectinases. In: J. Visser & A.G.J. Voragen (Eds). *Progress in Biotechnology,* vol. 14. Amsterdam, Netherlands: Elsevier Sicence.

In: Dietary Fiber
Editors: D. Betancur-Ancona, L. Chel-Guerrero et al.
ISBN: 978-1-62808-931-8

Chapter 2

Pectins: Sources, Properties and their Relationship to Health

Lúcia Cristina Vriesmann and Carmen Lúcia de Oliveira Petkowicz*
Universidade Federal do Paraná, Departamento de Bioquímica e Biologia Molecular, Curitiba-PR, Brazil

Abstract

Pectins are a family of complex, acid-rich polysaccharides present in the cell walls of all land plants. The main classes of pectins include homogalacturonan (HG) and rhamnogalacturonans (RG). The HG or 'smooth regions' have linear chains of (1→4)-linked α-D-galacturonic acid residues which can be partly methyl-esterified at the C-6 carboxyl, and sometimes O-acetylated at O-2 or O-3. The RG-I has repeating units of $[\text{-}\alpha\text{-D-galacturonic acid -1,2-}\alpha\text{-L-rhamnose-1,4-}]_n$. The rhamnose units being substituted at O-4 with neutral sugar chains, such as arabinans, galactans or arabinogalactans. RG-II is less abundant and has a backbone of HG with complex side-chains containing rare sugars. Pectins are largely used as gelling, thickening and stabilizing agents, mainly in the food industry. These properties are influenced by the structural features of the pectin leading to distinct applications. The composition and properties of pectin depends on the plant source and conditions used during pectin isolation and purification. In the last years progress has been made in the elucidation of the fine structure of pectins. Although pectins commonly occur in most plant tissues, the number of sources commercially used is quite limited and commercial pectins are almost exclusively derived from either citrus peels or apple pomace, both by-products from juice manufacturing. However due the crescent industrial demand for pectins many alternative sources are currently investigated. In the plants pectins are involved in many functions and undergo important changes during fruit ripening. Whether naturally present in vegetables and fruits or added as a food additive, pectins are present in the human diet. Pectins are not depolymerized by intestinal enzymes. As soluble dietary fibers, pectin intake assists in the proper functioning of the intestine and has several effects on human health, including

* Email: clop@ufpr.br.

interactions with bile acids or metal ions, lowering serum cholesterol and glucose, amongst others. Besides that, it has been shown that pectins can display other beneficial effects such as immunomodulatory and anti-cancer activity and their oligosaccharides can block the adherence of certain pathogenic microorganisms to the intestinal mucosa.

Introduction

In the last decades, the general perception about carbohydrates changed radically. Formerly described only as structural materials or energy sources, nowadays carbohydrates are recognized to perform a much broader biological role. They are involved in the immune response and inflammation, cell-cell recognition, infection by some pathogenic species and cancer pathology, among other biological process (Schepetkin and Quinn, 2006; Persin et al., 2011).

Carbohydrates are the most abundant organic compounds in nature and have emerged as a source for sustainable fuel, food, materials and medicine production. Polysaccharides have a central role in preparation of food products primarily as a carbohydrate source but also as thickener, gelling and emulsifier agents (Persin et al., 2011).

The main food carbohydrates can be divided into digestible (monosaccharides, disaccharides, dextrins and starch) and indigestible polysaccharides. Nondigestible polysaccharides that are contained in food products are referred to as dietary and many of them have been recognized as low calorie functional food ingredients and prebiotics (Wheeler and Pi-Sunyer, 2008; Persin et al., 2011). Plant polysaccharides have been investigated for their potential as health promoting food additive. Among the plant polysaccharides, this chapter focuses on pectins. Pectins are a group of structural polymers found in all higher plants thus being part of the natural human diet. However, the relative abundance and structural details of pectins differ between cell types and plant species. Besides to be a natural component of vegetables and fruits, pectins have been used as a food additive due to their thickening, gelling and stabilizing properties (Rolin, 1993; Voragen et al., 2009). It is regarded as an extremely safe food additive, and its composition and use is regulated under Food Additive law. It is also recognized under the international Codex Alimentarius (Voragen et al., 1995; IPPA, 2013). Next to their uses in the food industry, pectins have also been studied for pharmaceutical and medical applications and the pectin intake has beneficial effects on human health.

The discovery of pectins is attributed to Vauquelin (1790) that found an unidentified acidic material in the tamarind pulp. Later, Braconnot (1825) isolated a viscous acidic material from all the vegetables that he studied. He proposed the name pectic acid or pectin. The word pectin is derived from the Greek (πηχτος) where it means 'to congeal, solidify or curdle'. Braconnot (1825) was also the first to recognize that pectins were the fruit component responsible for gel formation (Willats et al., 2006). However, the assumption that pectins are polymers from galacturonic acid is atributted to Smolenski (1923).

The homemade jams and jellies have been produced at least since the 18th century. Recipes were published in 1750 which described jellies made from apple, currant, and quince, all fruits rich in gelling pectins. Pectin was first isolated in the 1820s, and shown to be the key to making jams and jellies with fruits which do not set jams well (IPPA, 2013).

The first commercial production of pectin was recorded in 1908 in Germany, and the process spread rapidly to the United States, where a patent was obtained (US Pat. 1.082,682, 1913). This was followed by a rapid growth of the pectin industry in the United States, and later in Europe. However, in the last years, the center of production has moved to Europe and to citrus-producing countries like Mexico and Brazil (IPPA, 2013).

At the beginning, pectin start to be commercialized as a liquid extract, however nowadays it is produced commercially as a white to light brown powder, extracted mainly from citrus peels or apple pomace (IPPA, 2013).

Although traditionally pectins are also defined by their extractability from the plant cell walls with chelating agents, the industrial process of production is based in the extraction using a hot diluted mineral acid. The extract is treated with alcohol (usually isopropanol) to precipitate the pectin. The precipitate is separated, washed with more alcohol to remove impurities and dried to afford the pectin powder (IPPA, 2013).

Plant Cell Walls and Pectins

In plant and animal cells, a plasma membrane encloses a cytosol containing several types of organelles. However, only plant cells are surrounded by a cell wall which provides strength and rigidity to the cell and also protects against desiccation and pathogens. Pectins are present in the cell walls of all living plants and are also found as the major adhesive material between cells (Willats et al., 2001). Pectins are complex polysaccharides from plant cell wall, present in combination with cellulose and hemicelluloses (xyloglucan, xylans, mannans and arabinogalactan), and also protein and aromathic substances. Constituting about one third of the dry material from cell wall of higher plants, they are found mainly in the primary wall and middle lamella of plant cells (O'Neill and York, 2003; Raj et al., 2012).

In the middle lamella, the region connecting neighboring cells, pectins are important for cell adhesion. In primary cell wall, present in growing cells, succulent tissue cells (as fruits) and meristhematic cells, pectins contribute to water retention and gel formation, influencing the mechanical properties of cell wall (O'Neill and York, 2003; Voragen et al., 2009).

Pectins play an important role in the formation of plant cell walls. They can form gels by crosslink with calcium ions, enabling a fine control of wall porosity. They influence the pH, ion balance, surface charge and porosity of cell wall. These properties in turn are likely to influence cell wall links and hydration status thus controlling the movement of molecules and ions, the access of cell wall-modifying enzymes to their substrate and the cell growth. They also can modify the growth and development of plant tissues, as well as they undergo structural modifications during these steps (O'Neill et al., 2001; Voragen et al., 2009).

The texture of fruits and vegetables during growing, ripening and storage is strongly influenced by the amount, composition and fine structure of the pectins (Voragen et al., 1995). One of the most important changes during ripening of fleshy fruits is the softening of their tissues which is due mainly to structural changes in the cell wall. The most common changes in the cell wall during ripening are related to pectin solubilization and depolymerization (Rose et al., 2003).

Desirable and undesirable changes in the properties of fruits and vegetables products during processing are also related to changes in the pectic components (Voragen et al., 1995).

Another function of pectins is related with plant defense against pathogens. Pectic oligosaccharides released by action of enzymes secreted by many plant pathogens activate several plant defense responses in diseased plants. These signalling oligomers, known as oligosaccharins, elicit the accumulation of phytoalexin which has anti-microbial activity, induces lignification and accumulation of protease inhibitors. Regulatory roles in non-diseased plants have also been proposed for pectic oligosaccharides (Dumville and Fry, 2000).

Composition and Chemical Structure of Pectins

Although pectin was discovered over 200 years ago, its composition and structure are not yet completely elucidated. Pectin may be composed out of as many as 17 different monosaccharides containing more than 20 different linkages. As pectin may alter during isolation from plants, and also during storage and processing of the plant material, its structure is very difficult to determine (Voragen et al., 2009; Raj et al., 2012).

Chemically, pectins encompass a family of complex polysaccharides rich in galacturonic acid and extremely diversified in their fine structure and molecular mass (Raj et al., 2012).

Structurally, pectic polysaccharides are classified as homogalacturonans (HGs), rhamnogalacturonans (RGs) and substituted galacturonans (O'Neill and York, 2003). Inside this classification, the three main blocks that compose pectins include homogalacturonan (HG), rhamnogalacturonan I (RG-I) and rhamnogalacturonan II (RG-II) (Willats et al., 2001).

Homogalacturonans (HG) are the main pectic polysaccharide in cell walls (60% of the total pectin amount). They constitute the 'smooth region' of pectin chain, being linear homopolymers composed by pyranosidic units of D-galacturonic acid (Gal*p*A) α-(1→4) linked in which some acidic groups are methyl-esterified. Depending on plant type, Gal*p*A units can carry *O*-acetyl at C-3 or C-2 (O'Neill and York, 2003; Voragen et al., 2009).

Rhamnogalacturonans constitute the 'hairy region' of pectins and can be rhamnogalacturonan I (RG-I) and rhamnogalacturonan II (RG-II). RG-I consists of a main chain with alternant pyranosidic units of D-Gal*p*A α-(1→4) linked and L-rhamnose (Rha) α-(1→2) linked. Although Gal*p*A units can present acetyl groups at *O*-2 or *O*-3, there was no evidence that they are methyl-esterified. Concomitantly, Rha units of main chain can be substituted (20-80%) at C-4 with side chains, as arabinans, galactans and arabinogalactans (O'Neill et al., 2001; Voragen et al., 2009).

Arabinans present a main chain of furanosidic units of L-arabinose (Ara) α-(1→5) linked, with branches attached to *O*-2 or *O*-3 of various Ara units from the main chain. They are present, for example, in apple and mustard seeds pectins (Voragen et al., 1995; Pérez et al., 2000).

Arabinogalactans occurs in two structurally different forms: type I and type II arabinogalactans. In the first type, they have a linear chain composed by pyranosidic units of D-galactose (Gal) β-(1→4) linked with 20-40% of furanosidic units of L-Ara α-(1→5) linked present as short side chains branched at *O*-3 from Gal units. Type I arabinogalactans were found in citric and tomato pectins (Pérez et al., 2000; Voragen et al., 1995). In contrast, type II arabinogalactanas are highly branched and more complex, composed by pyranosidic units of β-D-Gal joined by (1→3) and (1→6) linkages. The first predominate in internal chains and the second occurs mainly in external chains, which carry additional branches of furanosidic α-L-Ara units in (1→3) and/or (1→5) linkages (Voragen et al., 1995).

Other monosaccharides which can be present in side chains of RG-I are: D-xylose (Xyl), D-glucose (Glc), D-mannose (Man), L-fucose (Fuc), D-glucuronic acid (GlcA) and 4-*O*-methyl-D-glucuronic acid (2-*O*-Me GlcA) (Voragen et al., 1995). Phenolic acids, as ferulic acid and *p*-coumaric acid, also can be present in ester form in some side chains (O'Neill et al., 2001).

Ramnogalacturonan-II is the most complex pectic polysaccharide (Pellerin et al., 1996) and it is not structurally related to RG-I, being considered a substituted galacturonan (O'Neill et al., 2001). In the RG-II, the main galacturonan chain is formed by at least seven units of Gal*p*A α-(1→4) linked. Four complex side chains consisting by 12 different monosaccharides and 20 distinct linkages are connected in the main chain of Gal*p*A: two octasaccharides structurally distinct are linked at C-2 and two disaccharides structurally different are linked at C-3, although the localization of the side chains in relation to Gal*p*A units is not exactly known. Rare sugars are found among the monosaccharides of RG-II side chains, as aceric acid (3-*C*-carboxy-5-deoxy-β-L-xylose; Ace*f*A), apiose (Api*f*), 2-*O*-methyl-fucose (2-*O*-Me-Fuc*p*), 2-*O*-methyl-xylose (2-*O*-Me-Xyl*p*), 2-keto-3-deoxy-D-manno-octulosonic acid (Kdo) and 2-keto-3-deoxy-D-lyxo-heptulosaric acid (Dha). Apiose units of side chains from two RG-II chains are esterified with boric acid, forming RG-II dimers in primary plant cell walls. Even though the complexity, RG-II structure seems to be conserved in cell walls of higher plants (Pellerin et al., 1996; Pérez et al., 2000; O'Neill and York, 2003; Voragen et al., 2009).

Other substituted galacturonans include xylogalacturonans and apiogalacturonans. In xylogalacturonans, identified in soybean, pea, watermelon, carrot, lemon peel and apple, pyranosidic β-D-Xyl units are present as side chains composed by single units attached to C-3 of Gal*p*A from the main chain (O'Neill et al., 2001; Voragen et al., 1995; Willats et al., 2001). In apiogalacturonans, as those found in cell walls of some aquatic monocots (*Lemna* e *Zostera*), furanosidic β-D-Api is present as single unit in the side chains or as the disaccharide [β-D-Api*f*-(1→3')-β-D-Api*f*-(1→] linked at C-2 of Gal*p*A from the main chain (O'Neill et al., 2001). All pectin molecules have linear segments of Gal*p*A whose carboxylic groups can be esterified with methanol and Gal*p*A units also can have *O*-acetyl groups (O'Neill et al., 2001; Rolin, 1993). The proportion of methyl-esterified carboxylic groups in relation to the total carboxylic groups in pectins is termed as the degree of esterification (DE), and the proportion of *O*-acetyl groups in relation to the total Gal*p*A units is defined as degree of acetylation (DA). Depending on DE, pectins are classified in two groups: high-methoxyl pectins (HM pectins or 'pectin'), with DE higher than 50%, and low-methoxyl pectins (LM pectins or 'pectic acid'), with DE lower than 50% (Voragen et al., 1995; O'Neill and York, 2003). In general, native pectins have high DE (HM pectins) and low DA (Voragen et al., 1995). DE can vary depending on species, tissue, and maturity. Pectin seems be synthesized firstly in a highly esterified form, and decreases in the DE are often observed when cells mature (O'Neill and York, 2003; Raj et al., 2012). LM pectins can also be obtained by HM pectin deesterification using acid, alkali or enzyme treatments. If deesterification is made under alkaline conditions in the presence of ammonia, methyl-esterified groups are transformed in amide groups leading to the formation of 'amidated low methoxyl pectins' (Fraeye et al., 2010; Raj et al., 2012). A schematic representation of pectin structures is depicted in Figure 1. The plant sources as well the extraction conditions influence pectin characteristics (Rolin, 1993). Thus, they can present distinct compositions, DE, DA and physico-chemical characteristics, important parameters for their applicability.

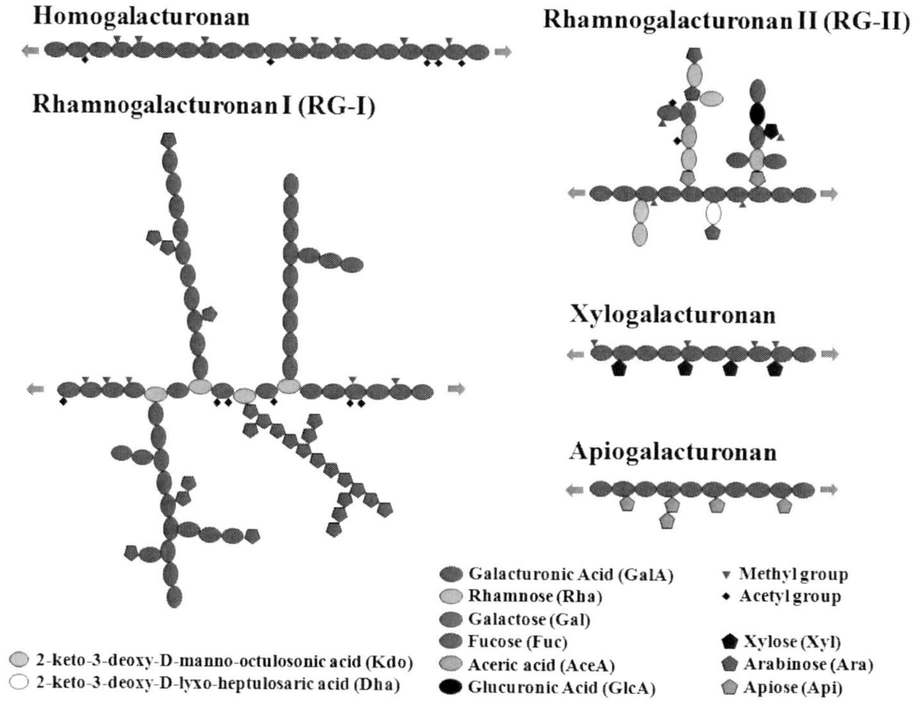

Figure 1. Schematic representation of pectin structures (Adapted from: Voragen et al., 2009 and Willats et al., 2006).

Functionalities and Application of Pectins

As previously stated, the name "pectin" is directly related to the ability of these polymers to form gel under certain conditions and also to improve liquid viscosity, properties that constitute the basis of their commercial use. Thus, pectin is considered an important additive in food, pharmaceutical and cosmetic manufactures, exhibiting specific functional properties depending on each application (Voragen et al., 1995; O'Neill et al., 2001; Fraeye et al., 2010).

In the food industry, pectin is one of the most commonly hydrocolloid employed. Due to its colloidal stabilizing and thickening properties, pectins are used as additives in jelly, mayonnaise, salad creams, dressings, concentrated juices, beverages and ice creams (Voragen et al., 1995). For stability at low pH values, pectins have applications in acidic food, stabilizing, for instance, yoghurts and milk drinks, and combinations thereof with fruit juices (Rolin, 1993; Fraeye et al., 2010).

The main application of pectin is as a gelling agent. Pectin gel is formed when homogalacturonan portions are associated to form a three dimensional network in which water and solutes are entrapped. Several factors determine the occurrence of pectin gelation and influence the gel characteristics, including the temperature, pectin concentration, pH, co-solute (sugar) and ion (Ca^{+2}) concentration (Rolin, 1993; Willats et al. 2006). The limits of these factors and the way in which they influence gelation are dependent on the molecular properties of pectins such as average molecular weight, degree of esterification and amidation (proportion of amide groups), presence of acetyl ester at C-2 and C-3 of *GalpA* units from galacturonan chain, presence and distribution of Rha (which causes twists in the pectin chain) and distribution (random or in block) of the charge and ester groups along the molecule (Rolin, 1993; Willats et al., 2006; Fraeye et al., 2010). Thus, pectins from different sources have variation in these factors, and consequently, their gelation capacities are distinct (Sato et al., 2004).

The gelation mechanism is different for HM and LM pectins (Rolin, 1993; Fraeye et al., 2010). Gelation of aqueous solution of HM pectins is frequently observed at acidic pH (lower than 3.5), in the presence of high amount of sugar and similar co-solutes (typically 60-65% sucrose), being this the procedure employed in conventional marmalade manufacture (Bulone et al., 2002; Raj et al., 2012).

The high co-solute concentration creates low water activity conditions, where chain-chain interaction predominates in relation to solvent-chain interactions, whereas acidic pH reduces carboxylic acid dissociation, resulting in less negative charges and thus minimizing electrostatic repulsion between chains. With the reduction of the repulsion and the availability of water for solvation of HM pectins, chains come together and form junction zones, which are stabilized by hydrophobic interactions between the methyl groups and hydrogen bonding between non-dissociated carboxylic groups and secondary alcohols (Figure 2) (Voragen et al., 1995; Raj et al., 2012).

Under similar conditions, HM pectins with higher molecular mass form stronger gels. High proportions of acetyl groups and hairy region (RG-I) disturb pectin gelation. The degree of esterification in HM pectins group determine the gelation rate: the time for gel formation may vary from 1-3 minutes to more than one hour, and the pH needed to reach gelation can decrease from 3.4 to 2.6 (Voragen et al., 1995).

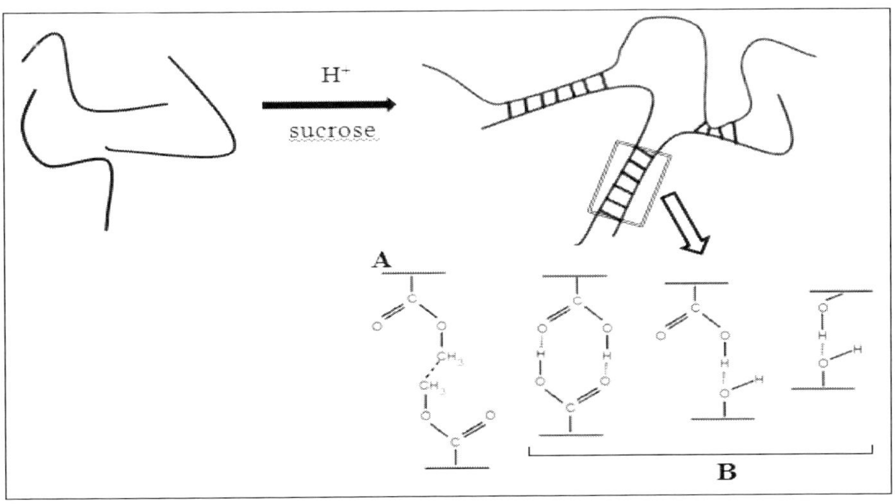

Figure 2. Mechanisms of gelation of HM pectin. A: hydrophobic interactions between the methyl groups, B: hydrogen bonds between non-dissociated carboxylic groups and secondary alcohols (Adapted from: Rinaudo, 1996 and Kastner et al., 2012).

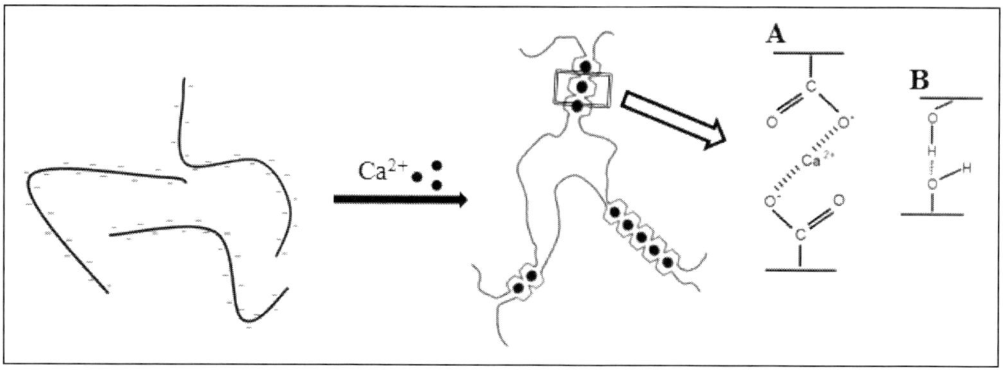

Figure 3. Mechanisms of gelation of LM pectin. A: ionic interactions between dissociated carboxylic groups through calcium ions ('egg box' model), B: hydrogen bonds (Adapted from: Rinaudo, 1996 and Kastner et al., 2012).

HM pectin gels are considerably important in food manufacture, as processed products containing fruit, such as jams and jellies, are acidic and contain a high sucrose concentration (O'Neill et al. 2001;), and thus, their characteristic and physicochemical properties are constantly analyzed.

In general, it has been observed that the formation of HM pectins gels occurs within a certain pH range, because very low pH values are critical and there is no gelation at pH> 3.5 (El-Nawawi and Heikel, 1997; Evageliou et al., 2000). Furthermore, the use of sucrose as co-solute in HM pectin gelation is recognized to form stronger gels (Tsoga et al., 2004).

In the case of LM pectins, sucrose is not necessary for the gelation, which occurs in the presence of divalent cations such as calcium ions, which act as a bridge between pairs of dissociated carboxylic groups from different pectin chains in a pH range between 2.5 and 6.0, forming junction zones between the homogalacturonan regions through ionic and electrostatic bonding, leading to gelation (Figure 3) (O'Neill et al., 2001; Fraeye et al., 2010; Raj et al., 2012).

This type of junction zones formation may be described by 'egg box' model, where pectate chains are double helices and in the junction areas, with their antiparallel arrangement, these chains form binding spaces, which entrap calcium ions which link the chains together. Apparently, the gelation involves two stages, being the first the dimers formation (egg box) and the second the condensation of dimmers in aggregates (many egg boxes are positioned) (Rolin, 1993; Fraeye et al., 2010).

In addition to the electrostatic interactions, the junction zones between two adjacent pectin chains are also stabilized by Van der Waals interactions and hydrogen bonding between the polar groups of pectin molecules (Fraeye et al., 2010). Because half of the carboxylic groups are guided out of the 'egg box', the presence of a limited number of methyl-esterified units does not preclude the formation of one junction (Fraeye et al., 2010).

Due the electrostatic nature of the chain junction zones, LM pectin gels are very sensitive to structural parameters that can modify the environment of the carboxylic groups, such as the nature, amount and distribution of substituents along the homogalacturonan chain. Thus, the presence of acetyl groups drastically reduces the affinity of pectin for calcium. Side branches in high proportion cause steric hindrance, which can hinder the interactions through calcium ions between adjacent chains of pectins and affect the gel. The presence of amide groups in

C-6 (amidation) improves the ability of LM pectins to form gels, especially at low pH values, due the additional contribution of hydrogen bonds between the amide groups. Additionally, less calcium is required for gelation of amidated pectins, which are also less susceptible to precipitation by high calcium content (Voragen et al., 1995; Lootens et al., 2003; Fraeye et al., 2010).

Furthermore, the gel forming ability of LM pectin increases with decreasing DE (because there are increasing numbers of deesterified Gal*p*A sequences) and the amount of the pectin required for the formation of such gel is lower. LM pectins with free carboxyl groups distributed in blocks are very sensitive to low calcium levels and form stronger gels than LM pectins with random distribution of free carboxyl groups (Voragen et al., 1995; Fraeye et al., 2010).

Gelation process of LM pectins also depends on external factors, such as temperature, pH, ionic strength and amount of calcium added. At excessive concentration of calcium, junction zones may consist of multiple interconnected HG chains, which may lead to precipitation (O'Neill et al. 2001; Fraeye et al. 2010).

If sugar is present in small amounts (10-20%), its effect combined with pH allows gelation at lower calcium levels by promoting chain-chain interactions, besides its presence leads to a tendency to decrease syneresis and adds desirable firmness of these LM pectin gels (Voragen et al., 1995; Raj et al., 2012). Increase in sucrose concentration favors the LM pectin gel formation (Fu and Rao, 2001; Cardoso et al., 2003; Iglesias and Lozano, 2004), as well as increases in the amount of pectin used (Fu and Rao, 2001; Cardoso et al., 2003). However, high sugar concentration (≥60%) may interfere with LM pectin gelation as the dehydration caused by sugar favors hydrogen bonding and decreases cross-linking by divalent ion forces (Raj et al., 2012).

Usual concentrations of HM pectin in gels vary from 2.0 to 4.0%, and of LM pectins from 0.1 to 4.0 % (Burey et al., 2008).

In most cases, a pectin gel is prepared under heating and then solidified by cooling. When cooled below the gelation temperature, systems containing LM pectins will gel almost instantaneously, whereas systems with HM pectins will gel after a certain time. Once formed, the HM pectin gel cannot be undone, but in most cases, a LM pectin gel can be undone and reconstituted repeatedly, in other words, is thermoreversible (Rolin, 1993).

By the characteristics of their gelling, LM pectin can be used in products with low sugar content, such as low calorie jellies, bakery, and other applications involving restriction in sugar content. The pH range where LM pectin gelation occurs allows its use in foods that require to form gel under less acidic conditions, e.g., to preserve flavors (Thibault and Ralet, 2001). The thermal reversibility of LM pectin gels allow their use in fillings and coatings of bakery and confectionery products that undergo pasteurization or sterilization procedures, or heating in a microwave (Iglesias and Lozano, 2004).

Commercial Sources of Pectin

Commercial pectin are usually obtained from apple pomace and citrus peel (lemon, lime, orange, and grapefruit), the by-products obtained after juice extraction by industries, and both pectins are primarily homogalacturonans (Rolin, 1993; Voragen et al., 2009). Apple pomace contains between 10 and 15% pectin on a dry matter basis, and citrus peels contain from 20 to 30% pectin. Both pectins are largely equivalent from an application point of view. However, apple pectins are often darker than citrus pectins, which are light tan or light cream in color. DE values for commercial HM-pectins typically range from 60 to 75% and those for LM-pectins range from 20 to 40% (Thibault and Ralet, 2001; Raj et al., 2012).

Pectins can be obtained from plant cell walls with hot water, buffer and chelating agent solutions, hot diluted acid, cold alkali solutions or with the use of enzymes (Voragen et al., 1995; O'Neill et al. 2001). By varying the extraction procedure, distinct molecules can be obtained.

Generally, commercial pectins are extracted from plant material with hot diluted mineral acid solutions, at pH from 1 to 3, time between 30 minutes to 24 hours and temperature from 50 to 100°C, and are recovered from extracts by alcoholic precipitation (Voragen et al., 1995; IPPA, 2013).

Although organic acids, as acetic, citric, lactic, malic and tartaric acids, can be employed for pectin extraction, there was a preference for mineral acids, as nitric, chloridric and sulphuric acids, mainly due their lower cost. For alcoholic precipitation, methanol, ethanol and 2-prophanol can be used. Normally, pectin precipitates in alcohol concentration of at least 45% (w/v). After precipitation, pectin is washed to remove contaminants. In the sequence, the precipitated pectin is collected, dried and milled. To constitute the form for commerce, pectins are standardized with sucrose, glucose or lactose until a degree of gelation of 150 °SAG U.S., to ensure always the same gel strength (Sakai et al., 1993; Voragen et al., 1995).

The Search for New Sources of Pectins

Considering that current commercial pectins are almost exclusively derived from citrus peel or apple pomace and that around the world there were several other plant by-products with potential to be exploited, new sources of pectin are constantly sought. The main of these include sugarbeet waste (Levigne et al., 2002), soy hulls (Kalapathy and Proctor, 2001), residues of sunflower seeds (Iglesias and Lozano, 2004) and fruit residues, as banana (Happi Emaga et al., 2008); cocoa (Vriesmann et al., 2011), passion fruit (Yapo, 2009) and mango (Koubala et al., 2008).

Depending on the starting material and the employed conditions, different yield and chemical and physicochemical properties are found for the pectin, which are directly involved in its applications. Furthermore, the presence of a large quantity of pectin in a plant material alone is not in itself enough to qualify that plant as a source of commercial pectin (Raj et al., 2012).

Besides the high content of pectin in sugar beet pulp, the main residue of sugar industry in Europe, the native pectins obtained from this source in general presented relatively low molecular mass and degree of esterification, and high content of acetyl and branches (Pippen et al., 1950; Thibault, 1986; Levigne et al., 2002), showing poor gelling properties in the native form (Pippen et al., 1950; Matthew et al., 1990). However, they were reported to exhibit surfactant and emulsifying properties (Yapo et al., 2007) and to be capable of forming a thermally stable covalently cross-linked gel through ferulic acid residues (Fraeye et al., 2010).

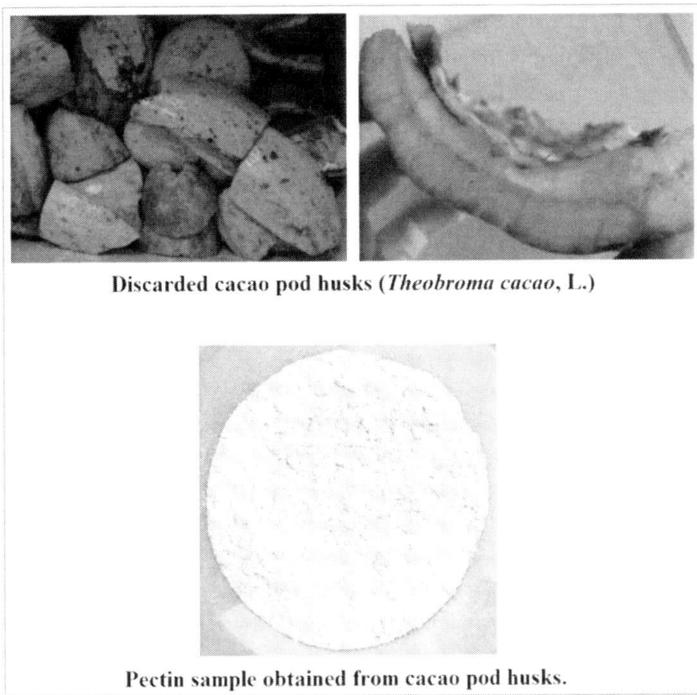
Discarded cacao pod husks (*Theobroma cacao*, L.)
Pectin sample obtained from cacao pod husks.

Figure 4. Cacao pod husk, a potential new source of pectin.

Soy hulls, banana and mango peels were suggested as potential pectin source (Kalapathy and Proctor, 2001; Happi Emaga et al., 2008; Koubala et al., 2008), however the physicochemical properties of their pectins and particularly their gelling properties were not known at present. For sunflower head residues pectins, gels were formed at high temperatures almost instantly in the presence of calcium ions (Iglesias and Lozano, 2004).

Yellow passion fruit peels, by-products obtained after juice extraction by industries in many tropical regions, LM and HM pectins rich in Gal*p*A were obtained and presented good gelling properties, suggesting their potential to exploitation (Yapo, 2009).

For cacao pod husks, the first and main by-product of cocoa exploitation, generated after cocoa beans are extracted from the mature cacao fruit, pectins with high content of acetyl were obtained (Figure 4) (Vriesmann et al., 2011), suggesting that gel formation would not be possible. However, gel was obtained at low pH and high sucrose content, indicating the potential use of the pectin as a gelling and thickening additive (Vriesmann and Petkowicz, 2013).

At the present, there was several suggested pectin with desirable properties from different available sources, but the pectins are not commercially employed, showing the need of research directed on their application in distinct products.

Pectins Contributing to Dietary Fiber

In the last years many attention has been given to the dietary fiber due the beneficial physiological effects that they may exert on health. Many authors have proposed chemical and physiological definitions for dietary fiber. One of the most accepted definition of dietary fiber is used for plant substances that are resistant to hydrolysis by human digestive enzymes. Dietary fiber escapes digestion in the small intestine and passes into large intestine, where it provides a substrate for the microflora of the large intestine (Dreher, 2001; Oakenfull, 2001).

The major portion of dietary fibers in foods came from plant cell walls (Dreher, 2001). Structural polysaccharides are the main components of plant cell walls and are usually categorized into cellulose, hemicellulose and pectins. Since all plant cells have cell walls, pectins are naturally present in fruits and vegetables in different amounts. It has been shown that fruits and vegetables have dietary fiber contents in the range of 1-2% and in a normal western diet around 5g of pectin are consumed by day (Voragen et al., 1995; Willats et al., 2006). However, it has been claimed that a consumption of at least 6 g/day of pectin is necessary to have a significant effect in cholesterol reduction (Sriamornsak, 2003).

Pectins are included in the soluble dietary fiber components and have a high water-holding capacity (Voragen et al., 1995; Oakenfull, 2001). They increase the volume of fecal material and assist in the proper functioning of the intestine. Soluble fibers are very accessible and ferment faster in the large intestine than insoluble fiber fractions. The pectins and are almost completely broken down by the microflora in the large intestine (Oakenfull, 2001). At least the portion RGII of pectins remain intact even in the large intestine, since the RGII side chains are resistant to glycanases secreted by microorganisms because they contain monomeric units and linkages that are not typically present in other cell wall polysaccharides (O'Neill and York, 2003).

The fermentation of polysaccharides by intestinal microbial flora in the large intestine leads to the production of short-chain fatty acids, which are used as an energy source by colonocytes and have a trophic effect on the colon wall. Pectins have been reported to stimulate short-chain fatty acids production, had a trophic effect on the different parts of the intestines, and greatly stimulated protein synthesis in those tissues (Pirman et al., 2007).

It has been pointed that high fiber foods induce a feeling of saciety thus reducing the food intake. It has been shown that soluble fibers, like pectins, reduce the appetite a longer time than insoluble (Oakenfull, 2001).

Although there are some controversial results, it is believed that viscous polysaccharides from dietary fibers inhibit transport across the small intestinal epithelia. Pectin reduces rates of digestion by immobilizing food components in the intestine and the viscous layer of the pectin make the contact between the intestinal enzyme and the food difficult (Sriamornsak, 2003).

It was demonstrated that pectins decreased post prandial hyperglycemia of diabetic patients (Jenkins et al., 1976). However, according to William et al. (1980), to reduce effectively the response in post-prandial glucose and insulin the pectin (and also other dietary fibers supplement) must be administered with the major carbohydrate content of the meal or that the timing of the fiber supplement in relation to the consumption of the remainder of the meal.

It is also frequently accepted that dietary fibers have ability to bind bile acids, thus lowering the cholesterol levels. It was observed that pectins increased the fecal excretion of bile acids. However, a study using supplementation with a commercially available product containing pectin and other dietary fibers provided modest shortterm benefits in reducing total and LDL-cholesterol, beyond that achieved by a standard cholesterol-lowering diet (Hosobuchi et al., 1999). In an earlier study, Mokady (1973) compared the effect of dietary pectin and alginate (a polysaccharide from algae) on blood cholesterol of growing rats fed with a cholesterol-free diet. The authors observed that pectin was found to lower blood cholesterol significantly while the effect of alginate was very small. It was shown that the level of endogenic cholesterol in rats was lowered by feeding them with highly viscous pectin which had a high content of methoxyl groups. By the other side, a high dietary intake of pectin was reported to decrease the availability of vitamin E in rats (de Lumen et al., 1982). According to the author, the effect is consistent with the hypothesis that pectins bind bile acids thus consequently decreasing the absorption of lipid-soluble components such as vitamin E.

Concerning the effect of pectins in cholesterol levels, it has been claimed that a daily intake of ~ three apples resulted in a decrease in total cholesterol of 5 - 8%. It seems likely that there is a reduction in total plasma and LDL cholesterol, and a considerable decrease in the risk of cardiovascular disease, after a daily intake of two-to-six apples; however the response may be more evident in hypercholesterolemic subjects (Jensen et al., 2009).

Polysaccharides have the ability to bind polar molecules and ions. In this way, diets high in fiber can reduce mineral availability. It seems that the number of free carboxyl groups and uronic acid contents are the major factor determining the ability to bind metal ions. Once pectins are rich in uronic acid (galacturonic) it is expected that pectins affect the mineral availability. However, it was shown that a highly esterified pectin with low molecular weight enhanced intestinal solubility and absorption of ferric and ferrous iron in rats (Kim, 1998). On the other hand, it has been reported that inclusion of pectins in to the human diet has been shown to reduce the uptake of toxic metals and actinides (Pellerin and O'Neill, 1998).

Pectins are solubilized during the processing of fruits and vegetables and are present in fruit-juices and fermented beverages including cider or wine. It has been demonstrate that dimers of RG II can form complex with heavy metals. Trace amounts of heavy metals, like lead, were found in red wines strongly associated with RG II, thus reducing its uptake (Pellerin and O'Neill, 1998).

Other Health Aspects of Pectins

Besides the properties associated to fiber ingestion, other aspects related with health have been investigated for pectins (Yamada, 1996).

Several authors have described the immunostimulating activity of pectic polysaccharides isolated from different plants (Kiyohara et al., 1988; Inngjerdingen et al., 2005; Nergard et al., 2005; Kiyohara et al., 2006; Grønhaug et al., 2011; Khramova et al., 2011).

Oral administration of pectic polysaccharides was reported to promote modulation of the intestinal immune system. It was shown that pectic polysaccharide fragments containing galactose expressed immunomodulating activity against Peyer's patch immunocompetent cells (Grønhaug et al., 2011).

The oral administration of a pectic polysaccharide from the stems of *Cirsium esculentum* was found to prevent induction of oral tolerance to ovalbumin, increase the levels of serum IgG2a, and down regulate serum IgE responses. When the polysaccharide was tested for anti-allergic properties the score of systemic anaphylactic reaction showed a decrease (Khramova et al., 2011). An oral adjuvant effect was observed for a pectic polysaccharide from *Lemna minor* L (Popov et al., 2006).

Pectic polysaccharides found in medicinal plants were described to activate the complement system through the classical and alternative pathways (Kiyohara et al., 1988). Two pectic polysaccharides isolated from a medicinal plant used against various types of illnesses related to the immune response were investigated and shown to exhibit potent dose-dependent complement fixating activities, and induced chemotaxis of macrophages, T cells and NK cells (Inngjerdingen et al., 2005). It was reported the presence of antibodies in normal human sera and human colostrum, which react with carbohydrate chains of pharmacologically active pectic polysaccharides from plants used in traditional medicine (Kiyohara et al., 2006).

The inhibitory effect of citrus pectins with different degrees of esterification on the expressions of inducible nitric oxide synthase (iNOS) and cyclooxygenase-2 (COX-2) in lipopolysaccharide (LPS)-activated macrophages was investigated (Chen et al., 2006). The pectin inhibited the protein and mRNA expressions of iNOS and COX-2 in LPS-activated macrophages, and DE90 pectin was the most-potent inhibitor. According to the authors, the pectin with DE 90 could bind with LPS, resulting in decreased binding of LPS to its receptor. These results suggest that modulation of iNOS and COX-2 expressions by dietary pectin may be important in cancer chemoprevention and anti-inflammation (Chen et al., 2006).

Citrus pectins with different degrees of esterification were also described to affect cytokine production by human peripheral blood cells (Salman et al., 2008). These authors observed that pectins induced inhibition or did not alter the secretion of pro-inflammatory cytokines and caused a dose-dependent increased secretion of the anti-inflammatory cytokines. The results indicated that citrus pectin possesses the capacity to exert an immunomodulatory response in human peripheral blood cells which may have a favorable effect on human health.

Several activities were described for a pectic polysaccharide from the roots of *Bupleurum falcatum* which have shown anti-complementary and anti-ulcer activities, induction of the proliferation and maturation of murine B lymphocytes in vitro and in vivo, increased non-specific immunoglobulin secretion from the B cells and stimulation of the secretion of interleukin 6 production of murine B cells and B cell lines (Guo et al., 2000).

Pectic polysaccharides and their lower molar mass fragments produced by enzymatic hydrolysis stimulated the *in vitro* differentiation of human keratinocytes (Gloaguen et al., 2008).

The potential gut health benefit of kiwifruit pectins was tested with respect to its influence on bacterial adhesion to intestinal epithelial cells (Caco-2) in vitro (Parkar et al., 2010). The authors observed that the most effective kiwifruit pectin was superior to inulin, a standard prebiotic in enhancing the adhesion of *Lactobacillus rhamnosus* and decreasing the adhesion of *Salmonella typhimurium* to Caco-2 cells.

Pectin-derived acidic oligosaccharides were found to be the active ingredient in the carrot soup used to alleviate childhood diarrhea. It have been demonstrated in animal models that pectin-derived acidic oligosaccharides improve the immune response and reduced disease parameters of allergic asthma. The pectin-derived acidic oligosaccharides have been proposed for use in infant formulae and medical nutrition. The genotoxic potential of these oligomers was evaluated and they were considered safe for human consumption for intended use (Garthoff et al., 2010).

Recently (Wang et al. 2010), it was proposed that polysaccharide portion from ginseng which contains pectins might have antidepressant effects.

Other activities attributed to pectins include antioxidant, anti-metastasis, anti-ulcer and anti-nephrosis (Dalonso and Petkowicz, 2012; Gan and Latiff, 2011; Yamada, 1996). It was also proposed that pectins can be used as vaccine for typhoid fever (Yamada, 1996).

It has been claimed that fragments of pectins obtained after chemical and/or enzymatic treatment that were called "modified pectin" (MCP) can act in the prevention and reduction of carcinogenesis. Usually these fragments are obtained from commercial citrus pectin by means of high pH and temperature treatment and are named "modified citrus pectin" also identified as MCP. The MCP has been shown to be effective either in vitro or in vivo, or both, against prostate carcinoma, colon carcinoma, breast carcinoma, melanoma, multiple myeloma, and hemangiosarcoma. One proposed explanation for such effects was that these pectin fragments, rich in galactans, contain structural elements that may bind to and inhibit the various actions of the pro-metastatic protein galectin-3 (GAL3). The animal studies into the effects of MCP on tumours and metastasis suggest that it is effectively absorbed into the bloodstream and thereby able to act upon GAL3 at its sites of action. It has been pointed that due to its anti-adhesive, apoptosis-promoting, and apoptosis-inducing properties, MCP is capable of targeting multiple critical rate-limiting steps involved in cancer metastasis. Although the evidences suggesting the potential use of MCP as an anti-cancer agent, the mechanisms involved are not completely known (Glinsky and Raz, 2009; Maxwell et al., 2012).

Pectins can also be used as a natural prophylactic substance against poisoning with toxic cations, due the ability to bind to toxic metals, as lead and mercury (Kohn, 1982).

In pharmaceutical area, pectins are studied as excipient in tablets (Liu et al., 2003), in formulations antireflux (Waterhouse et al., 2000), and to film formation (Hagesaether et al., 2009).

The pectin hydrogels can be used in tablet formulations as a binding agent and in controlled-release formulations (Sriamornsak, 2003). They have been suggested for the development of colon-specific therapeutic systems, in their native or modified forms, either alone or in combination with other natural or synthetic polymers (Ashford, 1993; Macleod et al., 1999; Sriamornsak, 2003; Maestrelli et al., 2008; Wong and Nurjaya, 2008). These systems are capable of retarding the release of tablet core materials until they reach the colon, where bacterial enzymes can degrade the pectins allowing drug release to occur (Macleod et al., 1999). Pectins display bioadhesive properties towards gastrointestinal tissues, which can contribute to their use as drug delivery device. The mucoadhesive properties of pectins can be improved by esterification with thioglycolic acid (Sharma and Ahuja, 2011). The range of applications of pectins in the health area is primarily attributable to their biodegradability and low oral toxicity (Wong and Nurjaya, 2008).

Conclusion

Pectins encompass a very diverse group of polysaccharides that are ubiquitous in plants. The functional properties of pectins are strongly dependent to their fine structures. Although commercial sources used for extraction of pectin are quite limited, promising new raw materials has been studied. Besides their use in food industry, an overview in their properties indicates a potential for wide range of applications in biomedical and pharmaceutical areas. The current status of research on pectins indicates that their biological actions in the human body can result in many beneficial health effects. Apart from the benefits from pectins intake as soluble fibers, considerable evidence from several studies suggests that pectins, native and modified, are involved in more sophisticated mechanisms than those usually associated to other soluble fibers. However, a proper application of the pectins and their derivatives requires a better understanding of the mechanisms underlying their effects.

References

Ashford, M.; Fell, J.; Attwood, D.; Sharma, H. & Woodhead, P. (1993). An evaluation of pectin as a carrier for drug targeting to the colon. *Journal of Controlled Release,* 26, 213–220.

Braconnot, H. (1825). Recherches sur un nouvel acide universellement répandu dans tous les végétaux. *Annales de Chimie et de Physique,* 28, 173-178.

Bulone, D.; Martorana, V.; Xiao, C. & Biagio, P. L. S. (2002). Role of Sucrose in Pectin Gelation: Static and Dynamic Light Scattering Experiments. *Macromolecules*, 35, 8147-8151.

Burey, P.; Bhandari, B. R.; Howes, T. & Gidley, M. J. (2008). Hydrocolloid Gel Particles: Formation, Characterization, and Application. *Critical Reviews in Food Science and Nutrition*, 48, 361-377.

Cardoso, S. M., Coimbra, M. A. & Silva, J. A. L. (2003). Temperature dependence of the formation and melting of pectin-Ca^{2+} networks: a rheological study. *Food Hydrocolloids*, 17, 801-807.

Chen C.H.; Sheu, M.T.; Chen, T.F.; Wang, Y.C.; Hou, W.C.; Liu, D.Z.; Chung, T.C. & Liang, Y.C. (2006). Suppression of endotoxin-induced pro-inflammatory responses by citrus pectin through blocking LPS signaling pathways. *Biochemical Pharmacology,* 72, 1001-1009.

Dalonso, N. & Petkowicz, C.L.O. (2012). Guarana powder polysaccharides: Characterisation and evaluation of the antioxidant activity of a pectic fraction. *Food Chemistry,* 134, 1804-1812.

de Lumen, B.O.; Lubin, B.; Chiu, D.; Reyes, P.S. & Omaye, S.T. (1982). Bioavailability of vitamin E in rats fed diets containing pectin. *Nutrition Research,* 2, 73-83.

Dreher, M.L. (2001), Dietary fiber overview. In: S.S. Cho & M.L. Dreher (Eds.), *Handbook of Dietary Fiber* (13-28). New York: Marcel Dekker.

Dumville, J. C. & Fry, S.C. (2000). Uronic acid-containing oligosaccharins: Their biosynthesis, degradation and signalling roles in non-diseased plant tissues. *Plant Physiology and Biochemistry,* 38, 125-140.

El-Nawawi, S. A., & Heikel, Y. A. (1997). Factors affecting gelation of high-ester citrus pectin. *Process Biochemistry*, 32, 381-385.

Evageliou, V., Richardson, R. K. & Morris, E. R. (2000). Effect of pH, sugar type and thermal annealing on high methoxyl pectin gels. *Carbohydrate Polymers*, 42, 245-259.

Fraeye, I.; Duvetter, T.; Doungla, E.; Loey, A. V. & Hendrickx, M. (2010). Fine-tuning the properties of pectin–calcium gels by control of pectin fine structure, gel composition and environmental conditions. *Trends in Food Science & Technology*, 21, 219-228.

Fu, J-T., & Rao, M. A. (2001). Rheology and structure development during gelation of low methoxyl pectin gels: the effect of sucrose. *Food Hydrocolloids*, 15, 93-100.

Gan, C-Y., & Latiff, A. A. (2011). Extraction of antioxidant pectic-polysaccharide from mangosteen (*Garcinia mangostana*) rind: Optimization using response surface methodology. *Carbohydrate Polymers*, 83, 600-607.

Garthoff, J.A.; Heemskerk, S.; Hempenius, R.A.; Lina, B.A.R.; Krul, C.A.M.; Koeman, J.H. & Speijers, G.J.A. (2010). Safety evaluation of pectin-derived acidic oligosaccharides (pAOS): Genotoxicity and sub-chronic studies. *Regulatory Toxicology and Pharmacology*, 57, 31–42.

Glinsky, V.V. & Raz, A. (2009). Modified citrus pectin anti-metastatic properties: one bullet, multiple targets. *Carbohydrate Research*, 344, 1788–1791.

Gloaguen, V.; Krausz, P.; Brudieux, V.; Closs, B.; Leroy, Y. & Guerardel, Y. (2008).

Structural patterns of rhamnogalacturonans modulating Hsp-27 expression in cultured human keratinocytes. *Molecules*, 13, 1207–1218.

Grønhaug, T.R.; Kiyohara, H.; Sveaass, A.; Diallo, D.; Yamada, H. & Paulsen, B.S. (2011). Beta-D-(1→4)-galactan-containing side chains in RG-I regions of pectic polysaccharides from Biophytum petersianum Klotzsch. Contribute to expression of immunomodulating activity against intestinal Peyer's patch cells and macrophages. *Phytochemistry* 72, 2139–2147.

Guo, Y.; Matsumoto, T.; Kikuchi, Y.; Ikejima, T.; Wang, B. & Yamad, H. (2000) Effects of a pectic polysaccharide from a medicinal herb, the roots of Bupleurum falcatum L. on interleukin 6 production of murine B cells and B cell lines. *Immunopharmacology*, 49, 307-316.

Hagesaether, E. Hiorth, M. & Sande, S. A. (2009). Mucoadhesion and drug permeability of free mixed films of pectin and chitosan: An *in vitro* and *ex vivo* study. *European Journal of Pharmaceutics and Biopharmaceutics*, 71, 325-33.

Happi Emaga, T.; Ronkart, S. N.; Robert, C.; Wathelet, B. & Paquot, M. (2008). Characterisation of pectins extracted from banana peels (Musa AAA) under different conditions using an experimental design. *Food Chemistry*, 108, 463-471.

Hosobuchi, C.; Rutanassee, L.; Bassin, S.L.; Wong, N.D. (1999). Efficacy of acacia, pectin and guar gum-based fiber supplementation in the control of hypercholesterolaemia. *Nutrition Research*, 19, 643 649.

Iglesias, M. T., & Lozano, J. E. (2004). Extraction and characterization of sunflower pectin. *Journal of Food Engineering*, 62, 215-223.

Inngjerdingen, K.T.; Debes, S.C.; Inngjerdingen, M.; Hokputsa, S.; Harding, S.E.; Rolstad, B.; Michaelsen, T.E.; Diallo, D. & Paulsen, B.S. (2005). Bioactive pectic polysaccharide from Glinus oppositifolius (L.) Aug. DC., a Malian medicinal plant, isolation and partial characterization. *Journal of Ethnopharmacology* 101, 204–214.

IPPA (2013). Available in: http://www.ippa.info. 3/21/2013.

Jenkins, D.A.; Leeds, A.; Wolever, T.S.; Goff, D.; George, K.; Alberti, M.M.; Gassull, M.; Derek,T. & Hockaday, R. (1976). Unabsorbable carbohydrates and diabetes: decreased post-prandial hyperglycaemia. *The Lancet*, 24, 172-174.

Jensen, E.N.; Buch-Andersen, T.; Ravn-Haren, G. & Dragsted, L.O. (2009). Mini-review: The effects of apples on plasma cholesterol levels and cardiovascular risk – a review of the evidence. *Journal of Horticultural Science & Biotechnology, ISAFRUIT Special Issue,* 34–41

Kalapathy, U., & Proctor, A. (2001). Effect of acid extraction and alcohol precipitation conditions on the yield and purity of soy hull pectin. *Food Chemistry*, 73, 393-396.

Kastner, H.; Einhorn-Stoll, U. & Senge, B. (2012). Structure formation in sugar containing pectin gels – Influence of Ca^{2+} on the gelation of low-methoxylated pectin at acidic pH. *Food Hydrocolloids*, 27, 42-49.

Khramova, D.S.; Golovchenko, V.V.; Shashkov, A.S.; Otgonbayar, D.; Chimidsogzol, A. & Ovodov, Y.S. (2011). Chemical composition and immunomodulatory activity of a pectic polysaccharide from the ground thistle *Cirsium esculentum* Siev. *Food Chemistry,* 126, 870–877.

Kim, M. (1998). Highly esterified pectin with low molecular weight enhances intestinal solubility and absorption of ferric iron in rats. *Nutrition Research,* 18, 1981-1994.

Kiyohara, H.; Matsumoto, T.; Nagai, T.; Kim, S.J. & Yamada, H. (2006). The presence of natural human antibodies reactive against pharmacologically active pectic polysaccharides from herbal medicines. *Phytomedicine,* 13, 494–500.

Kiyohara, H.; Cyong, J. & Yamada, H. (1988). Structure and anti-complementary activity of pectic polysaccharides isolated from the root of *Angelica acutiloba* Kitagawa. *Carbohydrate Research,* 182, 259-275.

Kohn, R. (1982). Binding of toxic cations to pectin, its oligomeric fragments and plant tissues. *Carbohydrate Polymers*, 2, 273-275.

Koubala, B. B.; Kansci, G.; Mbome, L. I.; Crepeau, M. J.; Thibault, J.-F. & Ralet, M.-C. (2008). Effect of extraction conditions on some physicochemical characteristics of pectins from "*Améliorée*" and "*Mango*" mango peels. *Food Hydrocolloids*, 22, 1345-1351.

Levigne, S., Ralet, M.C. & Thibault, J-F. (2002). Characterisation of pectins extracted from fresh sugar beet under different conditions using an experimental design. *Carbohydrate Polymers*, 49, 145-153.

Liu, L.; Fishman, M. L.; Kost, J. & Hicks, K. B. (2003). Pectin-based systems for colon-specific drug delivery via oral route. *Biomaterials*, 24, 3333-3343.

Lootens, D. (2003). Influence of pH, Ca concentration, temperature and amidation on the gelation of low methoxyl pectin. *Food Hydrocolloids*, 17, 237-244.

Macleod, G.S.; Fell, J.T.; Collet, J.H.; Sharma, H.L. & Smith A.M. (1999). Selective drug delivery to the colon using pectin: chitosan: hydroxypropyl methylcellulose film coated tablets. *International Journal of Pharmaceutics,* 187, 251-257.

Maestrelli, F.; Cirri, M.; Corti, G.; Mennini, N. & Mura, P. (2008). Development of enteric-coated calcium pectinate microspheres intended for colonic drug delivery. *European Journal of Pharmaceutics and Biopharmaceutics*, 69, 508-518.

Matthew, J. A.; Howson, S. J.; Keenan, M. H. J. & Belton, P. S. (1990). Improvement of the gelation properties of sugarbeet pectin following treatment with an enzyme preparation derived from Aspergillus niger - Comparison with a chemical modification. *Carbohydrate Polymers*, 12, 295-306.

Maxwell, E.G.; Belshaw, N.J.; Waldron, K.W. & Morris, V.J. (2012) Pectin – An emerging new bioactive food polysaccharide. *Trends in Food Science & Technology,* 24, 64–73.

Mokady S. (1973). Effect of dietary pectin and algin on blood cholesterol level in growing rats fed a cholesterol-free diet. *Nutrition and Metabolism* , 15, 290–294.

Nergard, C.S.; Matsumoto, T.; Inngjerdingen, M.; Inngjerdingen, K.; Hokputsa, S.; Harding, S.E.; Michaelsen, T.E.; Diallo, D.; Kiyohara, H.; Paulsen, B.S. & Yamada, H. (2005). Structural and immunological studies of a pectin and a pectic arabinogalactan from *Vernonia kotschyana* Sch. Bip. ex Walp. (Asteraceae). *Carbohydrate Research* 340, 115–130.

O'Neill, M. A. & York, W. S. (2003). The composition and structure of plant primary cell walls. In: J.K.C. Rose (Ed.), *The plant cell wall.Annual Plant Reviews series.* (1–54). Boca Raton, FL: Blackwell/CRC.

O'Neill, M. A., Darvill, A. G. & Albersheim, P. (2001). *Pectic substances.* Encyclopedia of Life Sciences, John Wiley & Sons.

Oakenfull, D. (2001), Physicochemical properties of dietary fiber: overview. In: S.S. Cho & M.L. Dreher (Eds.), *Handbook of Dietary Fiber* (195-206). New York: Marcel Dekker.

Parkar, S.G.; Redgate, E.L.; Wibisono, R.; Luo, X.; Koh, E.T.H. & Schroder, R. (2010). Gut health benefits of kiwifruit pectins: Comparison with commercial functional polysaccharides. *Journal of Functional Foods,* 2, 210-218.

Pellerin, P. & O'Neill, M.A. (1998). The interaction of the pectic polysaccharide Rhamnogalacturonan II with heavy metals and lanthanides in wines and fruit juices. *Analusis,* 26, 32-36.

Pellerin, P.; Doco, T.; Vidal, S.; Williams, P. & Brillouet, J-M. (1996). The pectic polysaccharide Rhamnogalacturonan II is a major component of the polysaccharides present in fruit-derived products. In: Visser, J., & Voragen, A. G. J. (Eds.), *Progress in Biotechnology:* Pectins and Pectinases (v. 14, pp. 67-78), Amsterdam: Elsevier.

Pérez, S. et al. (2000). The three-dimensional structures of the pectic polysaccharides. *Plant Physiology and Biochemistry*, 38, 37-55.

Persin, Z.; Stana-Kleinschek, K.; Foster, T.; Van Dam, J.E. G.; Boeriu, C.G. & Navard, P. (2011). Challenges and opportunities in polysaccharides research and technology: The EPNOE views for the next decade in the areas of materials food and health care. *Carbohydrate Polymers,* 84, 22–32.

Pippen, E. L., McCready, R. M. & Owens, H. S (1950). Gelation properties of partially acetylated pectins. *Journal of the American Chemical Society*, 72, 813-816.

Pirman, T.; Ribeyre, M.C.; Mosoni,L.; Rémond, D.; Vrecl, M.; Salobir, J. & Mirand, P.P. (2007). Dietary pectin stimulates protein metabolism in the digestive tract. *Nutrition,* 23, 69–75.

Popov, S.V.; Golovchenko, V.V.; Ovodova, R.G.; Smirnov, V.V.; Khramova, D.S.; Popova, G.Y. & Ovodov, Y.S. (2006). Characterisation of the oral adjuvant effect of lemnan, a pectic polysaccharide of *Lemna minor* L. *Vaccine,* 24, 5413–5419.

Raj, A. A. S.; Rubila, S.; Jayabalan, R. & Ranganathan, T.V. (2012). A Review on Pectin: Chemistry due to General Properties of Pectin and its Pharmaceutical Uses, 1:550 doi:10.4172/scientificreports.550.

Rinaudo, M. (1996). Physicochemical properties of pectins in solution and gel states. In: Visser, J., & Voragen, A. G. J. (Eds.), Progress in Biotechnology: Pectins and Pectinases (v. 14, pp. 20-33).

Rolin, C. (1993). Pectins. In: R. L. Whistler & J. N. BeMiller (Eds.), Industrial Gums: Polysaccharides and Their Derivatives (3 ed., 257-293). San Diego: Academic Press.

Rose, J.K.C.; Catalá, C.; Gonzalez-Carranza, Z. H. & Roberts, J. A. (2003). Cell wall disassembly. In: J.K.C. Rose (Ed.), The plant cell wall. Annual Plant Reviews series. (264-324). Boca Raton, FL: Blackwell/CRC.

Sakai, T.; Sakamoto, T.; Hallaert, J. & Vandarmme, E. J. (1993). Pectin, Pectinase, and Protopectinase: Production, Properties, and Applications. *Advances in Applied Microbiology*, 39, 213-294.

Salman, H.; Bergman, M.; Djaldetti, M.; Orlin, J. & Bessler, H. (2008). Citrus pectin affects cytokine production by human peripheral blood mononuclear cells. *Biomedicine & Pharmacotherapy,* 62, 579-582.

Sato, Y.; Kawabuchi, S.; Irimoto, Y. & Miyawaki, O. (2004). Effect of water activity and solvent-ordering on intermolecular interaction of high-methoxyl pectins in various sugar solutions. *Food Hydrocolloids*, 18, 527-534.

Schepetkin, A.I. & Quinn, M.T. (2006). Botanical polysaccharides: Macrophage immunomodulation and therapeutic potential. *International Immunopharmacology,* 6, 317-333.

Sharma, R & Ahuja, M. (2011). Thiolated pectin: Synthesis, characterization and evaluation as a mucoadhesive polymer. *Carbohydrate Polymers,* 85, 658–663.

Smolenski, K. (1923) Pectins. Rocznigi Chemki, 3, 86-152.

Sriamornsak P. (2003). Chemistry of pectin and its pharmaceutical uses: A review. *Silpakorn University International Journal,* 3, 206-228.

Thibault, J.-F. & Ralet, M.-C. (2001). Pectins, their origin, structure and functions. In: Mccleary, B. V., & Prosky, L. (Eds.). *Advanced Dietary Fiber Technology* (pp. 369-378), Hoboken, N.J.: Wiley-Blackwell.

Thibault, J.-F. (1986). Some physicochemical properties of sugar-beet pectins modified by oxidative cross-linking. *Carbohydrate Research*, 155, 183-192.

Tsoga, A.; Richardson, R. K. & Morris, E. R. (2004). Role of cosolutes in gelation of high-methoxyl pectin. Part 1. Comparison of sugars and polyols. *Food Hydrocolloids*, 18, 907-919.

Vauquelin, M. (1790). Analyse du tamarin. *Annales de Chimie,* 5, 92-106.

Voragen, A.G.J. ; Pilnik, W.; Thibault, J.F.; Axelos, M.A.V.; Renard, C.M.G.C. (1995). Pectins. In: A. M. Stephen (Ed.). *Food polysaccharides and their applications* (287-340). New York: Marcel Dekker.

Voragen, A.G.J.; Coenen, G-J.; Verhoef, R.P. & Schols, H.A. (2009). Pectin, a versatile polysaccharide present in plant cell walls. *Structural Chemistry,* 20, 263–275.

Vriesmann, L. C.; Teófilo, R. F. & Petkowicz, C. L. O. (2011). Optimization of nitric acid-mediated extraction of pectin from cacao pod husks (*Theobroma cacao* L.) using response surface methodology. *Carbohydrate Polymers*, 84, 1230-1236.

Vriesmann, L. C. & Petkowicz, C. L. O. (2013). Highly acetylated pectin from cacao pod husks (*Theobroma cacao* L.) forms gel. *Food Hydrocolloids*, 33, 58-65.

Wang, J.; Flaisher-Grinberg, S.; Li, S., Liu, H.; Sun, L.; Zhou, Y. & Einat, H. (2010). Antidepressant-like effects of the active acidic polysaccharide portion of ginseng in mice. *Journal of Ethnopharmacology,* 132, 65–69.

Waterhouse, E. T.; Washington, C. & Washington, N. (2000). An investigation into the efficacy of the pectin based anti-reflux formulation-Aflurax. *International Journal of Pharmaceutics*, 209, 79-85.

Wheeler, M. L. & Pi-Sunyer, F.X. (2008). Carbohydrate Issues: Type and Amount. *Journal of the American Dietetic Association,* 108, S34-S39.

Willats, W.G.T.; Knox, J.P. & Mikkelsen, J.D. (2006). Pectin: new insights into an old polymer are starting to gel. *Trends in Food Science and Technology,* 17, 97-104.

Willats, W.G.T.; McCartney, L.; Mackie, W. & Knox, J.P. (2001). Pectins: cell biology and prospects for functional analysis. *Plant Molecular Biology,* 47, 9-27, 2001.

Williams, D.R.R.; James, W.P.T. & Evans, I. E. (1980). Dietary fibre supplementation of a 'normal' breakfast administered to diabetics. *Diabetologia,* 18, 379-383.

Wong, T. W., & Nurjaya, S. (2008). Drug release property of chitosan-pectinate beads and its changes under the influence of microwave. *European Journal of Pharmaceutics and Biopharmaceutics*, 69, 176-188.

Yamada, H. (1996). Contribution of pectins on health care. In: J. Visser & A.G.J. Voragen (Eds.), *Pectins and Pectinases* (173-190). Amsterdam: Elsevier.

Yapo, B. M. (2009). Biochemical Characteristics and Gelling Capacity of Pectin from Yellow Passion Fruit Rind as Affected by Acid Extractant Nature. *Journal of Agricultural and Food Chemistry*, 57, 1572-1578.

Yapo, B. M.; Robert, C.; Etienne, I.; Wathelet, B. & Paquot, M. (2007). Effect of extraction conditions on the yield, purity and surface properties of sugar beet pulp pectin extracts. *Food Chemistry*, 100, 1356-1364.

In: Dietary Fiber
Editors: D. Betancur-Ancona, L. Chel-Guerrero et al.

ISBN: 978-1-62808-931-8

Chapter 3

Dietary Fiber as an Ingredient for the Meat Industry

Manuel Viuda-Martos, Juana Fernández-López and José A. Pérez-Alvarez*

IPOA Research Group (UMH-1 and REVIV-Generalitat Valenciana), AgroFood Technology Department, Escuela Politécnica Superior de Orihuela, Universidad Miguel Hernández, Orihuela Alicante (Spain)

Abstract

The prevailing diets of industrialized countries consist of foods that are calorie-dense, nutritionally-poor, phytochemically-depleted, highly processed and rapidly absorbable, with a deficiency of complex carbohydrates. Epidemiological research has demonstrated a relationship between a diet containing an excess of energy-dense foods rich in fats and sugar and the emergence of a range of chronic diseases, including colon cancer, obesity, cardiovascular diseases, and several other disorders. In this way, although meat and meat products are excellent sources of some essential fatty acids, oil soluble vitamins and minerals, and all these components have specific function to our body; a high consumption of meat and meat products have been implicated in diseases, especially in developed countries.

There is considerable evidence from epidemiological, clinical and biochemical studies that fiber exerts a strong positive influence on human health. The fiber may protect against cardiovascular disease, provide improvements in gastrointestinal health; provide improvements in glucose tolerance and the insulin response, reduce the risk of developing some cancers and influence lipid absorption, hence contributing to some degree of weight management. Nevertheless, dietary fiber intake in industrialized countries is currently estimated to be less than 25 g per person per day. However, nutritionists recommend intakes of 35 g per person per day. One way to increase the amount of fiber in the diet without radically changing of eating habits, which would be extremely difficult, is to consume foods enriched with fiber.

* Phone: +34 966749739; e-mail address: ja.perez@umh.es.

Due to the chemical structure and inherent fiber-specific properties dietary fiber shows functional effects that add important benefits to food and food processing. The fiber addition to meat products can be justified by three principal reasons. First, for their nutritional properties: products with fiber or fibers enrichment. Second, because of their technological properties: texture improvement, prevention of loss due to drying out, prevention of drying out due to juice loss during cooking, prevention of gel separation, rehydration capacity improvement, and freezing-thawing stability improvement. Third, for their characteristics as an ingredient without calories, which allow their use in low-energy meat products.

Introduction

The word population, mainly in USA and Europe, typically consumes diets high in meat and saturated fat and low in fruits, vegetables and whole grains. Meat and meat products continue to be an important food group in the diet for many consumers, particularly in the developed world (Bes-Rastrollo et al., 2006). These products are important sources for protein, fat, essential amino acids, minerals and vitamin and other nutrients (Biesalski, 2005). However, this dietary pattern increases the risk to development a great number of diseases. Recently, a number of epidemiological studies have associated red and processed meat consumption with the development of two of the major chronic diseases in the Western world; cardiovascular disease and colon cancer (Delgado, 2003). In order to mitigate such negative effects it has promoted the development of healthy meat products by removing, reducing or replacing undesirable ingredients or by addition of active ingredients. In addition, there are campaigns encourage people to have balanced diets, take regular physical exercise, and in general assume healthy habits. Such advice has been incorporated into many norms and laws by a variety of organizations whose aim is to promote the health and well-being of people.

On the other hand, the consumer demands for healthier meat and meat products with reduced level of fat, cholesterol, decreased contents of sodium chloride and nitrite, improved composition of fatty acid profile and incorporated health enhancing ingredients are rapidly increasing worldwide (Zhang et al., 2010). During the processing of meat and meat products, many functional compounds can be added such as, vitamins, bioactive compounds, proteins, minerals or fiber. Dietary fiber intake in industrialized countries is currently estimated to be less than 25 g per person per day. However, nutritionists recommend intakes of 35 g per person per day (Vuksan et al., 2008). One way to increase the amount of fiber in the diet without radically changing of eating habits, which would be extremely difficult, is to consume foods enriched with fiber. Different types of dietary fibers, such as carrots, apple, sugar beet, soy and citrus fibers, as well as inulin and gums, are now regularly incorporated into foods for their nutritional or functional and technological properties (Fernandez-Lopez et al., 2008; Eim et al., 2008; Beriain et al., 2011; Sayas-Barberá et al., 2012). Fiber in particular seems to be resonating substantially with consumers. They, in general, understand that fiber is a critical dietary component: in the Ingredion proprietary consumer survey, 81% of respondents who typically read product labels reported that they look for fiber content and fiber claims on product labels.

In the 2012 International Food Information Council Foundation (IFIC, 2012) survey, fiber ranked third—just behind caloric content and whole grains—among key components that consumers take into consideration in making purchase decisions about buying packaged foods or beverages; 62% of consumers surveyed reported that they take fiber content into consideration when buying processed foods. Fiber, in fact, ranked higher than other nutrients associated with health, like protein (56%) and calcium (46%). Furthermore, it appears from the survey that fiber content influences purchase decisions to a greater extent than even some of the high profile ingredients that consumers are often encouraged to reduce consumption of, like sodium/salt (60%), *trans* fats (56%), and saturated fats (55%).

Due to the chemical structure and inherent fiber-specific properties dietary fiber shows functional effects that add important benefits to food and food processing. The fiber addition to meat products can be justified by three principal reasons. First, for their nutritional properties: products with fiber or fibers enrichment. Second, because of their technological properties: texture improvement, prevention of loss due to drying out, prevention of drying out due to juice loss during cooking, prevention of gel separation, to manage moisture in the replacement of fat, to add color, as natural antioxidant rehydration capacity improvement, and freezing-thawing stability improvement (Viuda-Martos et al., 2010a). Third, for their characteristics as an ingredient "without" calories, which allow their use in low-fat meat products (Fernández-López and Pérez-Álvarez 2009). Larrauri (1999) described the "perfect fiber" as having the following characteristics: (i) It must not contain any components that are nutritionally offensive, (ii) to maximize its use, it must be of high concentrate in a small quantity, (iii) it should have no taste and no negative odor, color or texture effects, (iv) it should contain a balance between soluble and insoluble fiber with an acceptable presence of bioactive compounds, (v) its addition must not affect the food it is being added to, but it must also have a long shelf life (vi) it should work harmoniously with food processing, (vii) it should have a positive consumer image, (viii) it should contain the expected physiological effects (ix) it should be in an adequate price (Kunzek et al.,2002; Larrauri, 1999).

Dietary fiber concentrates, obtained after dehydration of fresh fruit and vegetables can be used in the food industry as functional ingredients with excellent results. Dietary fiber from cereals is more frequently used than fiber from fruit or vegetables. However, fruit and vegetable fiber has better quality due it's higher soluble dietary fiber content, better water and oil holding capacities and better colonic fermentability, as well as lower phytic acid contents and energy (Figuerola et al., 2005). This chapter examine current literature on effects of the dietary fiber addition to meat products from two points of view (i) the technological effects upon the meat products and (ii) the health benefits associated with meat products consumption, added with dietary fiber.

Fresh Meat Products Added with Dietary Fiber

Changes in socioeconomic factors in the recent years, such as increased women in the work force, have resulted in increased consumer's preference for ready-to-eat foods (Pérez-Alvarez, 2008). Thus, many efforts have been made to improve the quality and stability of these foods such as minced, meatballs, patties, burgers, fingers, etc. Most of these foods are rich in fats and sugar, but deficient in complex carbohydrates. For these reason, there is an interest in increasing the consumption of all foods that can increase daily fiber intake (especially insoluble fiber). Fiber addition to food products would help to overcome the current fiber deficit (Sanchez-Zapata et al., 2010). As mentioned above, there are a great amount of scientific studies that reported the addition of cereals and fruits fibers into fresh meat products (Table 1).

Table 1. Addition of fibers into fresh meat products

Meat product	Fiber	Technological effects	Reference
Meatballs	Wheat bran (5, 10, 15 and 20%)	Lower concentrations of total fat and total *trans* fatty acids. Lower moisture, salt content and weight losses.	Yilmaz (2005)
Meatballs	Corn flour (0, 2 and 4%)	Increased protein content but had no significant effect on fat content of cooked meatballs. Decreasing the fat content from 20% to 5%. Significantly increased cooking yield and fat retention	Serdaroglu and Degirmencioglu (2004)
Meatballs	Rice bran (1, 5, 10 and 15%)	Hardness, gumminess and chewiness decreased. No significant differences in proximate composition, cooking yield, color and sensory quality.	Huang et al., (2005)
Lower-fat patties	Inner pea fiber (10 and 14%)	Improved tenderness and cooking yield without having negative effects on juiciness and flavor	Anderson & Berry (2000)
Beef patties	Wheat bran (5-15%)	Protein and fat contents was decreased and increased, respectively as the amount of wheat bran increased. Lower addition resulted in higher acceptable product with respect to firmness, juiciness and overall quality properties.	Saricoban et al., (2009)
Reduced-fat pork patties	Brown seaweed powder (1, 3 and 5%)	Protein and fat contents, energy value, lightness, redness, cooking loss, reduction in diameter, reduction in thickness, hardness, gumminess, and chewiness of control samples were higher than reduced-fat pork patties	Choi et al., (2012)
Buffalo burgers	Decorticated legume flours	Lower thiobarbituric acid values before frying and organoleptically acceptable even after storage at -16 ºC for 4 months	Modi et al., (2003)
Beef burgers	Hazelnut pellicle (1, 2, 3 4 and 5%)	The cooking yield and reduction in diameter and thickness of beef burgers were improved	Turhan et al., (2005)
Pork burgers	Grape pomace (0.06%)	highest color stability, lipid oxidation inhibition and the best global acceptability after 6 days of storage than control	Garrido et al., (2011)
Pork burgers	arbutus-berries hawthorns dog roses, leaf blackberries (3%)	Fruit extracts significantly reduced the formation of protein carbonyls and inhibited color and texture deterioration during chilling storage	Ganhão et al., (2010)

Thus, in studies by Yilmaz (2004), rye bran was used as a fat substitute in the production of meatballs. The addition of rye bran to meatballs at the levels assayed (5% to 20%) improved their nutritional value and health benefits. The total *trans* fatty acid content was lower and the ratio of total unsaturated fatty acids to total saturated fatty acids was higher in the samples with added rye bran. The same samples were lighter and yellower than the control samples. The authors concluded that this type of fiber could be used as dietary fiber source. In other study, Yilmaz and Daglioglu (2003) studied the effect of oat bran addition (5, 10, 15 and 20%) on the fatty acid composition, *trans* fatty acids, total fat, some physicochemical and sensory properties of meatballs. These authors informed that meatballs made with 20% oat bran had the highest protein, salt and ash contents, lightness, yellowness, and the lowest moisture content and redness.

There was no significant difference ($p<0.05$) among the meatball samples with respect to sensory properties, and all samples had high acceptability. In a similar study, Serdaroglu et al., (2005) analyzed the addition of black-eye bean flour (BBF), chickpea flour (CF), lentil flour (LF) and rusk (R) at level of 10% in meatballs. BBF and LF resulted in greater cooking yield, fat retention and moisture retention values. Meatballs extended with LF were lighter than other samples. Meatballs formulated with BBF had the lowest reduction in diameter. Meatballs with BBF and CF had higher water holding capacity (WHC) than other treatment groups. All meatballs incorporating legume flours were tougher (lower penetration values) than the R treatment. According to sensory evaluation results all meatball treatments had high acceptability and received high scores. Sanchez-Escalante et al., (2003) analyzed the stabilization of color and odor of beef patties using lycopene-rich tomato fiber as a source of antioxidants, which they found exerted a significant antioxidative effect on the beef patties, depending on the lycopene concentration. These tomato products delayed meat deterioration to a varying extent, so that the shelf life of treated beef patties ranged between 8 and 12 days. Talukder and Sharma (2010) developed dietary fiber rich chicken meat patties by incorporating wheat and oat bran to chicken meat at 5, 10 and 15% levels. Oat bran contained higher amount of soluble dietary fiber and unsaturated fatty acids than wheat bran, whereas total dietary fiber, insoluble dietary fiber and saturated fatty acids were higher in wheat bran. Bran incorporation significantly increased the water holding capacity and emulsion stability. Oat bran showed better effect on water holding capacity and emulsion stability than wheat bran. Addition of bran resulted in significant increase in cooking yield, firmness, total dietary fiber, unsaturated fatty acids and reduction in sensory attributes, moisture, protein, fat and cholesterol content. Piñero et al., (2008) evaluated the effect of adding oat fiber source of β-glucan (13.45%) on beef patties. These authors informed of significant improvements in cooking yield and retentions of and moisture of low-fat patties. In addition, low-fat beef patties remained stable in microbiological quality during 60 days frozen storage. Yi et al., (2012) investigated if glutinous rice flour (GRF), at concentration of 1, 3 and 5%, could be a functional food additive to seasoned beef patties. They reported that GRF lowered texture profile values for hardness, gumminess, springiness, and chewiness of the patties, which are generally beneficial for this product and the beef patties with GRF were juicier and tenderer than the control. Bengtsson, Montelius and Tornberg (2011) reported that there was an increase in sensory measured firmness and compactness when potato pulp fiber added to produce a fresh low-fat sausage and this was due to the high content of insoluble fiber, which improve the texture of the sausage by creating a fibrous network while no effect on the meat protein network. Regarding the textural properties of the products, there was remarkably decreased with substitution of salt and addition of apple pulp. Sensory evaluation showed reduction in texture and overall acceptability scores of treatment products and the scores were in the range of very good.

Aleson-Carbonell et al., (2005), analyzed the incorporation of lemon albedo, at different concentration (2.5, 5 and 7.5%), to beef burger. These authors found that the type of albedo slightly influenced the lipid oxidation and pH of samples, while the cooking properties were significantly improved with average increments of 5.5-11% on treatment meat patties when compared with control samples. The tigernut fiber (TNF) was evaluated by Sanchez-Zapata et al., (2010). The authors included levels (5%, 10% and 15%) in the formulation of pork burgers. They reported that some of the negative changes in color (a* decrease and b* increase) and texture (chewiness and springiness increase) parameters were due to TNF addition. They, also, observed that raw burgers were masked by the stronger modifications due to the cooking process. Burgers with TNF were perceived as less greasy, less juicy, more grainy and with less meaty flavor than controls. In a similar study, Gök et al., (2011) investigated the use of ground poppy seed in formulation of meat burgers. They found that a strong decrease on the cholesterol content and saturated fatty acid contents of meat burgers with ground poppy seed addition was observed. Additionally, samples having 20% ground poppy seed had significantly better texture and juiciness score than any other sample. Kassem and Emara (2010), analyzed beef burger patties formulated with texture soy granules (1 and 2%). In corporation of textured soy significantly reduced the color, marbling, appearance, flavor, tenderness, juiciness, taste and overall acceptability in comparison with either control. Garcia et al., (2009) studied the addition of different amounts of dry tomato peel (0-6.0% w/w) to raw and cooked hamburgers. These authors reported that the addition of tomato peel to hamburgers at 4.5% showed a good overall acceptability and presented a final lycopene content of 4.9 mg/100 g of cooked hamburger. The addition of dry tomato peel increased the color characteristics (a* and b*) of raw and cooked hamburgers, decreased the pH values significantly in a concentration-dependent manner, and modified all the textural properties probably because of the presence of fiber.

Cooked Meat Products Added with Dietary Fiber

In general, cooked meat product may contain animal fat up to 30%. Fat, in these types of meat products, plays a major role in forming stable emulsions, reducing cooking loss, improving water holding capacity and binding properties, forming rheological and structural properties and providing juiciness and hardness to the products (Pietrasik and Duda, 2000). However, consuming high animal fat in meat products leads to high amounts of saturated fatty acids and cholesterol. Thus, the reduced fat content in meat products and substituting animal fat with dietary fiber, obtained from cereals or fruits should result in a healthier product (Choi et al., 2009). Many studies have been carried out on cooked meat products with fat partially replaced by dietary fiber, which helps to improve rheological properties and stability of these products (Table 2). The most popular cooked meat products are the Frankfurters and the bolognas sausage. Frankfurters and bolognas sausage are popular fast-foods which are easy to use and relatively cheap, but the questions raised about the influence of animal fats used in production of meat products on coronary heart disease have decreased the popularity of these types of products (Vural & Javidipour, 2002).

Frankfurters

As mentioned above, there are many studies where the additions of different types (obtained from cereals or fruits) of fiber were incorporated to frankfurters. Therefore, pigskin and wheat fiber mixture (PSFM) in frankfurter sausages were assessed by Choe et al., (2013) as fat replacers. They informed that the addition of PSFM increased the moisture and protein content in the sausage. The sausage sample containing 20% PSFM had 50% less fat, 32% fewer calories, and showed 39.5% less cooking loss than those of the control. Additionally, high PSFM content resulted in more stable meat emulsions and increased hardness, cohesiveness, gumminess, and chewiness.

Table 2. Addition of fiber into cooked meat products

Meat product	Fiber	Technological effects	Reference
Frankfurters	Wheat fiber	The combination of transglutaminase with wheat fiber led to harder, springier and chewier frankfurters with better water- and fat-binding properties emulsion stability and cooking loss	Jimenez-Colmenero et al., (2005)
Frankfurters	Seaweed (*Himanthalia elongata*) (5%)	Had little effect on the lipid and amino acid profiles. Constitute a means to produce low-sodium products with important dietary fiber content, with better Na/K ratios and rich in Ca.	López-López et al., (2009)
Frankfurters	Walnut (25%)	Frankfurter with walnut had a healthy polyunsaturated fatty acid profile, a lower ω6/ω3 ratio and lower indices of atherogenicity (0.10) and indices thrombogenicity (0.15).	Ayo et al., (2007)
Frankfurters	Konjac (1%, 2%) and gellan gum (0.25%, 0.5%)	Partial replacement of fat with Konjac/gellan gum mixed gel improved the overall sensory quality of reduced-fat frankfurter.	Lin and Huang (2003)
Frankfurters	Rice bran and walnut (2.5%)	The addition of rice bran led to an increase of cooking and fat exudates, indicating high emulsion instability. Walnut addition reported low cooking loss values, and a significant capacity for emulsion stabilization	Alvarez et al., (2011)
Bologna type sausage	Corn and potato starches	Modified starches affected emulsion stability and emulsion viscosity. The modification process was not significant for pH, WHC, jelly and fat separation	Aktas and Gençcelep (2006)
Bologna type sausage	Pomegranate peel fiber	Increased fiber content and decreased fat, improving its nutritional and sensorial characteristics	Ruiz-Navajas et al., (2011)
Bologna type sausage	Soy fiber	Higher soy fiber contents favored the formation of harder, chewier structures with improved fat and water binding properties	Cofrades et al., (2000)
Low-salt bologna type sausage	Carboxymethyl cellulose and carrageenan	The use of these ingredients decreased frying loss and increased saltiness	Ruusunen et al., (2003)
Light bologna type sausage	Oat fiber (3%)	The of oat fiber addition produced greater yields and a lighter red color	Steenblock et al., (2001)

No significant differences ($p > 0.05$) were observed in color, flavor, tenderness, juiciness, warm-off flavor, and overall acceptability between the control and sausage sample with PSFM. Özvural and Vural (2011) analyzed the addition of grape seed flour (GSF), at seven concentrations (0, 0.5, 1, 2, 3, 4, and 5%) with a total fiber concentration of 0, 0.43, 0.94, 1.60, 3.29, 4.62 and 4.71 g/100g respectively, into frankfurters. The color values of frankfurters generally decreased on account of the increasing amount of GSF. The utilization of this flour also led to a decline in the oxidation level of the products. The increment of GSF in the frankfurters enhanced the protein, total dietary fiber and water holding capacity of the treatments. The frankfurters containing the level up to 2% received scores above the average. Ayo et al., (2008) evaluated the physicochemical and sensory properties of healthier frankfurters with 25% added walnut versus low-fat frankfurters and traditional frankfurters. Results reveal that cooking losses were unaffected by the formulation of frankfurters. However, the addition of walnut led to higher redness and yellowness values. Additionally these samples presented higher hardness and chewiness values than low-fat and traditional frankfurters. Differences in composition were also accompanied by changes in the microstructure of the gel/emulsions. Deba et al., (2007) analyzed frankfurters (18% fat) produced with two levels of sodium nitrite, 0 and 150 mg/kg (0.015%), and seven levels (0, 2, 6, 8, 12 and 16%) of tomato paste with 12% soluble solids. As regards color these authors reported that the higher the tomato paste level the lower the values for lightness (L*) and hue (H*) values and the higher the redness (a*), yellowness (b*) and chroma (C*) values. Eyiler and Oztan (2011) analyzed the chemical properties including the nitrosomyoglobin content, lycopene content and the oxidation level, and the sensorial properties of frankfurters, which had been produced by both reducing the nitrite level and adding tomato powder. The pH of the frankfurters produced with tomato powder was reduced. The addition of 2% of tomato powder decreased the level of oxidation; however, 4% caused a slight increase compared with control samples. According to sensorial evaluations, tomato powder also improved consumer acceptability. The addition of tomato powder increased the internal and external color scores, and frankfurters were found to be more acceptable by the panelists. Jimenez-Colmernero et al., (2010) studied the effect of edible seaweed, Sea Spaghetti (*Himanthalia elongata*), on the physicochemical and sensory characteristics of reduced- and low-fat, low-salt frankfurters prepared with konjac gel as a fat substitute. These authors reported that Incorporation of a combination of Sea Spaghetti/konjac gel caused the formation of a more heterogeneous structure, in which the seaweed was integrated in the meat protein matrix. In addition, incorporation of a combination of Sea Spaghetti/konjac gel (accompanied by reduction in salt) increased cooking loss and reduced emulsion stability and produced a decrease of lightness (L*) and redness (a*) values and an increase of yellowness (b*) as compared to the other samples. Cierach et al., (2009) informed that carrageenan gels' texture depends on the type used and method of production, as well as the pH values of the solution. Carrageenan in low-fat frankfurters led to a reduction in cooking loss and purge during storage. The results of textural and sensorial analyses showed that addition of carrageenan to low-fat meat batters improved the quality of the frankfurters.

Bologna Sausage

As in the case of frankfurters, there are many researches that reported the addition of fiber, mainly of fruit source, into bolognas sausage. Thus, Sánchez-Zapata et al., (2011) added date palm fiber to a cooked pork sausage (bologna type). The addition of up to 15% date paste in the formulation of bologna-type products leads to the enhancement of the nutritional (lower fat content and higher fiber content than control) and technological quality (redder-colored and less hard, chewy and cohesive product than the control) together with a satisfactory sensory quality. Lemon albedo has also been incorporated in cooked products like bologna sausage. For example, Fernández-Ginés et al., (2003) reported that bologna sausage with added citrus fiber was improved nutritionally in fiber content and had decreased residual nitrite levels and a delay in the oxidation process as determined by thiobarbituric acid (TBA) values and red color. Only TBA values and redness were influenced by storage conditions (light and darkness) mainly due to the oxidant effect attributable to light. In both cases these effects were minimized by the citrus fiber. Citrus fiber at all concentrations made the products harder and less springy and chewy. All samples had similar satisfactory quality scores except bologna with 2% citrus fiber, which had the lowest scores. Similarly, Fernández-Ginés et al., (2004) analyzed the influence of different concentrations of raw and cooked lemon albedo on residual nitrite levels and concluded that (1) raw albedo is more effective than cooked, (2) reduction of residual nitrite levels is concentration dependent, and (3) the compounds responsible for these reductions are the bioactive compounds, although the researchers did not specify their nature (polyphenolic or otherwise). Viuda-Martos et al., (2010b) informed that the addition of orange fiber (1%) and oregano essential oil is a technologically viable alternative in fine paste meat products, since they improve their acceptance and have desirable effects as regards oxidative stability and reduced microbial growth, which contribute to prolonging their shelf life. Also maintain polyphenolic compounds, such as flavonoids, which may have a beneficial effect on human health since they have been linked with the prevention of various illnesses. In a similar study these authors Viuda-Martos et al., (2010c) analyzed the effect of adding orange dietary fiber (1%), rosemary essential oil (0.02%) or thyme essential oil (0.02%) and the storage conditions on the quality characteristics and the shelf life of *mortadella*, a bologna-type sausage. The moisture, fat, ash content and color coordinates lightness (L*) and yellowness (b*) were affected by the fiber content. The treatments analyzed lowered the levels of residual nitrite (57.56% and 57.61%) and the extent of lipid oxidation, while analysis of the samples revealed the presence of the flavonoids, hesperidin and narirutin. Sanjeewa et al., (2010) demonstrated that incorporation of chickpea flour at both levels (2.5% and 5%) into a low-fat pork bologna model system increased the product's cook yield, decreased water releasing properties, and increased the instrumental and sensory firmness without a biotype difference. For most flavor properties, bologna with chickpea flour performed similar to control, whereas panelists noted more foreign-flavors with addition of wheat and pea flour at 5%. Pietrasik and Janz (2010) reported that the addition of starch pea and fiber pea ingredients considerably improved the textural properties, restoring the values of the low fat samples to levels equivalent to regular fat bologna. All binder ingredients favorably affected hydration properties and thermal stability, yielding lower cooking and purge losses, and higher water holding capacity compared to low fat control bologna. Cava et al., [176] elaborated cooked chicken products with 1, 2 and 3% inulin compared with a control product without fiber added. The effect of fiber incorporation on (i) batters, (ii) cooked (30 min at 70 ◦C), and (iii) cooked and stored (for 10 d at 4 ◦C) chicken products were studied. The addition of the fiber to chicken meat products reduced the pH of chicken batters in proportional to the level of fiber addition. Fiber incorporation increased water-holding capacity. Inulin incorporation improved the instrumental texture properties and did not modify the color; but did not exhibit any antioxidant activity.

Dry-Cured Meat Products Added with Dietary Fiber

Dry fermented sausages are popular traditional meat products in many countries and are of great importance to the meat industry. However, these products present some negative health effects because of their high fat (25-45%) and energy content (300-450 kcal/100 g) and the fatty acid profiles of animal fat (Muguerza et al., 2004). Fat reduction is generally considered to be an important strategy for improving the fat content of foods, leading the meat industry to develop new formulations or modify traditional ones (Ruiz-Capillas et al., 2012). However, dry fermented sausage is one of the meat products where fat reduction is most difficult. Aside from its nutritional contribution, fat contributes to the quality and acceptability properties (flavor, texture, mouth-feel, etc.) of dry sausage (Ruiz-Capillas et al., 2012). A variety of non-meat adjuncts including carbohydrate-based substances including gums (alginate, xanthan, carrageenan), fibers (pea fiber, oat fiber, citrus fiber), starches (tapioca starch, modified food starches) and other carbohydrate compounds (pectin, micro-crystalline cellulose) have been assessed in low-fat meat products as fat replacers. Various types of fibers have been successfully used in processing of meat products: beet, wheat, oats, peas, carrots and among fruit fibers: peach, apple, pear, lemon and orange (Table 3). Thus, Sayas-Barberá et al., (2012) studied the combined addition of *Lactobacillus casei* and orange fiber (1%) for the production of Spanish non-fermented dry-cured sausage. They reported that the incorporation of 1% orange fiber favored the growth of lactic acid bacteria and accelerated the decline in pH and the release of organic acids and glycerol. Sausages containing both orange fiber and *L. casei* obtained the best sensory scores and provided the best guarantees of food safety, low pH and water activity, decreased counts of *Enterobacteriaceae* and reduced residual nitrite compared to the other type of sausages. In a similar study (Aleson-Carbonell et al., 2004), dry-cured sausages were treated with two types of dehydrated lemon albedo (raw and cooked) at five concentrations (0, 2.5, 5, 7.5 and 10%). The addition of albedo improved the nutritional properties as a result of fiber addition and may have beneficial effects due to the presence of active bio-compounds as evidenced by a decrease in residual nitrite levels and delayed oxidation (based on TBARS values). Fernández-López et al., (2008) analyzed Spanish dry-fermented sausages with three concentrations (0, 1 and 2%) of orange fiber. These authors reported that only residual nitrite level and micrococcus counts were affected by fiber addition during fermentation. pH, water activity, residual nitrite level and counts of *Micrococcaceae* were affected by fiber addition during dry-curing. Orange fiber decreases residual nitrite levels and favors micrococcus growth. Both effects have a positive impact on sausage safety and quality. Similarly, dry-cured sausages with orange fiber at five concentrations (0, 0.5, 1, 1.5 and 2%) were prepared and studied by Fernández-Lopez et al., (2007). TBARS values increased in all samples during drying, with lower increase in treatment samples than in control samples. The incorporation of orange fiber into sausages produced a significant decrease in residual nitrite level. García et al., (2002) studied the effect of adding cereal and fruit fibers on the sensory properties of reduced-fat, dry-fermented sausages. The cereal (wheat and oat) and fruit (peach, apple, and orange) dietary fibers were added at 1.5% and 3% concentrations. The addition of dietary fiber from cereals and fruits at 1.5% resulted in sausages with a final fiber content, after ripening, of about 2%, which represents an improvement in their nutritional properties and provides an acceptable sensory profile. Higher amounts of fiber (3%) increased the hardness, resulting in products with a lower sensory quality. The best results in this study were obtained with sausages containing 10% pork back fat and 1.5% fruit fiber. The orange fiber provides the best results with sensory properties similar to those of conventional sausage. Eim et al., (2008) investigated four formulations of a dry fermented sausage, known as *sobrasada*, containing different percentages of carrot dietary fiber (3, 6, 9, and 12%). Textural parameters, such as hardness and compression work, were significantly affected by the addition of over 3% of fiber. The lipolytic process, one of the major biochemical events, was only affected when relatively large percentages of fiber concentrate were incorporated. Mendoza et al., (2001) prepared low-fat, dry-fermented sausages with a fat content close to 50 and 25% of the original amount and supplemented with 7.5 and 12.5% of inulin. The results indicate that inulin impacts a softer texture and a tenderness, springiness, and adhesiveness very similar to that of conventional sausages. A low-calorie product (30% of the original) can be obtained with approximately 10% inulin.

Table 3. Addition of fiber into dry-cured meat product

Meat product	Fiber	Technological effects	Reference
Fermented sausages	Fructooligosaccharides (3, 6 and 9%)	Reduction in fat content (40%). There were no changes in technological and sensory properties	Alves-dos Santos et al., (2012)
Dry-cured sausage	Konjac gel	There was an increase in hardness and chewiness and a decrease in cohesiveness	Ruiz-Capillas et al., (2012)
Dry-fermented chicken sausage	Inulin	Inulin did not change the physicochemical or microbiological parameters and the acceptability of the products, but resulted in an altered texture profile and a tendency toward lighter and less reddish coloration	Zenaide Menegas et al., (2013)
Pamplona-style chorizo,	Inulin	The addition of inulin, 6%, resulted in a low-salt, reduced-fat product (20% less fat than control), while retaining sensory notes similar to those of the traditional chorizo used as a control and achieved a good acceptability rating	Beriain et al., (2011)
Sobrasada	Tigernut fiber	The addition of 5% decreased fat content and increased the total dietary fiber content. No significant changes in its physicochemical properties were found	Sanchez-Zapata et al., (2010)
Dry fermented sausage	Tomato peel fiber (0.6, 0.9 and 1.2%)	A slight losts of lycopene was detected after 21 days ripening, however, levels remained between 0.26 and 0.58 mg of lycopene/100 g of sausage. The sensory and textural properties and overall acceptability of all sausages were good	Calvo et al., (2008)
Sucuk (Turkish dry-fermented sausage)	Orange fiber (0, 2 and 4%)	Lactic acid bacteria and pH value were affected. Orange fiber caused a decrease in residual nitrite levels and an increase in the TBARS values. L* and b* values increased with the use of fiber. Fiber also decreased the cooking loss	Yalinkiliç et al., (2012).
Fermented sausages	Amorphous cellulose gel.	Sausages had significant reductions in fat and cholesterol, and the volatile compounds derived from lipid oxidation	Bastianello Campagnol et al., (2012)

Tsoukalas et al., (2011) studied fermented sausages produced with 0.84% and 1.68% freeze-dried leek powder (FDLP), providing 75 and 150 mg/kg $NaNO_3$. Sausages with FDLP were darker and yellower than the control. Lower FDLP levels resulted in higher sensory scores for external appearance, flavor and overall acceptability. No differences were found among the treatments with FDLP plus 75 or 150 mg/kg $NaNO_2$ in TBA value, lightness, redness (cross section), redness stability, yellowness, texture parameters and sensory firmness, flavor and overall acceptability. A study reported that in a low fat sausage, the greatest overall acceptability was attained when the hydrated oat-meal or tofu were at their 15% level and also improved the flavor and textural attributes compared to control sausage (Yang et al., 2007). Park and Lee (2012), study the effects of kimchi and freeze-dried kimchi-powder added to raw meat mixtures on the microbiological quality of fermented sausage. The results demonstrated that the lactic acid bacteria (LAB) integrated via the addition of kimchi as well as kimchi-powder were well adapted to the new habitat of fermenting sausage. In all kimchi and kimchi-powder sausages, the growth of Enterobacteriaceae was completely inhibited throughout the processing period. The sausage batches containing more than 10% kimchi and 2% kimchi-powder showed no growth of *Staphylococcus aureus*, whereas the control and another kimchi sausage batch reflected the growth of S. *aureus*.

Conclusion

Dietary fiber obtained from cereals and fruits are widely used by the food industry to improve the physic-chemical and technological properties of meat products, although their nutritional and functional properties make them suitable for other purposes, such as the enhancement of functional foods. Most people would like to eat a healthier diet without fundamentally changing their eating patterns. The unwillingness of the consumer to change dietary habits suggests that there is a great market potential for foods with altered nutritional characteristics but unchanged sensory attributes. However, despite the widely demonstrated beneficial effects of fiber on several diseases, including cancers and cardiovascular diseases more mechanistic studies and randomized controlled trials of large sample size are necessary to further confirm these effects.

References

Aktas, N. & H. Gençcelep, H. (2006). Effect of starch type and its modifications on physicochemical properties of bologna-type sausage produced with sheep tail fat. *Meat Science, 74,* 404-408.

Alesón-Carbonell, L., Fernández-López, J., Sendra, E., Sayas-Barberá, E. & Pérez-Alvarez, J. A. (2004). Quality characteristics of a non-fermented dry-cured sausage formulated with lemon albedo. *Journal of the Science and Food Agricultural, 84,* 2077-2084.

Alesón-Carbonell, L., Fernández-López, J., Pérez-Alvarez, J. A. & Kuri, V. (2005). Characteristics of beef burger as influenced by various types of lemon albedo. *Innovative Food Science and Emerging Technologies, 6,* 247- 255.

Álvarez, D., Delles, R. M., Xiong, Y. L., Castillo, M., Payne, F. A. & Laencina, J. (2011). Influence of canola-olive oils, rice bran and walnut on functionality and emulsion stability of frankfurters. *LWT-Food Science and Technology, 44,* 1435-1442.

Alves-dos Santos, B., Bastianello-Campagnol, P. C., Bertoldo-Pacheco, M. T. & Rodrigues-Pollonio, M. A. (2012). Fructooligosaccharides as a fat replacer in fermented cooked sausages. *International Journal of Food Science and Technology, 47,* 1183-1192.

Anderson, E. T. & Berry, B. W. (2000). Sensory. Shear and cooking properties of lower fat beef patties made with inner pea fiber. *Journal of Food Science, 65(5),* 805-810.

Ayo, J., Carballo, J., Serrano, J., Olmedilla-Alonso, B., C. Ruiz-Capillas, C. & Jiménez-Colmenero, F. (2007). Effect of total replacement of pork backfat with walnut on the nutritional profile of frankfurters. *Meat Science, 77,* 173-181.

Ayo, J., Carballo, J., Solas, M. T. & Jiménez-Colmenero, F. (2008). Physicochemical and sensory properties of healthier frankfurters as affected by walnut and fat content. *Food Chemistry, 107,* 1547-1552.

Bastianello Campagnol, P. C., Alves dos Santos, B., Wagner, R., Nascimento Terra, N. & Rodrigues Pollonio, M. A. (2012). Amorphous cellulose gel as a fat substitute in fermented sausages. *Meat Science, 90,* 36-42.

Bengtsson, H., Montelius, C., & Tornberg, E. (2011). Heat-treated and homogenized potato pulp suspensions as additives in low-fat sausages. *Meat Science, 88,* 75-81.

Beriain, M. J., Gómez, I., Petri, E., Insausti, K. & Sarriés, M. V. (2011). The effects of olive oil emulsified alginate on the physico-chemical, sensory, microbial, and fatty acid profiles of low-salt, inulin-enriched sausages. *Meat Science, 88,* 189-197.

Bes-Rastrollo, M., Sanchez-Villegas, A., Gomez-Gracia, E., Martinez, J. A., Pajares, R. M. & Martinez-Gonzalez, M. A. (2006). Predictors of weight gain in a Mediterranean cohort: the Seguimiento Universidad de Navarra Study 1. *American Journal of Clinical Nutrition, 83,* 362-370.

Biesalski, H. K. (2005). Meat as a component of a healthy diet - Are there any risks or benefits if meat is avoided in the diet?. *Meat Science, 70,* 509-524.

Cava, R., Ladero, L., Cantero, V. & Ramírez, M. R. (2012). Assessment of Different Dietary Fibers (Tomato Fiber, Beet Root Fiber, and Inulin) for the Manufacture of Chopped Cooked Chicken Products. *Journal of Food Science, 77(4),* 346-352.

Choe, J. H., Kim, H. Y., Lee, J. M., Kim, Y. J. & Kim, C. J. (2013). Quality of frankfurter-type sausages with added pig skin and wheat fiber mixture as fat replacers. *Meat Science, 93,* 849-854.

Choi, Y. S., Choi, J. H., Han, D. J., Kim, H. Y., Lee, M. A., Kim, H. W., & Kim, C. J. (2009). Characteristics of low-fat meat emulsion systems with pork fat replaced by vegetable oils and rice bran fiber. *Meat Science, 82,* 266-271.

Choi, Y. S., Choi, J. H., Han, D. J., Kim, H. Y., Kim, H. W., Lee, M. A., Chung, H. J. & Kim, C. J. (2012). Effects of Laminaria japonica on the physico-chemical and sensory characteristics of reduced-fat pork patties. *Meat Science, 91,* 1-7.

Cierach, M., Monika Modzelewska-Kapituła, M. & Kamil Szaciło, K. (2009). The influence of carrageenan on the properties of low-fat frankfurters. *Meat Science, 82,* 295-299.

Cofrades, S., Guerra, M. A., Carballo, J., Fernández-Martín, F. & Colmenero, F. J. (2000). Plasma protein and soy fiber content effect on bologna sausage properties as influenced by fat level. *Journal of Food Science, 65,* 281-287.

Deba, M. S., Bloukas, J. G. & Fista, G. A. (2007). Effect of tomato paste and nitrite level on processing and quality characteristics of frankfurters. *Meat Science, 76,* 501-508.

Delgado, C. L. (2003). Rising consumption of meat and milk in developing countries has created a new food revolution. *Journal of Nutrition, 133(11),* 3907-3910.

Eim, V. S., Simal, S., Rosselló, C. & Femenia, A. (2008). Effects of addition of carrot dietary fibre on the ripening process of a dry fermented sausage (*sobrassada*). *Meat Science, 80,* 173-182.

Eyiler, E. & Oztan, A. (2011). Production of frankfurters with tomato powder as a natural additive. *LWT-Food Science and Technology, 44(1),* 307-311.

Fernández-Ginés, J. M., Fernández-López, J., Sayas-Barberá, E., Sendra, E. & Pérez-Alvarez, J. A. (2003). Effect of storage conditions on quality characteristics of bologna sausages made with citrus fiber. *Journal of Food Science, 68,* 710-715.

Fernández-Ginés, J. M., Fernández-López, J., Sayas-Barberá, M. E., Sendra, E., Pérez-Alvarez, J. A. (2004). Lemon albedo as a new source of dietary fiber: application to bologna sausages. *Meat Sciemce, 67,* 7-13.

Fernández-López, J., Viuda-Martos, M., Sendra, E., Sayas-Barbera, M. E., Navarro, C., & Pérez-Álvarez, J. A. (2007). Orange fibre as potential functional ingredient for dry-cured sausages. *European Food Research and Technology, 226,* 1-6.

Fernández-López, J., Sendra, E., Sayas-Barbera, M. E., Navarro, C., & Pérez-Álvarez, J. A. (2008). Physico-chemical and microbiological profiles of "Salchichon" (Spanish dry-fermented sausage) enriched with orange fiber. *Meat Science, 80,* 410-417.

Fernández-López, J. & Pérez-Álvarez, J. A. (2009). Meat products as functional foods. In M. L. Passo, & C. P. Ribeiro (Eds.), Innovation in food engineering (pp. 579-600). Boca Raton, FL: CRC Press.

Figuerola, F., Hurtado, M., Estévez, A., Chiffelle, I. & Asenjo, F. (2005). Fibre concentrates from apple pomace and citrus peel as potential fibre sources for food enrichment. *Food Chemistry, 91*, 395-401.

Ganhão, R., Morcuende, D. & Estévez, M. (2010). Protein oxidation in emulsified cooked burger patties with added fruit extracts: Influence on colour and texture deterioration during chill storage. *Meat Science, 85,* 402-409.

García, M. L., Domínguez, R., Galvez, M. D., Casas. C. & Selgas, M. D. (2002). Utilization of cereal and fruit fibres in low fat dry fermented sausages. *Meat Science, 60,* 227-236.

García, M. L., Calvo, M. M., Selgas, M. D. (2009). Beef hamburgers enriched in lycopene using dry tomato peel as an ingredient. *Meat Science, 83,* 45-49.

Garrido, M. D., Auqui, M., Martí, N. & Linares, M. B. (2011).Effect of two different red grape pomace extracts obtained under different extraction systems on meat quality of pork burgers. *LWT-Food Science and Technology, 44,* 2238-2243.

Gök, V., Akkaya, L., Obuz, E. & Bulut, S. (2011). Effect of ground poppy seed as a fat replacer on meat burgers. *Meat Science, 89,* 400-404.

Huang, S. C., Shiau, C. Y., Liu, T. E., Chu, C. L. & Hwang, D. F. (2005). Effects of rice bran on sensory and physico-chemical properties of emulsified pork meatballs. *Meat Science, 70,* 613-619.

IFIC. 2012. Functional foods/foods for health consumer trending survey; International Food Information Council Foundation, Washington, D.C.

Jiménez Colmenero, F., Ayo, M. J. & Carballo, J. (2005). Physicochemical properties of low sodium frankfurter with added walnut: effect of transglutaminase combined with caseinate, KCl and dietary fibre as salt replacers. *Meat Science, 69*, 781-788.

Jiménez-Colmenero, F., Cofrades, S., López-López, I., Ruiz-Capillas, C., Pintado, T. & Solas, M. T. (2010). Technological and sensory characteristics of reduced/low-fat, low-salt frankfurters as affected by the addition of konjac and seaweed. *Meat Science, 84,* 356-363.

Kassem, M. A. G. & Emara, M. M. T. (2010). Quality and Acceptability of Value-Added Beef Burger. *World Journal of Dairy & Food Sciences, 5(1),* 14-20.

Kunzek, H., Müller, S., Vetter, S. & Godeck, R. (2002). The significance of physico chemical properties of plant cell wall materials for the development of innovative food products. *European Food Research and Technology, 214*, 361-376.

Larrauri, J. A. (1999). New approaches in the preparation of high dietary fibre powders from fruit by-products. *Trends in Food Science & Technology, 10(1),* 3-8.

Lin, K. W. & Huang, H. Y. (2003). Konjac/gellan gum mixed gels improve the quality of reduced-fat frankfurters. *Meat Science, 65,* 749-755.

López-López, I., Cofrades, S., Ruiz-Capillas, C. & Jiménez-Colmenero, J. (2009). Design and nutritional properties of potential functional frankfurters based on lipid formulation, added seaweed and low salt content. *Meat Science, 83,* 255-262.

Mendoza, E., García, M. L., Casas, C. & Selgas, M. D. (2001). Inulin as fat substitute in low fat, dry fermented sausages. *Meat Science, 57,* 387-393.

Modi, V. K., Mahendrakar, N. S., Rao, D. N. & Sachindra, N. M. (2003). Quality of buffalo meat burger containing legume flours as binders. *Meat Science, 66*, 143-149.

Muguerza, E., Gimeno, O., Ansorena, D. & Astiasarán, I. (2004). New formulations for healthier dry fermented sausages: A review. *Trends in Food Science & Technology, 15(9),* 452-457.

Özvural, E. B. & Vural, H. (2011). Grape seed flour is a viable ingredient to improve the nutritional profile and reduce lipid oxidation of frankfurters. *Meat Science, 88,* 179-183.

Park, Y. S. & Lee, J. Y. (2012). The effect of kimchi on the microbiological stability of fermented sausage. *Meat Science, 92,* 721-727.

Pérez-Alvarez, J. A. (2008). Overview of meat products as functional foods. In J. Fernández-López & J. A. Pérez-Alvarez (Eds.), Technological strategies for functional meat products development (pp. 1-18). Kerala, India: Transworld Research Network.

Pietrasik, Z. & Duda, Z. (2000). Effects of fat content and soy protein/carrageenan mix on the quality characteristics of comminuted, scalded sausages. *Meat Science, 56(2),* 181-188.

Pietrasik, Z. & Janz, J. A. M. (2010). Utilization of pea flour, starch-rich and fiber-rich fractions in low fat bologna. *Food Research International, 43*, 602-608.

Piñero, M. P., Parra, K., Huerta-Leidenz, N., Arenas de Moreno, L., Ferrer, M. Araujo S. & Barboza, Y. (2008). Effect of oat's soluble fibre (b-glucan) as a fat replacer on physical, chemical, microbiological and sensory properties of low-fat beef patties. *Meat Science, 80,* 675-680.

Ruiz-Capillas, C., Triki, M., Herrero, A. M., Rodriguez-Salas, L. & Jiménez-Colmenero, F. (2012). Konjac gel as pork backfat replacer in dry fermented sausages: Processing and quality characteristics. *Meat Science, 92,* 144-150.

Ruiz-Navajas, Y., Viuda-Martos, M., Pérez-Álvarez J. A., Sayas, E., Sendra, E. & Fernández-López, J. (2011). Effect of added pomegranate peel extract on the chemical and physic-chemical characteristics of a bologna sausage. In: Proceedings of 2011 EFFoST Annual Metting. Process-Structure-Function Relationships. pp: 3.49.

Ruusunen, M., Vainionpaa, J., Poulanne, E., Lyl, M., Lähteenmäki, L., Niemistö, M. & Ahvenainen, R. (2003b). Effect of sodium citrate, carboxymethyl cellulose and carrageenan levels on quality characteristics of low-salt and low-fat bologna type sausages. *Meat Science, 64,* 371-381.

Sánchez-Escalante, A., Torrescano, G., Djenane, D., Beltrán, J. A. & Roncalés, P. 2003. Stabilisation of colour and odour of beef patties by using lycopene-rich tomato and peppers as a source of antioxidants. *Journal of the Science and Food Agricultural, 83,* 187-94.

Sánchez-Zapata, E., Muñoz, C. M., Fuentes, E., Fernández-López, J., Sendra, E., Sayas, E., Navarro, C. & Pérez-Alvarez, J. A. (2010). Effect of tiger nut fibre on quality characteristics of pork burger. *Meat Science, 85*, 70-76.

Sánchez-Zapata, E., Fernández-López, J., Peñaranda, M., Fuentes-Zaragoza, E., Sendra, E., Sayas, E. & Pérez-Alvarez, J. A. (2011). Technological properties of date paste obtained from date by-products and its effect on the quality of a cooked meat product. *Food Research International, 44*, 2401-2407.

Sánchez-Zapata E., Viuda-Martos M., Fuentes-Zaragoza E., Fernández-López J., Sendra E., Sayas E., Navarro C., PérezÁlvarez J.A. (2010). Effect of tiger nut (*Cyperus esculentus*) fibre addition on color properties and quality of sobrasada (spanish dry fermented sausage). In: International Conference on Food Innovation. *Book of actas Food Innova* (pp 121). Valencia. Spain.

Sanjeewa, W. G. T., Wanasundara, J. P. D., Pietrasik, Z. & Shand, P. J. (2010). Characterization of chickpea (Cicer arietinum L.) flours and application in low-fat pork bologna as a model system. *Food Research International, 43,* 617-626.

Saricoban, C., Yilmaz, M. T. & Karakaya, M. (2009). Response surface methodology study on the optimisation of effects of fat, wheat bran and salt on chemical, textural and sensory properties of patties. *Meat Science, 83*, 610-619.

Sayas-Barberá, E., Viuda-Martos, M., Fernández-López, F., Pérez-Alvarez, J. A. &Sendra, E. (2012). Combined use of a probiotic culture and citrus fiber in a traditional sausage "Longaniza de Pascua". *Food Control, 27,* 343-350.

Serdaroglu, M. & Degirmencioglu, O. (2004). Effects of fat level (5%, 10%, 20%) and corn flour (0%, 2%, 4%) on some properties of Turkish type meatballs (koefte). *Meat Science, 68,* 291-296.

Serdaroglu, M., Yıldız-Turp, G. & Abrodímov, K. (2005). Quality of low-fat meatballs containing Legume flours as extenders. *Meat Science, 70*, 99-105.

Steenblock, R. L., Sebranek, J. G., Olson, D. G. & Love, J. A. (2001). The effects of oat fiber on the properties of light bologna and fat-free frankfurters. Journal of Food Science, 66(9), 1409-1415.

Talukder, S. & Sharma, D. P. (2010). Development of dietary fiber rich chicken meat patties using wheat and oat bran. *Journal of Food Science and Technology, 47(2),* 224-229.

Tsoukalas, D. S., Katsanidis, E., S. Marantidou, S. & Bloukas, J. G. (2011). Effect of freeze-dried leek powder (FDLP) and nitrite level on processing and quality characteristics of fermented sausages. *Meat Science, 87,* 140-145.

Turhan, S., Sagir, I. & Ustun, S. N. (2005). Utilization of hazelnut pellicle in low-fat beef burgers. *Meat Science, 71,* 312-316

Viuda-Martos, M., López-Marcos, M. C., Fernández-López, J., Sendra, E., López-Vargas, J. H. & Pérez-Alvarez, J. A. (2010a). Role of fiber in cardiovascular diseases: A review. *Comprehensive Reviews in Food Science and Food Safety, 9,* 240-258.

Viuda-Martos, M., Ruiz-Navajas, Y., Fernández-López, J. & Pérez-Álvarez, J. A. (2010b). Effect of orange dietary fibre, oregano essential oil and packaging conditions on shelf-life of bologna sausages. *Food Control, 21,* 436-443.

Viuda-Martos, M., Ruiz-Navajas, Y., Fernández-López, J. & Pérez-Álvarez, J. A. (2010c). Effect of added citrus fibre and spice essential oils on quality characteristics and shelf-life of mortadella. *Meat Science, 85,* 568-576.

Vuksan, V., Jenkins, A. L., Jenkins, D. A. J., Rogovik, A. L., Sievenpiper, J. L., & Jovanovski, E. (2008). Using cereal to increase dietary fiber intake to the recommended level and the effect of fiber on bowel function in healthy persons consuming North American diets. *American Journal of Clinical Nutrition, 88(5)*, 1256-1262.

Vural, H. & Javidipour, I. (2002). Replacement of beef fat in frankfurters by interesterified palm, cottonseed and olive oils. *European Food Research and Technology, 214*, 465-468.

Yalinkiliç, B., Kaban, G. & Kaya, M. (2012). The effects of different levels of orange fiber and fat on microbiological, physical, chemical and sensorial properties of sucuk. *Food Microbiology, 29,* 255-259.

Yang, H., Choi, S., Jeon, J., Park, G. & Joo, S. (2007). Textural and sensory properties of low fat pork sausages with added hydrated oatmeal and tofu as texture-modifying agents. *Meat Science, 75,* 283-289.

Yi, H. C., Cho, H., Hong, J. J., Ryu, R. K., Hwang, K. T. & Regenstein, J. M. (2012). Physicochemical and organoleptic characteristics of seasoned beef patties with added glutinous rice flour. *Meat Science, 92,* 464-468.

Yilmaz, I. & Daglioglu, O. (2003). The effect of replacing fat with oat bran on fatty acid composition and physicochemical properties of meatballs. *Meat Science, 65,* 819-823.

Yilmaz, I. (2004). Effects of rye bran addition on fatty acid composition and quality characteristics of low-fat meatballs. *Meat Science, 67,* 245-249.

Yilmaz, I. (2005). Physicochemical and sensory characteristics of low fat meatballs with added wheat bran. *Journal of Food Engineering, 69*, 369-373.

Zenaide Menegas, L., Colombo Pimentel, T. Garcia, S. & Prudencio, S. H. (2013). Dry-fermented chicken sausage produced with inulin and corn oil: Physicochemical, microbiological, and textural characteristics and acceptability during storage. *Meat Science, 93,* 501-506.

Zhang, W., Xiao, S., Samaraweera, H., Lee, E. J. & Ahn, D. U. (2010). Improving functional value of meat products. *Meat Science, 86,* 15-31.

In: Dietary Fiber
Editors: D. Betancur-Ancona, L. Chel-Guerrero et al.
ISBN: 978-1-62808-931-8

Chapter 4

Dietary Fiber in Meat Products: Functional and Bioactive Ingredient

Arun K. Verma*[*1] and Rituparna Banerjee[2]
[1]Goat Products Technology Laboratory
Central Institute for Research on Goats, Makhdoom, Farah, Mathura, India
[2]Department of Livestock Products Technology, NVC, Nagpur, India

Abstract

Meat consumption throughout the world, in particular developing countries is gradually rising. Additionally globalization and a rapid change in overall lifestyle have forced consumers to be dependent upon fast foods including meat products, which contain meager amount of dietary fiber. Many reports have revealed that regular intake of meat particularly red meat as well as meat products without dietary fiber may lead to colorectal cancer and associated problems. In order to prevent or mitigate the problems, meat consumers are advised to have sufficient amount of dietary fiber daily in their diet. Incorporation of various sources of dietary fiber in processed meat products seems a viable approach to supplement the consumers with adequate amount of dietary fiber along with meat. There are various components included in the term dietary fiber but they are broadly categorized into soluble and insoluble groups. The soluble fibres are generally present at high levels in fruits, oats, beans and vegetables. Basically, the soluble or easily digestible fibres including pectins, gums, starches and other storage polysaccharides produce viscous solutions that delay gastric emptying and absorption from the small intestine and tend to lower blood cholesterol level. Such substances are greatly accessible to bacterial enzymes and are rapidly fermented in the proximal colon hence; tend to have less impact on colonic transit. Insoluble fibres such as cellulose and lignins, by contrast, have much less effect on the viscosity of gut contents, tend to accelerate rather than delay small bowel transit and have more marked laxative effect than soluble fibre. Whole grains are a major food source for insoluble fibres. Addition of dietary fiber in meat products has been found to improve various physicochemical parameters besides beneficial physiological effects on consumer health. Physicochemical

* Email: arun.lpt2003@gmail.com.

characteristics of meat products including acidity, colour, amounts of moisture, protein, fat and fiber, texture and sensory attributes are affected by added sources of fiber. These effects depend upon pH value, colour, particle size, amount of ingredients and proportion of soluble and insoluble dietary fiber. Several purified as well as crude sources of dietary fiber have been incorporated in various meat products to reduce the fat and salt contents, improve fiber content along with total phenolics and shelf-life. Thus it is observed that dietary fiber may act as multifaceted ingredient in meat products resulting in improvement of quality characteristics and enrichment of consumer's health as well.

Introduction

Now, when most of the people are getting educated, they remain in regular touch with the information sources like television, print media, periodicals etc. This leads to the generation of awareness and interest among consumers about the nutritional and therapeutic aspects of the food they eat and directing new inquiries about the linkage between food and health. The basic tendency of human beings has always been to procure and consume "natural foods". However, the fast pace of modern life, changes in socioeconomic factors in the recent years, rapid urbanization, industrialization and globalization have kept consumers away from natural foods and, consequently, canned, packaged, and ready-to-eat foods including meat products have now moved into a central position and onto the tables of modern consumers. Most of these foods are rich in fats and sugar, but deficient in complex carbohydrates. Epidemiological research has demonstrated a relationship between this type of diet and the increase of a number of chronic diseases, including colon cancer, obesity, cardiovascular diseases and several other disorders (WHO/FAO, 2003). According to Kritchevsky (2000), research findings give enough association between dietary fiber intake and a healthier life style and fiber intake can be regarded as a marker of healthy diet. A generous intake of dietary fiber reduces the risk for developing coronary heart disease, stroke, hypertension, diabetes, obesity and certain gastrointestinal disorders. Furthermore, increased consumption of dietary fiber improves serum lipid concentrations, lowers blood pressure, improves blood glucose control in diabetes, promotes regularity, aids in weight loss and appears to improve immune function. The recommended acceptable intakes of dietary fiber for adults are 28–36 g/day, 70–80% of which must be insoluble fiber (Anderson et al., 2009).

Meat is considered as very nutritive food item. Its principal components, besides water, are proteins and fats, with a substantial contribution of vitamins and minerals of a high degree of bioavailability. However, regular consumption of meat and meat products which are lacking adequate amount of dietary fiber has also been implicated for development of certain kind of cancer. This problem can be ameliorated through tailoring of meat products with desired dietary fiber proportion and composition. Fiber is one of the valuable components that can be incorporated in meat products from health point of view. Moreover, dietary fibers in meat products can also impart many technological benefits attributed to inherent characteristics of fiber to bind water and fat as well as contribution of phenolic antioxidants (Choi et al., 2008; Sayago-Ayerdi et al., 2009).Various types of fibers have been studied either alone or combined with other ingredients for formulation of numerous kinds of comminuted meat products (Mansour and Khalil, 1999, Claus and Hunt, 1991). This chapter delineates about the dietary fibers their physiological and technological significance and application in various kinds of meat products.

Dietary Fiber

The link between the ingestion of unprocessed foods and good health is chronicled as far back as Hippocrates (4th century B.C.), who recommended the eating of wholemeal bread for its "salutary effects upon the bowels". This was mainly because whole meal is good source of dietary fiber. Many researchers attempted to define the dietary fiber time to time and a great deal of debate has existed over its definition, as well as methods for measuring its amount. This is principally because some people want to describe dietary fiber by its physiological attributes, and some by its chemical composition.

The term dietary fiber was used first by Hipsley (1953) to include lignin, cellulose and hemicellulose, and later broadened to include soluble substances (non-cell-wall derived materials) such as pectins, gums and mucilages (Trowell et al., 1976). This broad definition acknowledges the significance of fiber as a chemical and physiological component of the diet as compared with the static definition of crude fiber – 'the residue of plant food left after extraction with solvent, dilute acid, and dilute alkali' (Browne, 1940).

Trowell et al., (1976) adopted Hipsley's term in conjunction with a number of health-related hypotheses they were developing, referred to as their "dietary fiber hypotheses." The term was used to describe the remnants of plant components that are resistant to hydrolysis by human alimentary enzymes. Thus it was a physiological-botanical description, characterizing dietary fiber's indigestibility in the human small intestine, with plant cell walls being the major source of digestion-resistant material. The components included were cellulose, hemicellulose, lignin, and associated minor substances, such as waxes, cutin, and suberin. One widely accepted definition from the American Association of Cereal Chemists states: "Dietary fiber is the remnants of the edible parts of plants or analogous carbohydrates that are resistant to digestion and absorption in the human small intestine with complete or partial fermentation in the large intestine. According to this definition dietary fiber includes polysaccharides, oligosaccharides, lignin, and associated plant substances. Dietary fibers promote beneficial physiological effects including laxation, and/or blood cholesterol attenuation, and/or blood glucose attenuation" (AACC, 2001). These are an integral part of the foodstuffs we consume daily such as plants, vegetables, cereal grains, woody plants, fruits, legumes, leguminous plants, etc. (Meyer, 2004). The latest definition proposed by Codex Alimentarius includes carbohydrate polymers with a degree of polymerisation not lower than 3. They can be naturally present in or extracted from food raw material, or synthesised. The debate continues and some recent opinion has favoured a return to the original fiber definition along the lines that 'Dietary fiber consists of intrinsic plant cell wall polysaccharides'.

Based on their simulated intestinal solubility, dietary fiber is conventionally classified into two categories: soluble dietary fiber (SDF) such as pentosans, pectin, gums, and mucilage and insoluble dietary fiber (IDF) such as cellulose, part of hemicellulose, and lignin (Esposito et al., 2005). Basically, the soluble or easily digestible fibers, increase transit time through the digestive tract, delay gastric emptying, and slow glucose absorption so that the amount of starch reaching the colon is increased. The soluble fibers are generally present at high levels in fruits, oats, beans and vegetables (Anderson et al., 1994). Insoluble fibers, on the other hand, increase faecal bulk and excretion of bile acids, while decreasing intestinal transit time. Whole grains are a major food source for insoluble fibers (Welsh et al., 1994, Slavin et al., 1997).The various components of dietary fiber are given in Table 1.

Table 1. Proposed Constituents of Dietary Fiber (Tungland and Meyer, 2002)

Constituent	Main groups	Fiber components
Non-starch polysaccharides and oligosaccharides	Cellulose	
	Hemicellulose	Arabinogalactans, β-glucans, arabinoxylans, glucuronoxylans, xyloglucans, galactomannans, pectic substances
	Polyfructose	Inulin, oligofructans
	Gums & mucilages	Galactomannans, alginates, agar, carrageenan, psyllium, gum acacia, gum karaya, gum tragacanth,
	Pectins	
Carbohydrates analogues	Resistant starches and maltodextrins	
	Chemically synthesized	Polydextrose, lactulose, cellulose derivatives
	Enzymatically synthesized	Short chain fructo-oligosaccharides, Transgalactooligosaccharides, levon, xanthan gum, guar hydrolyzate, oligofructose, xylooligosaccharides, curdlan
Lignin	Lignin	
Substances associated with non-starch polysaccharides	Waxes, cutin, suberin	
Fibers of animal origin	Chitin, chitosan, collagen, chodroitin	

Health Benefits

Until the dietary fiber hypothesis was proposed by Burkitt and Trowell (1977), fiber was unable to get proper attention in our diet for several decades. This hypothesis signified the metabolic importance of dietary fiber in terms of reduction of diet related non-communicable chronic diseases such as obesity, cardiovascular disease, diabetes and cancer. Since then, many studies have been undertaken and the body of scientific data that supports a protective role for fiber in the prevention and management of chronic diseases continue to grow. The various physiological functions of dietary fiber as well as proposed mechanisms of action are presented in the Table 2.

Table 2. Health implications of dietary fiber and their mode of action

Effects	Mode of Action	References
Maintenance of gut health	Promotion of normal laxation by increasing stool weight.	Cummings (1993)
	Reduction of colonic transit time which in turn reduces impact of detrimental microflora associated characteristics viz. toxic nitrogenous compounds, H_2S & production of carcinogenic/genotoxic compounds	Gibson (2004)
	Short chain fatty acids (SCFA) from fiber fermentation, particularly butyrate, play a key role in the health of colon.	Wasan and Goodlad (1996)
	Inhibition of the growth of pathogenic organisms via SCFA production and lowering the pH of the colon.	Gray (2006), Scott et al., (2008)
	Acts as prebiotics to encourage health-promoting bacteria such as lactobacilli and bifidobacteria.	Roberfroid (2005)
Prevention of carcinogenesis	Reducing production of carcinogenic substances by decreasing number of pathogenic bacteria in colon	Rumney and Rowland (1995), Robertson et al., (1991)
	Decrease interactions between intestinal mucosa and faecal mutagens via increasing faecal bulk/diluting its contents and reducing intestinal transit time.	Harris and Ferguson (1993)
	Inhibitory effect on initiation and promotion stages in colon cancer formation through formation of SCFA particularly butyric acid.	Hague et al., (1993), Pierre et al., (1997)
	Protective effect against breast cancer through increased faecal losses of oestrogens.	Willett et al., (1992)
Prevention of cardiovascular diseases	Increase excretion of bile acids and cholesterol.	Bosaeus et al., (1986), Arjmandi et al., (1997)
	Delay absorption of carbohydrates, which lead to increased insulin sensitivity and decreased triacylglycerol concentrations.	Hallfrisch et al., (1995)
	SCFA, particularly propionate inhibit fatty acid metabolism, which plays a key role in the synthesis of cholesterol.	Nishina and Freeland (1990), Demignè et al., (1995)
Prevention of diabetes	Reduces absorption of carbohydrate in gastrointestinal (GI) tract.	Jenkins et al., (1978)
	Promotes gluconeogenic activity in the liver and lowers blood glucose and alters lipid metabolism.	Todesco et al., (1991)
	Improve whole body glucose disposal resulting in an improvement of insulin sensitivity.	Weickert et al., (2008)
	Stimulates post-prandial insulin release via accelerated secretion of glucose dependent incretin hormone.	Weickert et al., (2005)
	Reduction of post-prandial glucose response by SCFA production.	Ostman et al., (2002)
	Increases the expression of gut-derived pro-glucagon gene.	Massimino et al., (1998)
Enhanced Satiation	Adds bulk, which in turn alters energy density and palatability.	
	Form viscous colloidal dispersions when hydrated, which affects multiple aspects of GI function, such as gastric emptying, small bowel transit time, and digestion and absorption of nutrients, particularly fat and carbohydrate.	Vahouny et al., (1988), Schneeman and Tietyen (1994)
	Early satiation due to textural qualities of fibrous foods, increase in chewing effort and time required for mastication resulting in a variety of cephalic- and gastric-phase responses and signals.	Heaton (1980), Duncan et al., (1983), Sakata (1995)
Improvement in mineral utilization	Dissolve insoluble mineral salts such as calcium, magnesium, and iron by lowering of colon pH.	Brandt (2001), Manning and Gibson (2004)
	Stimulate proliferation of colon epithelial cells, increasing the absorptive capacity of the epithelium.	Scholz-Ahrens et al., (2001), Conway (2001),
	Increase the water content in the colon, thus increase the solubility of some minerals.	Kaur and Gupta (2002)

Technological Properties of Dietary Fiber

Dietary fibers also play significant role towards various physicochemical characteristics of foods including meat products besides improvement of various physiological and health values. These functions are contributed by different interlinked inherent attributes of fibers such as solubility, water and fat binding capacity as well as viscosity. Such properties of dietary fibers make them a vital ingredient while design and development of different meat products including the products with low salt and fat contents.

Solubility

It is considered as one of the major factors responsible for functional and nutritional properties of dietary fiber which is dependent upon the polysaccharide structure and stability. Most of the polysaccharides exist in some sort of helical shape (BeMiller and Whisler, 1996) while some polysaccharides have a structure in which the chains may adopt regular, ordered conformations and pack together into crystalline-solid assemblies. The polymer is likely to be more stable in solid state than in solution (Guillon and Champ, 2000). The chemical regularity of a chain increases the strength of the links, conferring insolubility thus leading to resistance to enzyme attack. Therefore, the polysaccharide with linear structure like cellulose may undergo limited enzymatic degradation. If the structure of polysaccharide is irregular such as in β-glucans, arabinoxylans, and/or branches are present, the links tend to be weaker and become prone to degradation. This kind of polysaccharide forms major chunk of dietary fiber in the nature and are regarded as soluble fibers, which enables rapid hydration. Solubility is also affected by temperature and ionic strength (Fleury and Lahaye, 1991; Mañas et al., 1994).

The soluble and insoluble nature of dietary fibers involves differences in their technological functionality and physiological effects (Jiménez-Escrig and Sánchez-Muniz, 2000). Soluble fibers are characterised by their capacity to increase viscosity, and to reduce the glycaemic response and plasma cholesterol (Abdul-Hamid and Luan, 2000). In food processing the soluble fraction of dietary fiber plays more vital technological role through improvement of viscosity, gelling capacity and emulsification without much influence on sensory characteristics, thus it is easier to incorporate in food and meat products. In the meat products soluble fibers supposed to contribute towards viscosity and other rheological behaviour of meat emulsion. Additionally soluble fiber affects various organoleptic and textural properties of meat products making them juicy and softer in texture. Insoluble fibers are characterised by their porosity, low density and ability to increase faecal bulk and decrease intestinal transit period. Cardoso et al., (2012) found that incorporation of chicory dietary fiber in the formulations of fish protein gels reduced elastic modulus (G'). According to Sánchez-Alonso et al., (2006) elastic modulus (G') of surimi with 6% wheat fiber found lower throughout thermal gelling. Under scanning electronic microscopy, gel samples with added wheat fiber presented uneven distribution of fiber. This induced the formation of a non-homogeneous protein network associated with lower gel strength, cohesiveness and water binding capacity (WBC). Later Sánchez-Alonso et al., (2007a) observed that wheat dietary fiber contributed towards reduced gel strength, hardness, cohesiveness and water binding capacity (WBC) of surimi gels. Sánchez-Alonso et al., (2006) noticed the differences in texture among surimi gels containing different proportions and types of wheat fiber and fiber with large particle sizes protected surimi from loss of gel strength and hardness during freezing.

Hydration Properties and Oil-Binding Capacity

The hydration properties of dietary fiber are characterized by the swelling capacity, solubility, water holding capacity (WHC) and water binding capacity (WBC). Alongside their hydration properties, fibers possess the capacity to hold oil. Dietary fiber swells to a variable extent in water depending upon the presence of hydrophilic or hydrophobic environment. Solubilisation is not possible in case of polysaccharides that adopt regular, ordered structures (e.g. cellulose), where the linear structure increases the strength of non-covalent bonds, which stabilize the ordered conformation. Under these conditions only swelling can occur (Thibault et al., 1992). WHC and WBC have been used interchangeably since both reflect the ability of a fiber source to incorporate water within its matrix. The ability of dietary fibers to hold water is strongly related to their source. Dietary fibers from algae have a greater affinity for water and oil than those from fruit juice by-products. Cereal derivatives present the lowest affinity. Structure of dietary fiber, presence and proportion of soluble fraction of fiber, availability of charged groups are the major factors determining their water and oil binding properties. Binding of water and oil by dietary fiber, WHC, swelling and oil holding capacity (OHC) suggest some possibilities about the use of fibers as ingredients in food products. Dietary fibers with high WHC can be used as functional ingredients for the development of meat products with less fat thus calories, as well as salt content. They also help to avoid syneresis and modify the viscosity and texture of the final product (Grigelmo-Miguel and Martina-Belloso, 1999). Water and fat binding capacity of dietary fibers can influence the meat emulsion stability, product yield, amount of moisture and fat as well as products juiciness.

Viscosity

Viscosity as related to dietary fiber refers to the ability of some polysaccharides to thicken or form gels when mixed with fluids or semisolid formulation resulting from physical entanglements among the polysaccharide constituents within matrix (Guillon and Champ, 2000). Water soluble fibers are the major component that increases the viscosity of a mix. Polysaccharides that form viscous solutions, such as gums and pectins, form thickened matrix depending on their unique chemical composition (Schneeman, 2001). Soluble fibers such as β-glucans, found in oats, and galactomannans are positively correlated with viscosity (Robinson et al., 1982). Viscosity is one of the most important physical properties of soluble dietary fiber not only from the perspective of food application but also regarding several physiological effects. With regard to connection of dietary fiber and viscosity in meat system, Choi et al., (2011) reported highest moisture content, myofibrillar protein solubility and water holding capacity in pork salt soluble proteins containing 1% rice bran fiber. The apparent viscosity indicated the improvement in water holding capacity and decreased texture due to added rice bran fiber.

Dietary Fibers in Meat Products

Low and Modified Fat, Fiber Rich Meat Products

Fats in meat products play important roles in stabilizing meat emulsions, reducing cooking loss, improving water holding capacity and providing juiciness and hardness (Pietrasik and Duda, 2000; Yoo et al., 2007). Hughes et al., (1997) found that fats have considerable effects on the binding, rheological and structural properties of meat products. However, high fat contents, in particular animal fats, provide great amounts of saturated fatty acids and cholesterol (Ozvural and Vural, 2008). Animal fat rich diets are associated with several types of problems like obesity, hypertension, cardiovascular diseases and coronary heart diseases (Serrano et al., 2007). Therefore, the reduction of fat content in meat products and the substitution of animal fat with vegetable oils should result in a healthier product. Dietary fibre has been added to different meat products to counteract the problems caused by fat reduction (Anonymous, 2001). Many studies have been carried out on low-fat meat products with fat partially replaced by dietary fibre, which helps to improve rheological properties and stability (Crehan et al., 2000; Hsu and Chung, 2001). Besides imparting to the technological characteristics of meat emulsion system, dietary fiber more importantly improve the nutritional and health value of meat and meat product as meat and meat products are very poor source of dietary fiber and their regular intake in daily diet needs additional fiber supplementation. Thus meat products themselves could be customized into more "healthier" form by adding ingredients considered beneficial for health such as fiber. Of late there is an increasing trend of fiber addition in meat products for technological reasons and benefits to human health (Vendrell-Pascuas et al., 2000). Development of low/modified fat, fiber rich meat products using variety of fiber ingredients has been summarized in Table 3.

Low Salt and Fortified Meat Products

Development and processing of meat products with low salt content is not an easy task as functionality of meat products such as water as well as fat binding capacity, batter stability, cooking yield and textural properties are severely affected due to less salt content in the formulation. A number of binding agents have been used to overcome property problems in low salt products, including water and fat-binding properties and texture (Collins, 1997; Monahan and Troy, 1997). Of late dietary fiber is being used to play significant role in the processing of low salt meat products. As nonmeat ingredients, dietary fibres are desirable not only for their nutritional properties but also for their functional and technological properties. Fibers can be used in cooked meat products (e.g. meat emulsions, patés) to increase the cooking yield thanks to their water- and fat binding properties, and to improve texture (Thebaudin et al., 1997). Additionally many dietary fiber ingredients are also either inherent source of bioactive ingredients such as phenolics or being combined with micronutrients. These ingredients can be included in various meat products to contribute towards functional and nutritional characteristics. Application of different dietary fiber ingredients in low salt and fortified meat products as well as their effects has been given in Table 4.

Table 3. Fiber ingredients in various low fat, high fiber meat products and their effects

Products	Dietary fiber ingredient	Effect on meat products	Reference
Pork meat batter	Rice bran fibre	Increase in moisture, protein, ash content, emulsion stability, pH values, yellowness value, hardness, cohesiveness, gumminess, chewiness and viscosity of meat batter; lower cooking loss.	Choi et al., (2009)
Low-fat frankfurters	Rice bran fibre	Increase in the moisture and ash content; increased pH, cooking yield and thiobarbituric acid (TBA) values; reduced-fat content, energy values, cholesterol and trans-fat levels; no effect on sensory attributes.	Choi et al., (2010)
Reduced-fat frankfurters	Makgeolli lees fibre	Higher moisture and ash content as well as lightness value.	Choi et al., (2013)
Frankfurters	Sugar beet fibre (SBF)	Significant increase in the total dietary fibre content and water-holding capacity (WHC); no significant effect on appearance, colour, texture, flavour or sensory scores.	Vural et al., (2004)
Turkish-type salami	Sugar beet fibre	SBF significantly increased the total dietary fiber content and water-holding capacity of salamis; no significant changes in appearance, colour, texture, flavour or sensory score.	Javidipour et al., (2005)
Frankfurters	Sugar beet fibre	SBF added frankfurters showed slightly lower sensory scores.	Özboy-Özbas et al., (2003)
Lower-fat beef patties	Inner pea fiber	Beef flavour intensity did not differ; improved tenderness and cooking yield without negative effects on juiciness and flavour.	Anderson and Berry (2000)
Low fat, dry fermented sausages	Inulin	Low calorie product; no difference in sensory attributes.	Mendoza et al., (2001)
Low-fat fish sausage	Dietary fiber from inner pea (Swelite®) and chicory powder (Fibruline®)	Swelite® favoured greater gel strength and hardness; high Fibruline® sausages were less cohesive and chewable but also exhibited greater gel strength; low-Fibruline® sausages presented almost all textural properties similar to the control, except hardness and gumminess.	Cardoso et al., (2008a)
Fish sausages	Chicory root inulin and extra hake mince	Higher gel strength and hardness; less elastic, cohesive, springy, and succulent; increase in saltiness and astringent after taste.	Cardoso et al., (2008b)
Beef patties	Soluble fiber inulin (Frutafit®)	Lower texture profile analysis (TPA) values except springiness than traditional beef patties.	Martínez et al., (2011)
Meatballs	Oat bran	Lower concentrations of total fat, and trans fatty acids; twenty percent oat bran in meatballs resulted in highest protein, ash contents, lightness, yellowness and lowest moisture as well as redness; no significant differences in the sensory properties.	Yilmaz and Daglioglu (2003)

Table 3. (Continued)

Products	Dietary fiber ingredient	Effect on meat products	Reference
Meatballs	Rye bran	Improvement in nutritional value and health benefits; reduction in the total trans fatty acid content and improvement in the ratio of total unsaturated fatty acids to total saturated fatty acids; lighter and yellower colour than control samples.	Yilmaz (2004)
Meatballs	Wheat bran	High ratio of total unsaturated fatty acids to total saturated fatty acids; low total trans fatty acids; lighter and yellower meat product.	Yilmaz (2005)
Low fat, high added water bologna	Duo Fiber®, oat fibre, pea fibre, wheat starch, Firm-tex®	Less firm product than high fat control but more firm than low fat control; more grainy and less juicy product.	Claus and Hunt (1991)
Low-fat beef burgers	Oat fibre	Limited effects on cooking yield and shear force value.	Desmond et al., (1998)
Light bologna, fat-free frankfurters	Oat fiber	Greater yield and a lighter red colour; reduction in purge but product hardness increased.	Steenblock et al., (2001)
Low-fat beef patties	Oat's soluble fibre (β-glucan)	Significant improvements in cooking yield, and retentions of fat as well as moisture of low-fat patties; lower degree of likeness in the taste but juicer than control; effect on appearance.	Piñero et al., (2008)
Beef patties	Oat flour	Decrease in moisture content in raw patties but increase in cooked patties; no change in the protein, fat and ash contents; improvement in cooking characteristics.	Serdaroglu (2005)
Low-fat high fibre mutton kofta	Wheat flour, oat flour, carrageenan	Oat flour and carrageenan significantly lowered fat content and increased water, protein, ash and carbohydrates; kofta containing carrageenan (0.5%) were softer in texture, had lower free fatty acids, Hunter redness and yellowness values and higher lightness values.	Modi et al., (2009)
Low fat, high dietary fibre frankfurters	Peach dietary fibre suspensions	Increase in viscosity of the meat batters; no change in protein and collagen content; effective retention of added water in the product.	GrigelmoMiguel and Martin-Belloso (1999)
Low fat dry fermented sausages	Cereal (wheat and oat) and fruit (peach, apple and orange) dietary fibres	Reduction in energy value of the final products (35%) and increase in dietary fiber; harder and more cohesive product with 3% dietary fiber; sausage with 1.5% fruit fibre found best.	García et al., (2002)
Low-fat beef burgers	Wheat fibers	Significantly higher moisture, protein, carbohydrate and ash contents and lower fat contents; decrease in the energy value, cholesterol content; improvement in the cooking yield and reduction in diameter; red and white wheat fiber in the product improved textural properties; no effect on colour traits, tenderness, juiciness, connective tissue amount, beef flavour intensity and overall palatability.	Mansour and Khalil (1999)

Products	Dietary fiber ingredient	Effect on meat products	Reference
Ultra-low-fat pork bologna sausages	Hull-less waxy barley and normal starch barley	Better purge control and water holding capacity during storage with 4% hull-less waxy barley; firmer texture and better sensory properties.	Shand (2000)
Poultry meat sausages	Hydrated barley	Improved juiciness and biological value by 25–30%.	Titov et al., (1994)
Low-fat beef burger	Hazelnut pellicle	Improvement in the reduction in cooking yield, diameter and thickness of beef burgers.	Turhan et al., (2005)
Low fat bologna	Pea flour, starch and fiber	Pea starch and fibre restored texture profile values of low fat samples to high fat levels; low cooking and purge losses, and increased water holding capacity; no effect on consumer acceptability.	Pietrasik and Janz (2010)
Pig liver paté	Enzymatically extracted dietary fibers 1 (9% DM, w/w), 2 (7.7% DM, w/w) and 3 (spray dried) from potato pulp, dry potato pulp and Potex®	Very hard patties with a high level of deformation energy, gumminess, and modulus due to fiber 1 and 2 that had a detrimental effect on pate texture and flavour; fiber 3 resulted in patties with a very delicious texture and flavour but darker, redder and less yellow colour; lowest baking loss for patties processed using fiber 3; 4 to 6.2% total dietary plant fiber in liver patties.	Kaack et al., (2006)
Low-fat meatballs	Dietary fibre suspensions from olive mill wastewater and carrot fiber	Improvement in cooking properties due to water soluble alcohol insoluble residue and carrot fibres; restriction in oil uptake thereby giving rise to meatballs with sustained reduced fat content.	Galanakis et al., (2010)
Kung-wan, an emulsified pork meatball	Rice bran	Protein, fat and white index of meatballs decreased; decrease in hardness, gumminess and chewiness; sensory score not affected up to 10% level.	Huang et al., (2005)
Restructured fish products	Inner pea fiber (Swelite®) or chicory root inulin (Fibruline INSTANT)	Increase in hardness at 4% dietary fibre level and up to 2% carrageenan; colour of product redder and more yellow.	Cardoso et al., (2007)
Cooked sausages, raw fermented sausages and cooked ham	Wheat fiber (VITACEL®)	-	Lander (2004)
High fiber camel meat patties	Soy hulls	Significant effect on chemical composition, calorific content, flavour, cooking yield, reduction in thickness, fat and water retention and shear force values.	Al-Khalifa and Atia (1997)
Low salt, low fat and high fiber chicken nuggets	Chickpea hull flour (CHF)	Decrease in emulsion stability, cooking yield, moisture, protein, ash, colour values, total cholesterol and glycolipid contents; increase in dietary fiber and textural parameters.	Verma et al., (2012a)

Table 3. (Continued)

Products	Dietary fiber ingredient	Effect on meat products	Reference
Restructured fish products	Wheat fiber	Increase in water holding capacity and water binding capacity; decrease in rigidity, cohesiveness, cooking loss; no effect on sensory attributes up to 3%.	Sánchez-Alonso et al., (2007b)
Low salt, low fat and high fiber chicken nuggets	Pea hull flour, gram hull flour, apple pulp and bottle gourd	Reduction in pH, emulsion stability, cooking yield, protein, ash and TPA values; increase in dietary fiber; effect on product colour; no effect on sensory properties of up to 10%.	Verma et al., (2009)
Bologna sausage	Citrus fiber	Improvement in dietary fiber, oxidative stability and colour; negative effect on textural properties; no effect on sensory parameters below 2% level.	Fernández-Ginés et al., (2003)
Sausage	Lemon albedo	Increase in moisture, fiber and protein content; decrease in fat; no effect on sensory attributes.	Fernandez-Gines et al., (2004)
Breakfast sausages	Citrus fiber extract, β-glucan rich ingredient, wheat rusk	Reduction in cooking loss and shrinkage; increased lightness and overall acceptability.	Aleson-Carbonell et al., (2005)
Dry fermented sausage (sobrassada)	Carrot dietary fiber	Above 3% level of fiber led unsuccessful fermentation; critical effect on pH, hardness and compression work.	Eim et al., (2008)
Low salt, low fat chicken nuggets	Bottle gourd (*Lagenaria siceraria* L.)	Increase in pH values, moisture and dietary fiber; decrease in TPA values, cholesterol and cooking yield; negative effect on products flavour and texture at higher level.	Verma et al., (2012b)
Low salt, low fat chicken nuggets	Apple pulp	Low pH value, moisture, dietary fiber and colour parameters; lower batter stability and cooking yield; significant reduction in texture and overall acceptability scores (in the range of very good).	Verma et al., (2010)
Pork burgers	Tiger nut fiber	Higher fiber content, cooking yield, fat retention and moisture retention; negative changes in colour such as redness and yellowness; increase in texture parameters like chewiness and springiness; no effect on acceptability.	Sánchez-Zapata et al., (2010)

Table 4. Fiber ingredients in various low salt and fortified meat products and their effects

Products	Dietary fiber ingredient	Effect on meat products	Reference
Low salt frankfurters	Wheat fibre	Harder, springier and chewier frankfurters with better water- and fat-binding properties.	Jiménez Colmenero et al., (2005)
Low salt pork sausages	Carrot fibre and potato starch	Marked increase in whitening; more impact on textural properties than the level of salt; improvement in water binding capacity to the same level as high salt sausages.	Grossi et al., (2012)
Dry cured sausage	Orange fiber	Chromatographic analysis of orange fiber detected numerous peaks, most of them matched with phenolic compounds; lower increase in thiobarbituric acid reacting substances (TBARS) number in sample with orange fiber during drying; significant decrease in residual nitrite level in sausage.	Fernández-López et al., (2007)
Horse mackerel minced muscle	Grape antioxidant dietary fiber (GADF)	Addition of red grape fiber considerably delayed lipid oxidation during the first 3 months of frozen storage.	Sánchez-Alonso et al., (2007c)
Horse mackerel minced muscle	Grape antioxidant dietary fiber	Bound water after thawing and cooking of minced samples was proportional to the amount of GADF used; softness and loss of cohesiveness were dependent on the amount of GADF; inhibition of lipid oxidation during frozen storage.	Sánchez-Alonso and Borderías (2008)
Raw and cooked chicken breast hamburger	Grape antioxidant dietary fiber	A significant reduction in lightness and yellowness and a significant increase in redness value; significantly improvement in the concentration dependent oxidative stability and the radical scavenging activity; no effect on product's acceptability.	Sáyago-Ayerdi et al., (2009)
Sheep meat nuggets	Guava (*Psidium guajava* L.) powder	Guava powder: rich source of dietary fiber, phenolics and possessed good radical scavenging activity as well as reducing power; significant reduction in pH of emulsion and nuggets, emulsion stability, cooking yield and moisture content of nuggets; increase in total phenolics, total dietary fiber (TDF), ash content and redness value in the product; no effect on sensory attributes and textural properties of the product except springiness and shear force value; reduced lipid peroxidation as measured by TBARS number during refrigerated storage.	Verma et al., (2013)
Pork meatballs	Wheat fiber	Wheat fiber was found to be more effective in limiting iodine losses during thermal processing.	Waszkowiak and Szymandera-Buszka, (2008)

Miscellaneous Meat Products with Dietary Fiber

In addition to the above specific applications of dietary fiber in meat products, fiber has also found a significant place for the development of some meat products to get desired physicochemical and functional characteristics. Besbes et al., (2008) used pea fiber concentrate (PFC) at 0.5% and wheat fiber concentrate (WFC) at 0.5%, 1% and 1.5% levels in beef burger. Both the fibers presented similar water binding capacity, whereas a higher oil-binding capacity was observed for WFC. The water holding capacity of raw beef burger was significantly higher with the addition of fibers and fibers improved the cooking yield and decrease the shrinkage, and minimize production cost without degradation of sensory properties.

The effect of adding orange dietary fiber (1%), rosemary essential oil (0.02%) or thyme essential oil (0.02%) and the storage conditions on the quality characteristics and the shelf-life of mortadella, a bologna-type sausage was studied (Viuda-Martos et al., 2010a). The moisture, fat, ash content, lightness and yellowness were affected by the fiber content. The treatments analysed lowered the levels of residual nitrite and the extent of lipid oxidation, while analysis of the samples through HPLC revealed the presence of the flavonoids, hesperidin and narirutin. No enterobacteria or psychotropic bacteria were found in any of the treatments. The treated samples stored in vacuum packaging showed the lowest aerobic and lactic acid bacteria count. The products containing fiber and rosemary essential oil and stored under vacuum was most appreciated upon sensory evaluation.

Further Viuda-Martos et al., (2010b) observed the effects of 1 % orange dietary fiber (ODF), 0.02% oregano essential oil (OEO) and the storage conditions on the shelf-life of bologna sausage. Lowest oxidation as measured by TBARS number, lowest aerobic and lactic acid bacteria counts was found in samples with ODF + OEO stored in vacuum. The sensory evaluation scores were similar for samples with ODF + OEO and stored either in air or vacuum packaging.

Conclusion

In the era of modernization, urbanization and globalization number of fast foods and ready-to-eat products including meat products have made their universal presence even in our kitchen. Such food products lack adequate amount of dietary fiber and their intake in daily diet should not be considered wise as diet lacking in enough fiber content poses many health related problems. Incorporation of dietary fiber in meat products either in conventional or non-conventional forms could be an intelligent step toward supply of healthier meat products to the consumers. Besides several physiological benefits, addition of fiber in meat products also imparts technological advantages resulting in development of low fat, low salt, high fiber and fortified functional meat products. Awareness among meat consumers are creating demand for more and more dietary fiber enriched meat products and it is expected that the day would come when such functional foods will be ubiquitous and make part in our day to day diet.

References

Abdul-Hamid, A. & Luan, Y. S. (2000). Functional properties of dietary fiber prepared from defatted rice bran. *Food Chemistry, 68,* 15–19.

Aleson-Carbonell, L., Fernández-López, J., Pérez-Alvarez, J. & Kuri, V. (2005). Functional and sensory effects of fiber-rich ingredients on breakfast fresh sausages manufacture. *Food Science and Technology International, 11(2),* 89-97.

Al-Khalifa, A. & Atia, M. (1997). Effect of soy hull and fat on camel meat patties. *Alexandria Science Exchange, 18,* 303–311.

American Association of Cereal Chemists (2001). The definition of dietary fiber. Report of the Dietary Fiber Definition Committee to the Board of Directors of the AAC, 1, 10.

Anderson, E. & Berry, B. (2000). Sensory, shear, and cooking properties of lower-fat beef patties made with inner pea fiber. *Journal of Food Science, 65(5),* 805-810.

Anderson, J. W., Baird, P., Davis, R. H., Jr., Ferreri, S., Knudtson, M., Koraym, A., et al., (2009). Health benefits of dietary fiber. *Nutrition Reviews,* 67, 188–205.

Anderson, J.W., Smith, B.M. & Gustafson N.J. (1994). Health benefits and practical aspects of high-fiber diets. *American Journal of Clinical Nutrition, 1242S*–1247S.

Anonymous (2001). The definition of dietary fiber. Report of the dietary fiber definition committee to the board of directors of the American association of cereal chemists. American Association of Cereal Chemists Report. *Cereal Foods World, 46,* 112–126.

Arjmandi, B.H., Sohn, E., Juma, S., Murthy, S.R. & Daggy, B.P. (1997). Native and partially hydrolyzed psyllium have comparable effects on cholesterol metabolism in rats. *Journal of Nutrtion, 127,* 463–469.

BeMiller, J. N. & Whisler, R. L. (1996). Carbohydrates. In O. R. Fennema (Ed.), In *Food Chemistry* (pp 157-224). New York, Marcel Dekker Inc.

Besbes, S., Attia, H., Deroanne, C., Makni, S. & Blecker, C. (2008). Partial replacement of meat by pea fiber and wheat fiber: Effect on the chemical composition, cooking characteristics and sensory properties of beef burgers. *Journal of Food Quality, 31(4),* 480-489.

Bosaeus, I., Carlsson, N.G., Sandberg, A.S. & Andersson, H. (1986). Effect of wheat bran and pectin on bile acid and cholesterol excretion in ileostomy patients. *Human nutrition. Clinical nutrition, 40 (6),* 429–440.

Brandt, L. A. (2001). Prebiotics enhance gut health. *Prepared Foods, 170(9),* 7–10.

Browne, C. A. (1940). The origin and application of the term nitrogen-free extract in the valuation of feeding stuffs. *Journal of the Association of Official Analytical Chemists, 23,* 102–108.

Burkitt, D. P. & Trowell, H. C. (1977). Dietary fiber and western diseases. *Irish Medical Journal, 70(9),* 272–277.

Cardoso, C., Mendes, R. & Nunes, M. L. (2007). Effect of transglutaminase and carrageenan on restructured fish products containing dietary fibers. *International Journal of Food Science & Technology, 42(11),* 1257-1264.

Cardoso, C., Mendes, R. & Nunes, M. L. (2008a). Development of a healthy low-fat fish sausage containing dietary fiber. *International Journal of Food Science & Technology, 43(2),* 276-283.

Cardoso, C., Mendes, R., Pedro, S. & Nunes, M. L. (2008b). Quality changes during storage of fish sausages containing dietary fiber. *Journal of Aquatic Food Product Technology, 17(1),* 73-95.

Cardoso, C., Ribeiro, B. & Mendes, R. (2012). Effects of dietary fiber and microbial transglutaminase addition on the rheological and textural properties of protein gels from different fish species. *Journal of Food Engineering, 113(4),* 520-526.

Choi, Y. S., Choi, J. H., Han, D. J., Kim, H. Y., Lee, M. A., Jeong, J. Y., Chung, H.J. & Kim, C.J. (2010). Effects of replacing pork back fat with vegetable oils and rice bran fiber on the quality of reduced-fat frankfurters. *Meat Science, 84(3)*, 557-563.

Choi, Y., Choi, J., Han, D., Kim, H., Lee, M., Lee, E., et al., (2008). Effects of rice bran fiber on quality of low-fat tteokgalbi. *Food Science and Biotechnology, 17(5),* 959−964.

Choi, Y., Park, K., Kim, H., Hwang, K., Song, D., Choi, M., Lee, S., Paik, H. & Kim, C. (2013). Quality characteristics of reduced-fat frankfurters with pork fat replaced by sunflower seed oils and dietary fiber extracted from makgeolli lees. *Meat Science, 93(3),* 652-658.

Choi, Y.S., Choi, J.H., Han, D.J., Kim, H.Y., Lee, M.A., Kim, H.W., Jeong, J.Y. & Kim, C.J. (2011). Effects of rice bran fiber on heat-induced gel prepared with pork salt-soluble meat proteins in model system. *Meat Science, 88(1),* 59-66.

Choi, Y.S., Choi, J.H., Han, D.J., Kim, H.Y., Lee, M.A., Kim, H.W., Jeong, J.Y. & Kim, C.J. (2009). Characteristics of low-fat meat emulsion systems with pork fat replaced by vegetable oils and rice bran fiber. *Meat Science, 82(2),* 266-271.

Claus, J. & Hunt, M. (1991). Low-fat, High Added-water Bologna Formulated with Texture-modifying Ingredients. *Journal of Food Science, 56(3),* 643-647.

Collins, J. E. (1997). Reducing salt (sodium) in processed meat, poultry and fish products. In A. M. Pearson & T. R. Dutson (Eds.), *Production and processing of healthy meat, poultry and fish products. Advances in meat research series* (Vol. 11, pp. 282–297). London, Chapman & Hall.

Conway, P. L. (2001). Prebiotics and human health: The state-of-the-art and future perspectives. Scand. *Journal of Nutrition, 45,* 13–21.

Crehan, C. M., Jughes, E., Troy, D. J. & Buckley, D. J. (2000). Effects of fat level and maltodextrin on the functional properties of frankfurter formulated with 5, 12 and 30% fat. *Meat Science, 55,* 463–469.

Cummings, J.H. (1993). The effect of dietary fiber on faecal weight and composition. In G.A. Spiller (Ed), *Handbook of dietary fiber in human nutrition* (p 263). Boca Raton, FL, CRC Press.

Demigne, C., Morand, C., Levrat, A.M., Besson, C., Moundras, C. & Remesy, C. (1995). Effects of propionate on fatty acid and cholesterol synthesis and on acetate metabolism in isolated rat hepatocytes. *British Journal of Nutrition, 74,* 209–219.

Desmond, E., Troy, D. & Buckley, D. (1998). The effects of tapioca starch, oat fiber and whey protein on the physical and sensory properties of low-fat beef burgers. *LWT-Food Science and Technology, 31(7),* 653-657.

Duncan, K. H., Bacon, J. A. & Weinsier, R. L. (1983). The effects of high and low energy density diets on satiety, energy intake, and eating time of obese and non-obese subjects. *American Journal of Clinical Nutrition, 37,* 763–767.

Eim, V. S., Simal, S., Rosselló, C. & Femenia, A. (2008). Effects of addition of carrot dietary fiber on the ripening process of a dry fermented sausage (sobrassada). *Meat Science, 80(2),* 173-182.

Esposito, F., Arlotti, G., Maria Bonifati, A., Napolitano, A., Vitale, D. & Fogliano, V. (2005). Antioxidant activity and dietary fiber in durum wheat bran by-products. *Food Research International, 38(10),* 1167-1173.

Fernández-Ginés, J. M., Fernández-López, J., Sayas-Barberá, E., Sendra, E. & Pérez-Alvarez, J. (2003). Effect of storage conditions on quality characteristics of bologna sausages made with citrus fiber. *Journal of Food Science, 68(2),* 710-714.

Fernández-Ginés, J., Fernández-López, J., Sayas-Barberá, E., Sendra, E. & Pérez-Álvarez, J. (2004). Lemon albedo as a new source of dietary fiber: application to bologna sausages. *Meat Science, 67(1),* 7-13.

Fernández-López, J., Viuda-Martos, M., Sendra, E., Sayas-Barberá, E., Navarro, C. & Pérez-Alvarez, J. (2007). Orange fiber as potential functional ingredient for dry-cured sausages. *European Food Research and Technology, 226(1-2),* 1-6.

Fleury, N. & Lahaye, M. (1991). Chemical and physico-chemical characterisation of fibers from *Lamiaria digitata* (Kombu Breton): A physiological approach. *Journal of the Science of Food and Agriculture, 55,* 389–400.

Galanakis, C. M., Tornberg, E. & Gekas, V. (2010). Dietary fiber suspensions from olive mill wastewater as potential fat replacements in meatballs. *LWT-Food Science and Technology, 43(7),* 1018-1025.

Garcıa, M., Dominguez, R., Galvez, M., Casas, C. & Selgas, M. (2002). Utilization of cereal and fruit fibers in low fat dry fermented sausages. *Meat Science, 60*(3), 227-236.

Gibson, G.R. (2004). Fiber and effects on probiotics (the prebiotic concept). *Clinical Nutrition Supplements, 1,* 25–31.

Gray, J. (2006). Dietary Fiber: Definition, Analysis, Physiology and Health. International Life Sciences Institute, Brussels.

Grigelmo-Miguel N. & Martín-Belloso, O. (1999). Comparison of dietary fiber from by-products of processıng fruits and greens and from cereals. *LWT Food Science and Technology, 32(8),* 503-508.

Grossi, A., Søltoft-Jensen, J., Knudsen, J. C., Christensen, M. & Orlien, V. (2012). Reduction of salt in pork sausages by the addition of carrot fiber or potato starch and high pressure treatment. *Meat Science, 92,* 481-489.

Guillon, F. & Champ, M. (2000). Structural and physical properties of dietary fibers and consequences of processing on human physiology. *Food Research International, 33,* 233-245.

Hague, A., Manning, A.M., Hanlon, K., Hutschtscha, L.I., Hart, D. & Paraskeva, C. (1993). Sodium butyrate induces apoptosis in human colonic tumor cell lines in 53-independent pathway: implications for possible role of dietary fiber in the prevention of large bowel cancer. *International Journal of Cancer, 55,* 498–505.

Hallfrisch, J., Scholfield, D. J. & Behall, K. M. (1995). Diets containing soluble oat extracts improve glucose and insulin responses of moderately hypercholesterolemic men and women. *The American Journal of Clinical Nutrition, 61(2),* 379-384.

Harris, P. J. & Ferguson, L. R. (1993). Dietary fiber: its composition and role in protection against colorectal cancer. *Mutation Research, 290(1),* 97-110.

Heaton, K. W. (1980). Food intake and regulation by fiber. In G. A. Spiller & R. M. Kay, (Eds.), *Medical Aspects of Dietary Fiber* (pp. 223–238). New York.

Hipsley, E.H. (1953). Dietary fiber and pregnancy toxaemia. *British Medical Journal, 2,* 420–422.

Hsu, S. Y. & Chung, H. Y. (2001). Effects of *k*-carrageenan, salt, phosphates and fat on qualities of low fat emulsified meatball. *Journal of Food Engineering, 47,* 115–121.

Huang, S., Shiau, C., Liu, T., Chu, C. & Hwang, D. (2005). Effects of rice bran on sensory and physico-chemical properties of emulsified pork meatballs. *Meat Science, 70(4),* 613-619.

Hughes, E., Cofrades, S. & Troy, D. J. (1997). Effects of fat level, oat fiber and carrageenan on frankfurters formulated with 5, 12 and 30% fat. *Meat Science, 45(3),* 273–281.

Javidipour, I., Vural, H., Özbaş, Ö. Ö. & Tekin, A. (2005). Effects of interesterified vegetable oils and sugar beet fiber on the quality of Turkish-type salami. *International Journal of Food Science & Technology, 40(2),* 177-185.

Jenkins, D., Wolever, T., Leeds, A. R., Gassull, M. A., Haisman, P., Dilawari, J., Goff, D. V., Metz, G. L. & Alberti, K. (1978). Dietary fibers, fiber analogues, and glucose tolerance: importance of viscosity. *British Medical Journal, 1(6124),* 1392-1394.

Jimenez Colmenero, F., Ayo, M. & Carballo, J. (2005). Physicochemical properties of low sodium frankfurter with added walnut: effect of transglutaminase combined with caseinate, KCl and dietary fiber as salt replacers. *Meat Science, 69(4),* 781-788.

Jiménez-Escrig, A. & Sánchez-Muniz, F. J. (2000). Dietary fiber from edible seaweeds: Chemical structure, physicochemical properties and effects on cholesterol metabolism. *Nutrition Research, 20,* 585–598.

Kaack, K., Lærke, H. N. & Meyer, A. S. (2006). Liver paté enriched with dietary fiber extracted from potato fiber as fat substitutes. *European Food Research and Technology, 223(2),* 267-272.

Kaur, N. & Gupta, A. K. (2002). Applications of inulin and oligofructose in health and nutrition. *Journal of Biosciences, 27(7),* 703-714.

Kritchevsky, D. (2000). Dietary Fiber in Health and Disease. In B.V. McCleary & L. Prosky (Eds.), *Proceedings of the 1st International Conference on Dietary Fiber*; Dublin, Ireland. Oxford, UK, Blackwell Science.

Lander, S. (2004). VITACEL® wheat fiber- highly functional in meat products. *Innovations in Food Technology,* 23–32, 34.

Mañas, E., Bravo, L. & Saura-Calixto, F. (1994). Sources of error in dietary fiber analysis. *Food Chemistry, 50(4),* 331-342.

Manning, T. S. & Gibson, G. R. (2004). Prebiotics. *Best Practice & Research Clinical Gastroenterology, 18(2),* 287-298.

Mansour, E. H. & Khalil, A. H. (1999). Characteristics of low-fat beefburgers as influenced by various types of wheat fibers. *Journal of the Science of Food and Agriculture, 79(4),* 493-498.

Martínez, B., Miranda, J. M., Franco, C. M., Cepeda, A. & Vázquez, M. (2011). Evaluation of transglutaminase and caseinate for a novel formulation of beef patties enriched in healthier lipid and dietary fiber. *LWT-Food Science and Technology, 44(4),* 949-956.

Massimino, S. P., McBurney, M. I., Field, C. J., Thomson, A. B. R., Pospisil, L., Keelan, M., Hayek, M. G. & Sunvold, G. D. (1998). Fermentable fiber increases GLP-1 secretion and improves glucose homeostasis despite increased intestinal glucose transport capacity in healthy dogs. *Journal of Nutrition, 128,* 1786–1793.

Mendoza, E., Garcıa, M., Casas, C. & Selgas, M. (2001). Inulin as fat substitute in low fat, dry fermented sausages. *Meat Science, 57(4),* 387-393.

Meyer, P. D. (2004). Non-digestible oligosaccharides as dietary fiber. *Journal of the Association of Official Analytical Chemists International, 87(3),* 718–726.

Modi, V., Yashoda, K. & Mahendrakar, N. (2009). Low-fat mutton kofta prepared by using carrageenan as fat replacer: quality changes in cooked product during storage. *Journal of Food Science and Technology, 46(4),* 316-319.

Monahan, F. J. & Troy, D. J. (1997). Overcoming sensory problems in low fat and low salts products. In A. M. Pearson & T. R. Dutson (Eds.), *Production and processing of healthy meat, poultry and fish products. Advances in meat research series* (Vol. 11, pp. 257–281). London, Chapman & Hall.

Nishina, P. M. & Freedland, R. A. (1990). Effects of propionate on lipid biosynthesis in isolated rat hepatocytes. *The Journal of Nutrition, 120(7),* 668-673.

Östman, E. M., Elmståhl, H. G. L. & Björck, I. M. (2002). Barley bread containing lactic acid improves glucose tolerance at a subsequent meal in healthy men and women. *The Journal of Nutrition, 132(6),* 1173-1175.

Özboy-Özbas, Ö., Vural, H. & Javidipour, I. (2003). Effects of sugarbeet fiber on the quality of frankfurters. *Zuckerindustrie, 128(3),* 171-175.

Ozvural, E. B. & Vural, H. (2008). Utilization of interesterified oil blends in the production of frankfurters. *Meat Science, 78(3),* 211–216.

Pierre, F., Perrin, R., Champ, M., Bornet, F., Meflah, K. & Menanteau J. (1997). Short-chain fructooligosaccharides reduce the occurrence of colon tumors and develop gut-associated lymphoid tissue in Min mice. *Cancer Research, 57,* 225–228.

Pietrasik, Z. & Duda, Z. (2000). Effects of fat content and soy protein/carragenan mix on the quality characteristics of comminuted, scalded sausages. *Meat Science, 56,* 181–188.

Pietrasik, Z. & Janz, J. (2010). Utilization of pea flour, starch-rich and fiber-rich fractions in low fat bologna. *Food Research International, 43(2),* 602-608.

Pinero, M., Parra, K., Huerta-Leidenz, N., Arenas de Moreno, L., Ferrer, M., Araujo, S. & Barboza, Y. (2008). Effect of oat's soluble fiber (β-glucan) as a fat replacer on physical, chemical, microbiological and sensory properties of low-fat beef patties. *Meat Science, 80(3),* 675-680.

Roberfroid, M. B. (2005). Introducing inulin-type fructans. *British Journal of Nutrition, 93(1),* 13-26.

Roberton, A. M., Ferguson, L. R., Hollands, H. J. & Harris, P. J. (1991). Adsorption of a hydrophobic mutagen to five contrasting dietary fiber preparations. *Mutation Research, 262(3),* 195-202.

Robinson, G., Ross-Murphy, S. B. & Morris, E. R. (1982). Viscosity-molecular weight relationships, intrinsic chain flexibility, and dynamic solution properties of guar galactomannan. *Carbohydrate Research, 107(1),* 17-32.

Rumney, C. & Rowland, I. (1995). Non-digestible oligosaccharides—potential anticancer agents? *Nutrition Bulletin, 20(3),* 194-203.

Sakata, T. (1995). A Very-low-calorie conventional Japanese diet: Its implications for prevention of obesity. *Obesity Research, 3(S2),* 233s-239s.

Sánchez-Alonso, I. & Borderías, A. J. (2008). Technological effect of red grape antioxidant dietary fiber added to minced fish muscle. *International Journal of Food Science & Technology, 43(6),* 1009-1018.

Sánchez-Alonso, I., Haji-Maleki, R. & Borderías, A. J. (2006). Effect of wheat fiber in frozen stored fish muscular gels. *European Food Research and Technology, 223(4),* 571-576.

Sánchez-Alonso, I., Haji-Maleki, R. & Borderias, A. J. (2007b). Wheat fiber as a functional ingredient in restructured fish products. *Food Chemistry, 100(3),* 1037-1043.

Sánchez-Alonso, I., Jiménez-Escrig, A., Saura-Calixto, F. & Borderías, A. (2007c). Effect of grape antioxidant dietary fiber on the prevention of lipid oxidation in minced fish: evaluation by different methodologies. *Food Chemistry, 101(1),* 372-378.

Sanchez-Alonso, I., Solas, M. T. & Javier Borderias, A. (2007a). Technological implications of addition of wheat dietary fiber to giant squid (Dosidicus gigas) surimi gels. *Journal of Food Engineering, 81(2),* 404-411.

Sánchez-Zapata, E., Muñoz, C., Fuentes, E., Fernández-López, J., Sendra, E., Sayas, E., Navarro, C. & Pérez-Alvarez, J. (2010). Effect of tiger nut fiber on quality characteristics of pork burger. *Meat Science, 85(1),* 70-76.

Sáyago-Ayerdi, S., Brenes, A. & Goñi, I. (2009). Effect of grape antioxidant dietary fiber on the lipid oxidation of raw and cooked chicken hamburgers. *LWT-Food Science and Technology, 42(5),* 971-976.

Schneeman, B. O. & Tietyen, J. (1994). Dietary fiber. In M. E. Shills, J. A. Olson & M. Shike, (Eds.), Modern *Nutrition in Health and Disease*, (8th edn., pp. 89–100). Philadelphia, PA, Lea and Febiger.

Schneeman, B.O. (2001). Dietary fiber and gastrointestinal function. In B.V., McCleary & L. Prosky (Eds.), *Advanced Dietary Fiber Technology* (*pp.*168–176). Ames, IA, Blackwell Sciences.

Scholz-Ahrens, K. E., Schaafsma, G., van den Heuvel, E. G. & Schrezenmeir, J. (2001). Effects of prebiotics on mineral metabolism. *The American Journal of Clinical Nutrition, 73(2),* 459s-464s.

Scott, K.P., Duncan, S.H. & Flint, H.J. (2008). Dietary fiber and the gut microbiota. *Nutrition Bulletin, 33,* 201–211.

Serdaroğlu, M., Yıldız-Turp, G. & Abrodímov, K. (2005). Quality of low-fat meatballs containing legume flours as extenders. *Meat Science, 70(1),* 99-105.

Serrano, A., Librelotto, J., Cofrades, S., Sanchez-Muniz, F. J. & Jimenez-Colmenero, F. (2007). Composition and physicochemical characteristics of restructured beef steaks containing walnuts as affected by cooking method. *Meat Science, 77(3),* 304–313.

Shand, P. (2000). Textural, water holding, and sensory properties of low-fat pork bologna with normal or waxy starch hull-less barley. *Journal of Food Science, 65(1),* 101-107.

Slavin, J., Jacobs, D. & Marquart, L. (1997). Whole-grain consumption and chronic disease: protective mechanisms. *Nutrition and Cancer, 27(1),* 14-21.

Steenblock, R. L., Sebranek, J., Olson, D. & Love, J. (2001). The effects of oat fiber on the properties of light bologna and fat-free frankfurters. *Journal of Food Science, 66(9),* 1409-1415.

Thebaudin, J. Y., Lefebvre, A. C., Harrington, M. & Bourgeois, C. M. (1997). Dietary fibers: nutritional and technological interest. *Trends in Food Science and Technology, 8(2),* 41–48.

Thibault, J. F., Lahaye, M. & Guillon, F. (1992). Physicochemical properties of food plant cell walls. In T. F. Schweiger & C. A. Edwards (Eds.), *Dietary fiber: A Component of Food. Nutritional Function in Health and Disease* (pp. 21-39). London, Springer.

Titov, E.I., Mitaseva, L.F., Kulishev, U.V. & Medkova, E.V. (1994). Utilization of plant raw materials in production of poultry meat products. *Myasnaya-Promyshlennost, 1,* 13–15.

Todesco, T., Rao, A. V., Bosello, O. & Jenkins, D. J. A. (1991). Propionate lowers blood glucose and alters lipid metabolism in healthy subjects. *American Journal of Clinical Nutrition, 54,* 860–865.

Trowell, H.C., Southgate, D.A.T., Wolever, T.M.S., Leeds, A.R., Gassull, M.A. & Jenkins, D.J.A. (1976). Dietary fiber redefined. *The Lancet, 1,* 967.

Tungland, B. & Meyer, D. (2002). Nondigestible Oligo-and Polysaccharides (Dietary Fiber): Their Physiology and Role in Human Health and Food. *Comprehensive Reviews in Food Science and Food Safety, 1(3),* 90-109.

Turhan, S., Sagir, I. & Sule Ustun, N. (2005). Utilization of hazelnut pellicle in low-fat beef burgers. *Meat Science, 71(2),* 312-316.

Vahouny, G., Satchithanandam, S., Chen, I., Tepper, S., Kritchevsky, D., Lightfoot, F. & Cassidy, M. (1988). Dietary fiber and intestinal adaptation: effects on lipid absorption and lymphatic transport in the rat. *The American Journal of Clinical Nutrition, 47(2),* 201-206.

Vendrell-Pascuas, S., Castellote-Bargallo, A. & Lopez-Sabater, M. (2000). Determination of inulin in meat products by high-performance liquid chromatography with refractive index detection. *Journal of Chromatography A, 881(1),* 591-597.

Verma, A. K., Rituparna, B. & Sharma, B. (2012a). Quality of Low Fat Chicken Nuggets: Effect of Sodium Chloride Replacement and Added Chickpea (*Cicer arietinum* L.) Hull Flour. *Asian-Australasian Journal of Animal Science, 25(2),* 291-298.

Verma, A. K., Sharma, B. & Banerjee, R. (2010). Effect of sodium chloride replacement and apple pulp inclusion on the physico-chemical, textural and sensory properties of low fat chicken nuggets. *LWT-Food Science and Technology, 43(4),* 715-719.

Verma, A. K., Sharma, B. D. & Banerjee, R. (2012b). Quality characteristics of low-fat chicken nuggets: effect of common salt replacement and added bottle gourd (*Lagenaria siceraria* L.). *Journal of the Science of Food and Agriculture, 92(9),* 1848-1854.

Verma, A., Sharma, B. & Banerjee, R. (2009). Quality characteristics and storage stability of low fat functional chicken nuggets. *Fleischwirtschaft International, 24,* 52-57.

Verma, A.K., Rajkumar, V., Banerjee, R., Biswas, S. & Das, A.K. (2013). Guava (Psidium guajava L.) powder as an antioxidant dietary fiber in sheep meat nuggets. *Asian-Australasian Journal of Animal Sciences,* http://dx.doi.org/10.5713/ajas.2012.12671.

Viuda-Martos, M., Ruiz-Navajas, Y., Fernandez-Lopez, J. & Perez-Alvarez, J. (2010a). Effect of added citrus fiber and spice essential oils on quality characteristics and shelf-life of mortadella. *Meat Science, 85(3),* 568-576.

Viuda-Martos, M., Ruiz-Navajas, Y., Fernández-López, J. & Pérez-Álvarez, J. (2010b). Effect of orange dietary fiber, oregano essential oil and packaging conditions on shelf-life of bologna sausages. *Food Control, 21(4),* 436-443.

Vural, H., Javidipour, I. & Ozbas, O. O. (2004). Effects of interesterified vegetable oils and sugarbeet fiber on the quality of frankfurters. *Meat Science, 67(1),* 65-72.

Wasan, H.S. & Goodlad, R.A. (1996). Fiber-supplemented foods may damage your health. *The Lancet, 348,* 319–320.

Waszkowiak, K. & Szymandera-Buszka, K. (2008). The application of wheat fiber and soy isolate impregnated with iodine salts to fortify processed meats. *Meat Science, 80(4),* 1340-1344.

Weickert, M. O. & Pfeiffer, A. F. (2008). Metabolic effects of dietary fiber consumption and prevention of diabetes. *The Journal of Nutrition, 138(3),* 439-442.

Weickert, M. O., Mohlig, M., Koebnick, C., Holst, J., Namsolleck, P., Ristow, M., Osterhoff, M., Rochlitz, H., Rudovich, N. & Spranger, J. (2005). Impact of cereal fiber on glucose-regulating factors. *Diabetologia, 48(11),* 2343-2353.

Welsh, S., Shaw, A. & Davis, C. (1994). Achieving dietary recommendations: Whole-grain foods in the food guide pyramid. *Critical Reviews in Food Science & Nutrition, 34(5-6),* 441-451.

WHO/FAO (2003). Diet nutrition and the prevention of chronic diseases. Report of the joint WHO/FAO experts consultation. WHO Technical Report Series, n° 916.

Willett, W. C., Hunter, D. J., Stampfer, M. J., Colditz, G., Manson, J. E., Spiegelman, D., Rosner, B., Hennekens, C. H. & Speizer, F. E. (1992). Dietary fat and fiber in relation to risk of breast cancer. *The Journal of the American Medical Association, 268(15),* 2037-2044.

Yılmaz, İ. & Dağlıoğlu, O. (2003). The effect of replacing fat with oat bran on fatty acid composition and physicochemical properties of meatballs. *Meat Science, 65(2),* 819-823.

Yılmaz, I. (2004). Effects of rye bran addition on fatty acid composition and quality characteristics of low-fat meatballs. *Meat Science, 67(2),* 245-249.

Yılmaz, I. (2005). Physicochemical and sensory characteristics of low fat meatballs with added wheat bran. *Journal of Food Engineering, 69(3),* 369-373.

Yoo, S. S., Kook, S. H., Park, S. Y., Shim, J. H. & Chin, K. B. (2007). Physicochemical characteristics, textural properties and volatile compounds in comminuted sausages as affected by various fat levels and fat replacers. *International Journal of Food Science & Technology, 42,* 1114–1122.

In: Dietary Fiber
Editors: D. Betancur-Ancona, L. Chel-Guerrero et al.
ISBN: 978-1-62808-931-8

Chapter 5

Antioxidant Dietary Fiber: Sources and Applications

Isabel Goñi [*]
Nutrition and Gastrointestinal Unit,
Department of Nutrition I, UCM, Madrid, Spain,
Facultad de Farmacia, Universidad Complutense de Madrid,
Ciudad Universitaria, Madrid, Spain

Abstract

Intake of dietary fiber (DF) has been included as an essential dietary indicator to define a healthy dietary pattern, but intake values underestimate a major part of the non-digestible compounds that escape the action of digestive enzymes and enter the colon.

There is a general tendency to extend the concept of DF to include all indigestible food constituents. This is the concept of total food indigestible fraction, defined as the part of plant foods that is not digested nor absorbed in the small intestine, reaching the colon where it is a substrate for the fermentative microflora. As such, it comprises non-starch polysaccharides, lignin and other compounds of proven resistance to the action of digestive enzymes, including phytochemicals.

A major proportion of phytochemicals are antioxidants (polyphenols and carotenoids) and a substantial portion of these, mainly polymeric pholyphenols or polyphenols trapped in the fiber matrix, traverse the small intestine bonded to DF and may be released into the colon by the action of microbiota, producing active metabolites and an antioxidant environment. Both DF and dietary antioxidants are major components of fruits and vegetables. Despite healthy effects and recommendations, the consumption of fruits and vegetables is currently low, and consequently DF and antioxidants are generally deficient in most diets around the world. This is one important reason why these compounds are widely used as functional ingredients in processed foods. The market in this field is competitive and the development of new types of fibers is a challenge for the food industry. Against this background, a study of sources of antioxidant dietary fibers is clearly justified.

* e-mail: igonic@ucm.es.

Then again, plant food processing industries produce large amounts of waste and residues (leaves, stems, wastewaters, etc.) that are good sources of DF and antioxidant compounds. Several fruit and vegetable by-products meet the definition of antioxidant in fat and, in addition dietary fiber. These materials can be used as food ingredients to increase DF content and to prevent lipid oxidation. Moreover, there are good prospects for the use of these materials as dietary supplements for intestinal health, including prevention of gastrointestinal cancer and reduction of cardiovascular disease risk factors.

Introduction

Plant foods, particularly fruits and vegetables, have been consistently identified in epidemiological research as the key components of dietary patterns that reduce risk for the development of chronic and degenerative diseases. These foods are generally high in water, vitamins, minerals, and contain significant amounts of DF and phytochemicals – mainly polyphenols and carotenoids - with significant biological properties, including antioxidant activity. The potential health benefits of fruit and vegetable are mainly attributed to the effects of DF and antioxidants (Saura-Calixto & Goñi, 2009).

Phytochemicals or phytonutrients are bioactive substances that can be found in foods derived from plants and are not essentials for life. DF of fruit and vegetable transports a significant amount of polyphenols and carotenoids linked to the fiber matrix through the human gut (Saura-Calixto et al., 2006, 2007). Thus, phytochemicals may be considered DF constituents in view of the similarity of their properties in terms of resistance to digestive enzymes and colonic fermentability (Saura-Calixto et al., 2006, 2007).

The capacity of the fiber matrix to act as a carrier of antioxidant compounds is an essential physiological function of DF. Therefore, DF and antioxidants could be approached jointly in nutrition and health studies, combining the properties of both DF and antioxidants in a single material, defined as *antioxidant dietary fiber* (Saura-Calixto, 1998).

Several fruits and vegetables are good sources of antioxidant dietary fiber and several fruit and vegetable byproducts from food processing industries also meet the criteria of antioxidant dietary fiber definition. They are certain to be an excellent source of DF and natural antioxidants and they coul be used as high-quality ingredients in functional foods or dietary supplements.

Dietary Fiber versus Indigestible Fraction

The role of DF in nutrition and health is well defined. Numerous clinical and epidemiological studies have addressed the essential role of DF in intestinal health, prevention of cardiovascular disease and cancer, obesity, and diabetes (Murphy et al. 2012). DF intake has recently been included as an essential indicator for definition of a healthy dietary pattern such as the Mediterranean Diet (Saura-Calixto & Goñi, 2009). The recommended daily intake of DF is 25-35 g/person (Buttriss & Stokes, 2008). Despite the importance of DF to human health, the intake in Western diets is deficient. DF intake in European countries (Elmadfa, 2009) and the USA (USDA, 2010) accounts for only about 20 and 15 g/person/day respectively.

DF intake is usually estimated from food composition tables, and these data may be of limited value since they can lead to significant conceptual and methodological errors (Saura-Calixto & Goñi, 2004). On the one hand, it is known that DF data include only a part of indigestible food components (Saura-Calixto et al. 2000). On the other hand, DF data do not usually refer to foods as eaten, since they are obtained in non-physiological analytical conditions.

Definitions of DF in national and international recommendations generally conform and relate to methods of analysis of the Association of Official Analytical Chemists (AOAC). However, some errors associated with this analytical procedure have been reported (Mañas & Saura, 1995). Moreover, following the AOAC procedure, only non-digestible carbohydrates and lignin can be quantified. And yet the characteristics of the primary DF constituents—resistance to hydrolysis by human digestive enzymes and fermentation in the large intestine—can be found in other non-digestible food constituents contained in many plant foods (Figure 1). It is important to note at this point that the importance of defining and quantifying DF in foods lies in physiological effects that are associated with the consumption of such dietary components, which include, among others, reduced intestinal transit time and increased stool bulk, reduction of total and/or LDL blood cholesterol levels, and reduction of post-prandial blood glucose and/or insulin levels. These physiological effects of DF are distinct from those of indigestible carbohydrates considered in the first definition of DF (EFSA, 2007).

DF is a nutritional concept that combines botanical, chemical and physiological considerations, which accounts for the threefold debate on definition - analytical method - physiological effects. The main problem is how to define DF taking into account only physiological attributes or only chemical composition, for both aspects are closely related to the concept of fiber. Therefore, with growing knowledge, the definition of fiber has evolved into a broader concept that takes more account of physiological behaviour.

Carbohydrates	Polysaccharides	Non starch Polysaccharides	Cellulosics	Cellulose Hemicelluloses
			Non Cellulosics	Hemicelluloses β-glucans Pectins Gums and mucilages Others (galactomannan; alginates; arabinoxylan; carrageenan)
		Resistant starch		
	Resistant oligosaccharides			
Non Carbohydrates	Lignin			
	Resistant macronutrients (protein; lipid)			
	Bioactive Compounds	Polyphenols		
		Carotenoids		
		Fitosterols		
		Others		

Figure 1. Components of the indigestible fraction of foods.

From a physiological and nutritional standpoint DF may be considered as a heterogeneous complex whose physicochemical characteristics and physiological properties are derived from its components, which in turn depend on the type and amount of food consumed in the whole diet (EFSA, 2007). Figure 1 lists the non-digestible components of foods, including non-digestible carbohydrates, klason lignin and other associated compounds.

Plant foods contain a wide range of non-digestible components. Some are nutrients such as starch, protein, fat, etc., and others are non-nutrients such as bioactive compounds (Figure 1). Both groups satisfy the physiological condition of not being digested in the small intestine by the digestive enzymes. Therefore, they reach the large intestine largely in association with the classical fiber components (non-starch polysaccharides and lignin) and can be degraded by the enzymatic activity of microbiota. The set of all non-digestible food components is known as the total indigestible fraction (TIF) of foods and has been defined as "*the part of plant foods that is neither digested nor absorbed in the small intestine, reaching the colon where it is a substrate for fermentative microflora*" (Saura-Calixto et al. 2000). Recently, TIF was proposed as a good alternative to DF for nutritional and epidemiological studies (Saura-Calixto & Goñi, 2004) and has been proposed as one of the four indicators defining a healthy dietary pattern (Saura-Calixto & Goñi, 2009).

According to the definition of TIF, phytochemicals may be considered DF constituents in view of the similarity of their properties in terms of resistance to digestive enzymes and colonic fermentability (Goñi et al. 2006; Saura-Calixto et al. 2007).

More than 8000 phenolic compounds have been reported, and they are widely dispersed throughout the plant kingdom. They may be classified according the number of phenol rings that they contain and according to the structural elements that are bound to each one of them (Manach et al. 2005). Polyphenols can be classified according to chemical structure as flavonoids (anthocyanins, chalcones and dihydrochalcones, flavanols or catechins, flavanones, flavones, flavonols, isoflavones and proanthocyanidins or condensed tannins) and non-flavonoids (benzoic acids, cinnamic acids and cinnamic acid conjugates, such as chlorogenic acid, and gallic acid esters or hydrolysable tannins). Flavonoids, the largest group of plant phenolics, contain compounds in a wide range of molecular weights. In addition to flavonoids and non-flavonoids there are "derived polyphenols", substances that are characteristic of many traditionally processed foods and beverages but which do not occur in healthy intact plant tissue (Williamson & Clifford, 2010).

Otherwise, polyphenols may be classified on the basis of their capacity to be extracted from plant foods using aqueous organic solvents. They may be extractable polyphenols, which are compounds with low or intermediate molecular mass, or non-extractable polyphenols, which remain in the residues from aqueous organic extraction due to the ability to form macromolecules as well as to bind to polysaccharides, protein and cell walls. Non-extractable polyphenols may contain polymeric polyphenols or low molecular weight polyphenols bound to other components of the food matrix.

Non-Digestible Dietary Substrates and Microbiota

Colonic microbiota play an important role in human digestive physiology and contribute significantly to homeostasis in the large bowel. The large gut is an open system where non-digestible substrates of the diet, microbiota and epithelial colonic cells interact. The gastrointestinal tract is home to between some 10 and 100 trillion microbes (Bäckhed et al. 2005), approximately 10 times as many cells as found in the human body (Savage et al. 1996). The majority of the organisms are located at the distal site, where the concentration of some 500 bacterial species may reach $10^{11} - 10^{12}$ colony forming units per g of intestinal content, and account for some 35 – 50 % of the contents (Salminen et al. 1996).

The anaerobic breakdown of substrates by metabolic activity of colonic microorganisms is known conventionally as colonic fermentation, and this process generates active metabolites, various end compounds with biological activity, energy and biomass.

The relationships between the microbial community, food metabolism and intestinal health have direct consequences for human health. The metabolites produced by gut microbiota from food constituents are often better absorbed than the original compounds and can be responsible for the health benefits associated with a given food product. In addition, food constituents modulate gut microbiota composition.

Colonic dietary substrates comprise non-digestible carbohydrates such as non-starch polysaccharides, resistant starch and oligosaccharides, and also other non-carbohydrate compounds such as lignin, resistant protein, and other associated compounds of nutritional importance such as phytochemicals.

The bacterial degradation of carbohydrates is well-known. Short-chain fatty acids (SCFA), predominantly acetate, propionate and butyrate, are the principal metabolites generated during the catabolism of carbohydrates. Most SCFA are absorbed from the gut and metabolized in various body tissues, making a relatively small but significant contribution to the daily energy requirements of the body. Proteins may be substrates for colonic microbiota. They also generate SCFA and other nitrogen catabolites usually associated with the growth of potential pathogens (Bauer et al. 2006).

According to the definition of TIF, phytochemicals are substrates for colonic fermentation. A significant amount of phytochemicals (mainly polyphenols) (Saura-Calixto et al. 2010 a) linked to the complex food matrix interacts with microbiota; however, they not produce SCFA but instead a wide range of active metabolites. Selma et al (2009) have summarized the current information about microbial degradation metabolites and their formation pathways obtained from the different groups of dietary phenolic compounds, identifying their differences and similarities.

Interactions, competition and synergistic effects between bacterial enzymes and dietary substrates may be expected. The relative amount and type of polysaccharides and polyphenols and other compounds reaching the human colon may affect the type and concentration of metabolites in the intestinal ecosystem. Be it noted that polyphenols represent only about 5 % of the total amount of substrates available for human colonic fermentation, but they are attached to other non-digestible substrates. Few studies have considered the possible synergistic effect of DF and polyphenols present in whole plant foods. However, the colonic fermentation of phenolic compounds together with different amounts of DF or polysaccharides has shown that DF may enhance the yield of polyphenolic metabolites, probably due to an increase of bacterial activity. Therefore, microbiota interact with bioactive food components to modify their bioavailability and activity, and along with fiber constitute the main energy source for colonic fermentation (Tuohy et al. 2012; Pozuelo et al. 2012).

Certain non-digestible components may affect the growth and survival of the beneficial bacteria by influencing their growth and enzymatic activities. A part of the products of fermentation is utilized by bacteria, yielding energy and carbon necessary for synthesis and growth of the microbiota. Another part is eliminated in the stool or rectal gases, but the major part is absorbed by the colonic mucosa.

Consequently, the composition of the diet can influence the profile and metabolic activity of the microbial ecology in the gut. Some of these issues will be discussed in a later section.

A number of factors are likely to affect the utilization of fermentable substrates in the colon, such as factors involving digestive motility, individual differences in microflora, and the solubility of substrates in the intestinal medium. Usually, soluble compounds are readily degraded by the microbiota because they are more accessible to hydrolytic enzymes, whereas insolubles are more resistant to bacterial degradation. However, there are important exceptions such as alginates or carrageenans that are soluble but poorly fermented. Water solubility therefore does not always predict the physiological effects. The FAO/WHO (1998) proposed phasing out the distinction between soluble and insoluble fiber. Nevertheless, this distinction based on the solubility of the non-digestible compounds in the intestinal environment is still used.

There is another argument in support of the indigestible fraction of foods versus the classical concept of DF. On the basis of bacterial growth, it has been estimated that up to 60 g of substrates reaching the colon would be necessary to maintain the daily bacterial cell turnover (Cummings & Macfarlane, 1991). However, DF intake in Western countries only accounts for about 20 g of non starch polysaccharides (Chuang, 2012), which leaves a "carbohydrate gap" of 40 g/day.

Taking into account the concept of TIF as defined above, this gap would reflect an incorrect quantification of available food substrates in the large intestine as a consequence of conceptual and methodological errors concerning DF, discussed above.

The comparison of DF intakes in specific populations (data derived from food composition tables or from analytical data) with the values calculated from the quantification of TIF would support the above contentions.

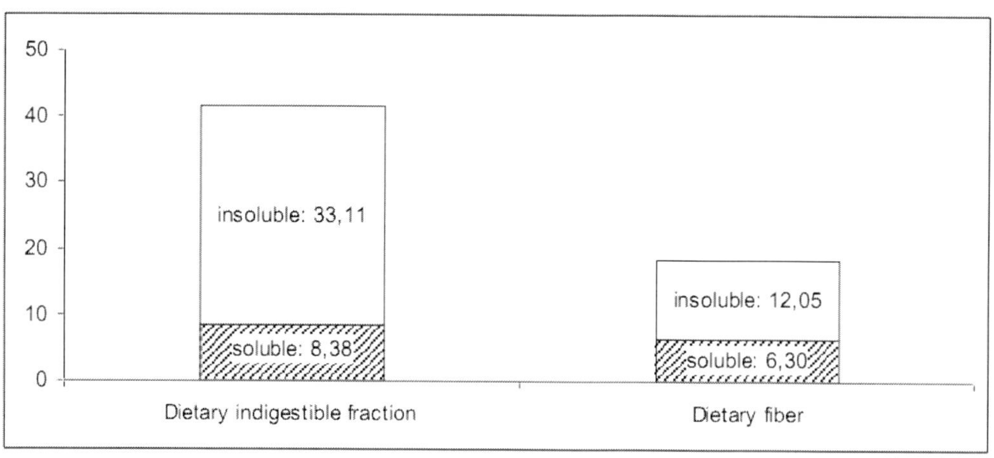

Figure 2. Intake of dietary indigestible fraction and dietary fiber in Spanish diet (adapted from Saura-Calixto & Goñi, 2004).

Figure 2 shows the comparison of total DF and TIF intakes in the whole Spanish diet. In this case, analytical values of DF in Spanish plant foods were determined following the

AOAC method with minor modifications to avoid methodological errors (Mañas & Saura-Calixto, 1995). The intake was 18.3 g of DF/person/day. However, the total amount of non digestible dietary substrates (TIF) was 41.5 g/person/day (Saura-Calixto & Goñi, 2004). TIF was determined by a procedure that combines treatments with digestive enzymes and subsequent separation of digestible compounds by dialysis using physiological conditions (Saura Calixto et al. 2000). These results indicate that DF intake values underestimate a major part of the dietary substrates that reach the colon, while TIF figures are more realistic, being closer to the intestinal microflora and energy needs than the corresponding DF intakes.

Microbiota and Bioavailability of Polyphenols

Health benefits of polyphenols have been widely reported and are associated with numerous physiological effects (Hervert-Hernández & Goñi, 2011; Del Rio et al. 2010; Chong et al. 2010; Selma et at, 2009). In addition to their antioxidant properties, polyphenols may have other specific biological effects in the prevention of age-related diseases, including cardiovascular disease and cancer. To exert their biological properties, polyphenols have to be available to some extent in the target tissue. Therefore, the biological properties of dietary polyphenols may depend on intake, bioaccessibility and bioavailability. Only polyphenols released from the food matrix are bioaccessible. A small amount of polyphenolic compounds in food are free, but most are attached to the food matrix and need to be released prior to absorption. The release of polyphenols may occur in the small or the large intestine, or it may not take place at all.

The bioavailability of dietary polyphenols and their healthy effects depend very much on their transformation by components of the gut microbiota. Phytochemicals and/or their metabolic products may inhibit pathogenic bacteria while stimulating the growth of beneficial bacteria, exerting prebiotic-like effects. Therefore, the intestinal microbiota are both a target for nutritional interventions and a factor influencing the biological activity of other food compounds.

The intestinal tract harbours a complex bacterial community which has an enormous impact on the nutritional and heath status of the host. Overall, a balanced gut microbiota composition confers benefits on the host, while microbial imbalances are associated with metabolic and immune-mediated disorders. The composition of the gut microbiota is influenced by endogenous and environmental factors. The diet is considered a major driver for changes in gut diversity that may affect its functional relationships with the host.

Then again, as indicated above, the total food indigestible fraction is a mixture of non-digestible compounds with different chemical structures that are potential substrates for microflora. A substantial part of the dietary polyphenols bound to DF may become fermentable substrates for bacterial microflora, along with other non-digestible components of DF.

Therefore, it is of particular interest to study the reciprocal interaction between the gut microbiota and dietary polyphenols: 1) The microflora transforms polyphenols. The polyphenols are metabolized to a large extent by gut microbiota, producing metabolites such as phenylacetic, phenylpropionic and phenylbutyric acids, urolithin A and urolithin B, which may be absorbed and exert systemic effects (Hervert-Hernández & Goñi, 2011; Williamson &

Clifford, 2010; Selam et al. 2009). Moreover, non-absorbable metabolites and non-fermented polyphenols remain in the colonic lumen, where they can contribute to a healthy antioxidant environment by scavenging free radicals and counteracting the effects of dietary pro-oxidants; 2) Polyphenols modulate the bacterial population and the enzymatic activity of the microflora. Intestinal microbiota composition can be modulated by living micro-organisms, and non-digestible components of the diet (Hervert-Hernandez & Goñi, 2011; Selam et al. 2009). Extensive research into interaction among phenolic compounds and intestinal bacteria has centred on the following aspects: Degradation of polyphenols and generated metabolites (Tulipani et al. 2012; Del Rio et al. 2009; Selma et al. 2009); systemic effects derived from absorbed polyphenols (pattern and metabolites) (Williamson & Clifford, 2010; Chong et al. 2010; Clifford, 2004); antimicrobial properties against pathogenic bacteria and the stimulatory role of polyphenols on beneficial microorganisms (Pozuelo et al. 2012; Hervert-Hernández et al. 2009).There are two main reciprocal interactions between the gut microbiota and polyphenols. On the one hand, dietary polyphenols undergo a complex metabolism after ingestion and interact with human and microbial enzymes, leading to the production of a large number of circulating and excreted polyphenol metabolites and catabolic products. On the other hand, polyphenols and their metabolites can influence and induce a modulation of the gut microbiota composition by means of several interactions. It is clear that polyphenols may confer health benefits through interactions with and hence modulation of the gut microbiota. Intestinal microbial ecology can be modulated by living microorganisms and non-digestible dietary compounds, including plant secondary phytochemicals. In this regard, polyphenols may exert a double positive effect: inhibiting pathogenic bacteria and stimulating beneficial bacteria. Recently-published reviews extensively discuss the current information on these subjects (Hervert-Hernández & Goñi, 2011; Selma et al. 2009).

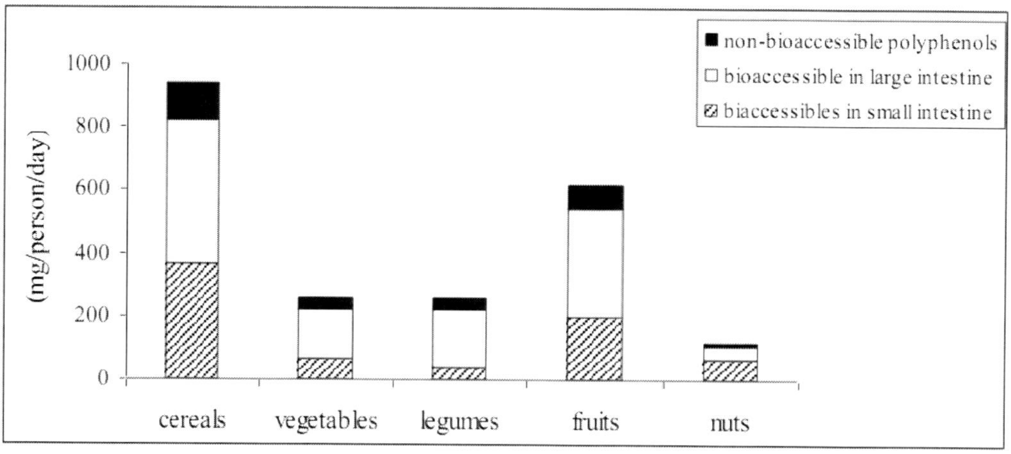

Figure 3. Estimation of the intestinal bioaccessibility of polyphenols from plant foods in the Spanish diet (adapted from Saura-Calixto et al. 2007).

The Microflora Transforms Polyphenols

The health benefits of phenolic consumption derive from polyphenols, their bioactive metabolites and also the modulation of the intestinal bacterial population by phenolic compounds.

Bacteria–host interactions may be viewed in terms of a continuum between mutualism and pathogenicity. In addition to their direct beneficial effect on the human tissues, unabsorbed dietary phenolics and their metabolites exert significant effects on the intestinal environment through modulation of the microbiota (Lee et al. 2006). For these effects to materialize, it is essential to take into account the solubility of the compounds concerned in the intestinal medium.

Polyphenols can be classified in physiological terms according to their solubility in the intestinal medium: a) polyphenols solubilized and b) polyphenols not solubilized in the small intestine. The first are polyphenols present in food that are solubilized in the small intestine along with other phenolic compounds released from the food matrix by the action of digestive enzymes, which are also solubilized in the small intestine. The others constitute a substantial portion of dietary polyphenols (mainly polymeric polyphenols and low molecular weight polyphenols linked to DF and/or trapped in cores of the fiber matrix along with minor amounts of carotenoids and others). These pass undissolved and/or unaltered through the upper intestine in association with DF and reach the colon, where they become fermentable substrates for bacterial microflora along with non-digestible carbohydrates and other compounds, producing active metabolites susceptible of being absorbed at the colon level (Williamson & Manach, 2005).

To our knowledge only the intestinal microflora is able to disrupt the DF matrix and release some associated compounds under mild physiological conditions (Saura-Calixto et al. 2010b). The human microflora can hydrolyse, reduce or decarboxylate polyphenols, producing several metabolites (dyhydroxyphenyl acids, urolithin, equol and others). This enormous capacity to extract and transform non-digestible polyphenols, which greatly outstrips physicochemical and biotechnological treatments, is a consequence of the genomic complexity and variety of the human microflora.

Intestinal bioaccessibility is defined as the amount of a food constituent that is present in the gut as a consequence of the release of this constituent from the solid food matrix and may be able to pass through the intestinal barrier. Only polyphenols released from the food matrix by the action of digestive enzymes (small intestine) and enzymatic activity of microflora (large intestine) are bioaccessible in the gut and therefore potentially bioavailable. Polyphenols solubilized in the stomach and small intestine can be absorbed at least partially through the small intestinal mucosa, followed by metabolic and systemic effects. However, only between 5 and 10 % of bioaccessible polyphenols in the small intestine are bioavailable (Clifford, 2004). Therefore, in addition to polyphenols associated with the TIF, a major part of the polyphenols that are bioaccessible in the small intestine may also reach the colon because of their low bioavailability (Saura-Calixto et al. 2007). The major part of dietary polyphenols (non-extractable polyphenols) travel through the gastrointestinal tract as insoluble substrates. They reach the colon, where some of them may be released from the fiber matrix by the action of bacterial enzymes and become bioaccessible in the large intestine. The microbial catabolites are often better absorbed than the parent compounds because of the mechanism of absorption, the large absorptive area available in the colon and the high concentrations in the colonic lumen (Williamson & Clifford, 2010).

These could be responsible for a significant proportion of the biological activity derived from consumption of fruits, vegetables and other plant derived products such as fruit drinks, coffee, tea, and others (Williamson & Clifford, 2010).

Briefly then, polyphenols may be bioavailable in the human intestine, both in the small intestine (due to the action of digestive enzymes) and in the large intestine (due to the enzymatic activity of the human microbiota). Colonic fermentation of some polyphenols generates intermediate metabolites and fermentation end products that have local and/or systemic healthy effects on the host. The biological activity of these microbial catabolites would be in addition to the biological activity of any absorbed parent compounds and their mammalian metabolites (Williamson & Clifford, 2010).

Major parts of food polyphenols are associated with the food components not solubilized in the intestinal medium. These are non-extractable polyphenols, which paradoxically are usually ignored in studies on bioavailability and metabolism and in clinical and observational studies. However, they may be partially degraded by microbiota, and both metabolites and parent compounds may exhibit antioxidant activity. Non-extractable polyphenols or proanthocyanidins (condensed tannins) are oligomers and polymers of (+)-catechin and (-)-epicathechin and other related flavonoids, mainly associated by either B-type or A-type linkages. They are widely present in human diets and constitute a major part of dietary polyphenols. Their consumption has been found to be inversely related to a decreased risk of colorectal cancer (MacDonald & Wagner, 2012; Rosi et al. 2010; Theodoratou et al. 2007). Deprez et al (2000) reported that human microbiota degrade proanthocyanidins to low molecular weight phenolic compounds, suggesting that absorption of the parent compounds is unlikely. However, Ottaviani et al (2012) demonstrated that dietary procyanidins do not contribute to the systemic pool of flavonols in humans. Choy et al (2012) indicated that proanthocyanidins remained in the colon as the intact parent compounds, while Saura-Calixto et al (2010) showed the presence of proanthocyanidin metabolites from colonic fermentation in human plasma. Thus, the metabolism of oligomeric and polymeric proanthocyanidins in the colon is unclear.

Phenolic compounds with more than three subunits may be more resistant to degradation due to their chemical structure, and therefore higher levels may be observed in the colon. Conversely, other flavonoids, including anthocyanins, are rapidly metabolized in the gut to simple phenolic acids and related metabolites (Choy et al. 2012). Proanthocyanidins and their bioavailable metabolites exhibit significant biological activity associated with gastrointestinal health and potential systemic effects. The presence of larger proanthocyanidins in the colon would allow these compounds to exert local beneficial biological actions, particularly on the colon epithelial cells and on gut microbiota. In addition, the recovery of parent proanthocyanidins in faeces is partial, indicating that proanthocyanidins undergo extensive but incomplete biotransformations by the gut microbiota during transit through the intestinal tract. Thus, these important dietary polyphenols may directly contribute to the health status of the colon.

Dietary intake of fiber and polyphenols, taking into account their bioavailability in the human gut, is a key factor in assessing their significance for human health. However, there are few studies on intestinal bioaccessibility of dietary polyphenols in whole diets. The mean daily intake of polyphenols (including extractable and non-extractable polyphenols or highly polymerized polyphenols) in the Spanish whole diet was recently estimated at between 2590 and 3016 mg/day, using an *in vitro* system (Saura-Calixto et al. 2007) (Figure 2). Despite the limitations of an *in vitro* method, the results could be indicative of the situation *in vivo*. One interesting finding is that 48 % of dietary polyphenols were bioaccessible in the small intestine, while 42 % became bioaccessible in the large intestine. About 10 % of dietary polyphenols were inaccessible and remained in the food matrix after the complete digestion process. This is quite important because these data confirm that a large amount of indigestible polyphenols from diet remains unabsorbed in the intestinal ecosystem, in contact with microbiota and colonic epithelium cells.

It is clear that polyphenols may confer health benefits by interaction with gut microbiota and modulation of the latter. In this regard, polyphenols may exert a twofold healthy effect, on the host by enhancing antioxidant status at systemic and local level, and on the bacterial population by inhibiting pathogenic bacteria and stimulating beneficial bacteria.

Polyphenols Modulate the Population and the Enzymatic Activity of the Microbiota

The composition of the human colonic microbiota is usually considered to be fairly stable over the long term. However, it is possible to influence the growth of certain bacterial species by dietary manipulation.

Gut microbiota support a large variety of physiological functions and possess enzymatic and metabolic activities which impact on host nutrition and health. Gut microbiota are strongly influenced by both endogenous (intestinal mucines, enzymes, gut hormones, mucosa cells) and exogenous substrates. Certain non-digestible components such as recognized prebiotics may affect the growth and survival of beneficial bacteria by influencing their growth and metabolites. Consequently, the composition of the diet can influence the profile and metabolic activity of the gut microbial ecology.

Several fruit polyphenols have been shown to inhibit the growth and adhesion of Salmonella to a human gut cell line and to enhance the proliferation and adhesion of *lactobacillus rhamnosus* (Parker et al. 2008). In this connection, polyphenols extracted from grape pomace have been found to stimulate beneficial *Lactobacillus acidophilus* growth (Hervert-Hernández et al. 2009). Indeed, the prebiotic effect may be enhanced when a substantial amount of polyphenols is associated with DF (Pozuelo et al. 2012).

The effect of various phenolic compounds on modulation of growth of intestinal bacteria isolates has been studied. The action mechanisms of food phytochemicals and their metabolites are not well known, but there are a number of results that demonstrate their role as antiadhesion agents, that is to say, they have an inhibitory effect on pathogenic bacteria (Selma et al. 2009).

The gut microbial ecology is composed of a broad spectrum of highly metabolically active species. Bacterial cells are predominantly located in the large intestine. *Bifidobacterium, Eubacterium, Clostridium, Peptococcus, Peptostreptococcus* and *Ruminococcus* are the predominant species of colonic microbiota, while the subdominant group is composed of *Escherichia, Enterobacter, Enterococcus, Klebsiella, Lactobacillus,* and *Proteus*. The composition of this bacterial ecosystem is dynamic and susceptible to changes driven by dietary factors and diverse disease conditions (Laparra & Sanz, 2009).

Dietary polyphenols and their metabolites contribute to the maintenance of gastrointestinal health, to a large extent by modulation of gut microbial balance with simultaneous inhibition of pathogens and stimulation of beneficial bacteria. In the past, the concept of prebiotics was limited to non-digestible carbohydrates, but the latest evidence strongly suggests that polyphenols have the ability to exert prebiotic action. Indeed, the prebiotic effect could be enhanced when a substantial amount of polyphenols is associated with DF (Pozuelo et al. 2012; Herver-Hernández et al. 2009).

Non-digestible components of the diet modify the number and type of bacteria and enzymatic activity developed by the microflora. The growth of beneficial bacteria such as *Lactobacillus* spp., and inhibition of pathogenic bacteria (Staphylococcus aureus, *Eschrichoa coli, Candida albicans*) by the action of dietary polyphenols and their metabolites, have been reported in this connection (Herver-Hernández et al. 2009; Herver-Hernández & Goñi, 2011).

Therefore, the regular consumption of a diet rich in plant foods with high polyphenol contents may beneficially balance the gut microbial ecology, helping to prevent gastrointestinal disorders and thus enhancing the health of the host.

Dietary Fiber, Carrier of Bioactive Compounds

DF does not constitute a defined chemical group but a combination of chemically heterogeneous substances, as explained below. The physiological and physicochemical effects of dietary fibers are determined by the relative amount of individual non-digestible components, and the combination of these with one other and with the food matrix.

DF transports phytochemicals linked to the fiber matrix through the human gut (Goñi et al. 2006; Saura-Calixto et al. 2007; Goñi & Harvert-Hernández, 2011). Therefore, the presence of phytochemicals associated with DF may significantly affect the physiological properties and healthy effects attributed to DF compounds.

Phytochemicals or phytonutrients are bioactive substances that can be found in foods derived from plants and are not essential for life, at least for now. The human body cannot produce them. Bioactive compounds are not considered as nutrients, but much of the disease prevention potential of fruits and vegetables in human health is thought to be provided by these compounds (Palafox-Carlos et al. 2011). The main dietary phytochemicals are polyphenols, carotenoids and phytosterols. Of these, polyphenols are the largest group. Carotenoids and polyphenols are powerful antioxidants and polyphenols are most abundant in quantitative terms.

Vitamins (A, C, and E), phenolic compounds (flavonoids, phenolic acids, stilbenes and tannins) and carotenoids (carotenes and xanthophylls) are recognized as the main groups of antioxidants present in beverages and plant foods. Vitamins are single molecules, and their metabolism and allowances are well-known, but polyphenols and carotenoids are made up of hundreds of compounds with a wide range of structures and molecular masses, and the knowledge of their intakes, metabolism, and bioavailability is currently partial and incomplete.

Dietary polyphenols are found in plant foods, and fruits and vegetables are the most important sources of polyphenols in Western diets (Saura-Calixto, 2007). They are chemically and biologically active plant secondary metabolites. In addition to their diversity, polyphenols may be associated with various carbohydrates and organic acids as well as with one another (Manach et al. 2004; Tapiero et al. 2004).

DF and antioxidants are healthy food constituents and functional ingredients that are generally addressed separately in both chemical and nutritional studies. However, it has been proven that a substantial proportion of the antioxidant polyphenols (Saura-Calixto et al., 2007) and carotenoids (Goñi et al. 2006; Serrano et al. 2005) contained in plant foods are linked to DF, and that they are a substantial part of the total antioxidants in the diet. It therefore seems logical to suppose that the association between antioxidants and DF compounds may contribute significantly to the health effects, and that some of the postulated benefits of the fiber intake can be attributed to the DF-antioxidants complex.

This capacity of the fiber matrix to act as a carrier of antioxidant compounds is an essential physiological function of DF. The release of some antioxidant compounds in the colon improves antioxidant status (Goñi & Serrano, 2005) and yields different metabolites with potential systemic effects (Williamson & Clifford, 2010; Selma et al. 2009). Therefore, DF and antioxidants could be approached jointly in nutrition and health studies, combining the properties of both DF and antioxidants in a single material. In this approach, the concept of antioxidant dietary fiber has been defined as a product containing significant amounts of natural antioxidants associated with the fiber matrix. As such it complies with requirements relating to the content of DF and quantification of intrinsic antioxidant activity derived from the natural constituents of the material, and not from added antioxidants or from constituents released by previous chemical or enzymatic treatments (Saura-Calixto, 1998).

In this regard, DF with exceptional antioxidant capacity, defined as antioxidant dietary fiber, has been found in mango peel (Larrauri et al. 1996), pineapple shell (Larrauri et al. 1997), grape pomace (Pérez-Jimenez et al. 2008), cabbage outer leaves (Nilnakara et al. 2009), asparagus by-products (Fuentes-Alventosa et al. 2009) and others (Table 5).

The concept of antioxidant dietary fiber may be useful to differentiate DF-rich materials with significant antioxidant capacity from those with negligible activity. Furthermore, the antioxidant capacity measured in the whole material is derived from the cumulative synergistic antioxidant activity of polyphenols and other constituents. This parameter provides an integrated measurement that may represent the amount of antioxidant units carried by DF in the human gut.

A Healthy Dietary Pattern Based on Plant Foods

UNESCO has included the Mediterranean Diet in the Intangible Cultural Heritage, as offering important benefits for the health, quality of life and well-being of communities. The Mediterranean dietary pattern offers a nutritional model enriched by diverse cultures which over centuries has essentially maintained the same food structure and the same proportions: olive oil, fresh fruits and vegetables, grains and derivatives, fish, and to a lesser extent nuts, dairy products and meat. There is also moderate consumption of wine, coffee and tea during meals while respecting religious rules and beliefs. The Mediterranean Diet is not just a diet (mixture of food), it means a lifestyle (UNESCO, 2010).

The traditional definition of the Mediterranean Diet is based mainly on consumption of foods. An inverse association between low mortality and high intakes of food groups rich in bioactive compounds such as fruits and vegetables or fruits and nuts has been described (Trichopoulou, 2003). However, despite this robust inverse association, it is not clear which food constituents of this dietary pattern contribute most to its health effects.

The intake of DF is similar in Mediterranean and non-Mediterranean countries, around 20 g/person/day (Elmadfa, 2009). However a high proportion of DF in Mediterranean countries comes from fresh fruits and vegetables, while in non-Mediterranean regions DF comes more from cereals. This qualitative difference could have a direct bearing on the low mortality from cardiovascular diseases and cancer associated with the Mediterranean dietary pattern and is probably related to the presence of a significant amount and variety of antioxidants in plant foods that are characteristic of this healthy dietary pattern.

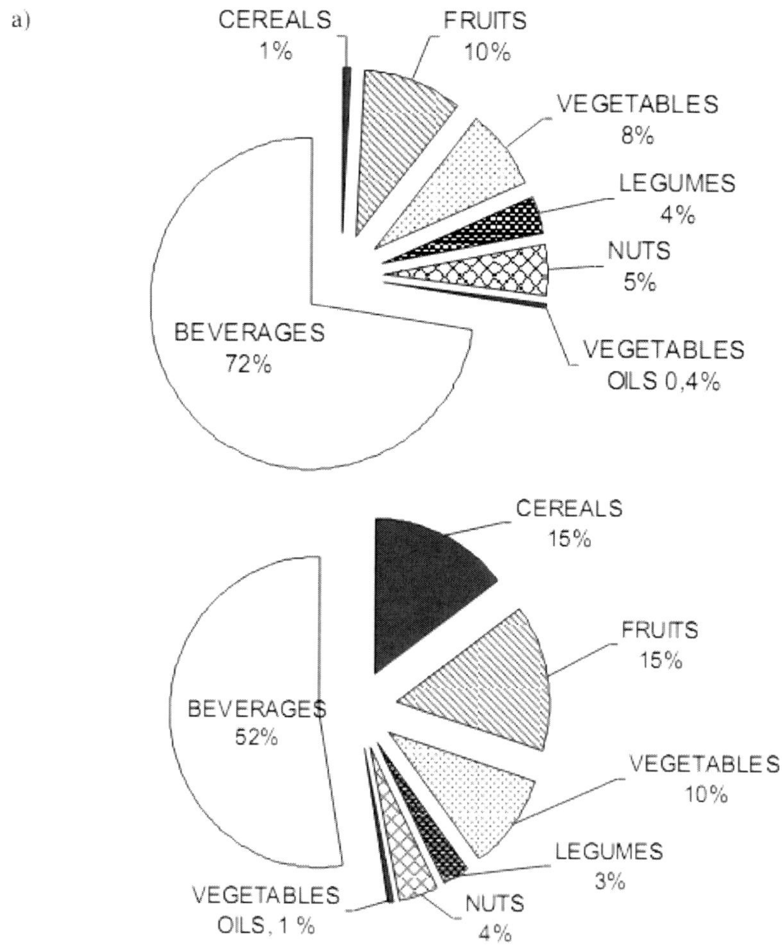

Figure 4. Total antioxidant capacity (a) and polyphenol intake (b) per capita daily in the Spanish diet. Total antioxidant capacity: 3549 μmol trolox equivalent, by ABTS method; Total polyphenols: 1172 mg, non-extractable polyphenols not included. (adapted from Saura-Calixto & Goñi, 2006).

The total dietary antioxidant capacity (TDAC) of the Mediterranean Diet is probably higher than in other countries that present a higher incidence of chronic diseases. Dietary antioxidants may be critical mediators of the beneficial effects of the Mediterranean Diet. This is why TDAC has recently been proposed as an essential indicator to define the Mediterranean dietary pattern (Saura-Calixto & Goñi, 2009). It has been defined as the antioxidant capacity of all plant foods and beverages consumed daily in a diet. TDAC represents the amount of antioxidant units present daily in the human gut. Figure 4a shows the contribution of each food group to the TDAC in the Spanish diet. The largest contributors to TDAC were beverages (about 72 %) and fruits and vegetables (about 18 %), while the contribution of cereals (about 1 %) and vegetable oils (0.4 %) was very low. Nuts and legumes accounted for nearly 8 % of TDAC despite low consumption, because this food group contains a high percentage of compounds with antioxidant activity. Obviously, the contribution of each specific food to the TDAC was dependent on both food intake and food antioxidant capacity. Studies on individual foods may overestimate their potential effects within a whole diet. Individual foods that present high antioxidant capacity may contribute very little to the TDAC of the whole diet, as is the case of olive oil in the Spanish diet.

It would be very hard for a single food or for a mixture of a small number of foods to supply theDF, antioxidant or otherwise, necessary for health, because it is known that a healthy diet has to have a wide variety of foods and the sum of the antioxidant capacity of each food in the diet would probably not equal the TDAC. Therefore, the estimation of TDAC intake seems to be a good indicator of dietary quality.

Plant foods, and in particular fruits and vegetables, have been recognized as important sources for a wide array of non-digestible components and phytochemicals that may contribute synergistically, individually or in combination, to the nutritional and health benefits of these food commodities.

Studies addressing total polyphenols in a whole diet are scarce, but it is known that polyphenols are quantitatively the main dietary antioxidants and even possess higher in *vitro* antioxidant capacity than vitamins and carotenoids. The recommended daily intake of vitamin C (60 mg) plus vitamin E (12 mg) represents only about 10 % of the TDAC in the Spanish diet, and the contribution of carotenoids is negligible. TDAC correlates closely with polyphenol content (Saura-Calixto & Goñi, 2006).

Most literature data on food polyphenols concern only compounds dissolved in aqueous organic extracts (extractable polyphenols), but this approach may be limited by the extraction techniques, since some polyphenols (non-extractable polyphenols) may escape the standard extraction methods. It is important not to ignore this fact because there are much more non-extractable than extractable polyphenols in all food groups (Figure 5).

The mean total intake of polyphenols (extractable plus non-extractable) in the Spanish diet ranges from 2590 to 3016 mg/person/day. Even though the estimated non-extractable polyphenol content of the diet is almost double that of extractable polyphenols, their physiological effects are closely associated with their degree of bioavailability, and they must be released from the food matrix by digestive enzymes or by bacterial enzymatic activities to be susceptible of absorption through the gut barrier. Polyphenols bound to the DF matrix account for a substantial part of total polyphenols in foods (Figure 6) For instance, fruits and vegetables provide a daily intake of 700 – 1000 mg of polyphenols/person/day in the Spanish diet, and a major fraction (600 mg/person/day) is associated with DF (Saura-Calixto et al. 2007).

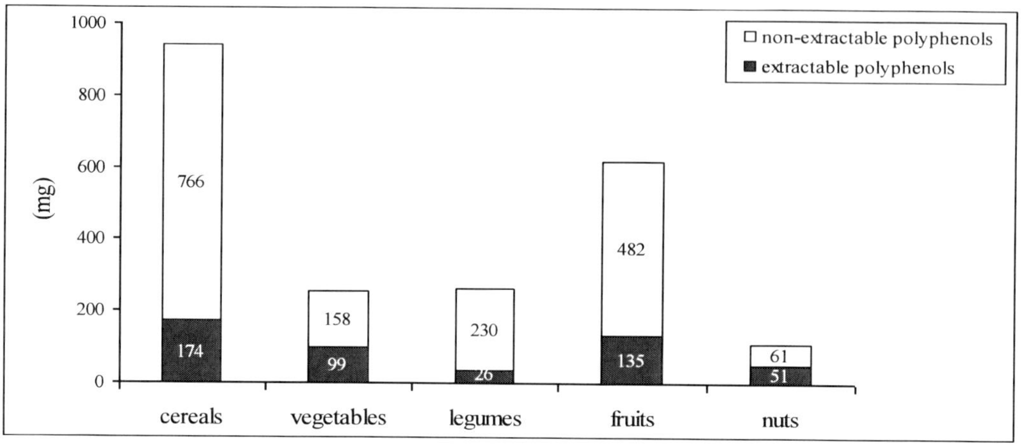

Figure 5. Total polyphenol intake from plant foods in the Spanish diet (adapted from Saura-Calixto et al. 2007).

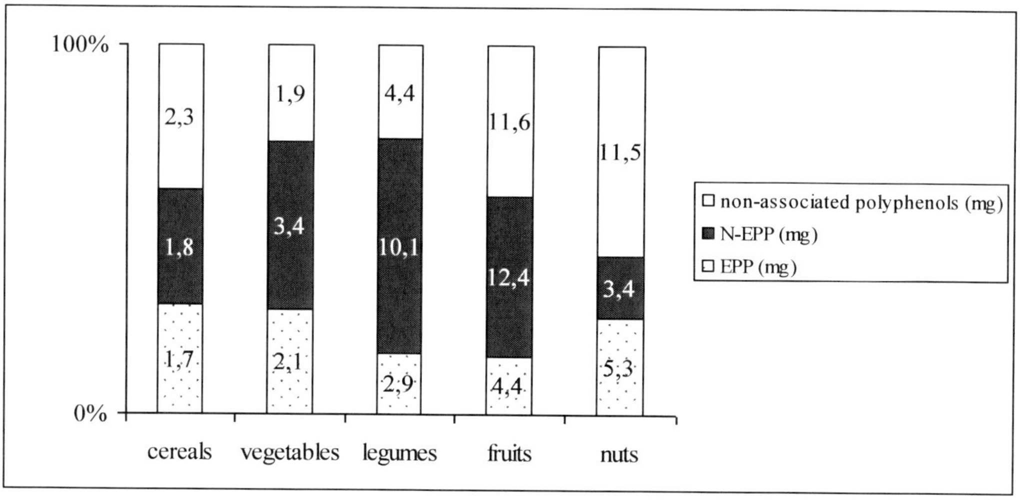

Figure 6. Polyphenols associated and not associated with the fiber matrix of foods; N-EPP, non-extractable polyphenols; EPP, extractable polyphenols.

Although cereals present the lowest polyphenol content (mg/g of original sample), because of the proportion of cereals in the Spanish diet, they are the principal food source of polyphenols in the diet, followed by fruits and vegetables (Figure 5). However, as shown in Figure 3, the percentage of polyphenols that are bioaccessible in the small and large intestine depends on the food group.

Dietary Fiber, Polyphenols and Antioxidant Activity in Agri-Food by-Products

There is abundant scientific evidence for the health benefits of DF and antioxidants. In addition, there are national and international campaigns to promote high consumption of varied plant foods, specifically fruits and vegetables. However, plant food consumption is low and consequently the intake of fiber and antioxidants is usually deficient in most diets worldwide. Nowadays DF and antioxidant bioactive compounds are widely used as functional ingredients in processed foods. The market in this field is competitive and the development of new types of fibers is a challenge for the food industry. There is a trend towards a search for new sources of functional ingredients, such as plant food by-products that have traditionally been undervalued.

The plant food processing industry produces large volumes of waste, both solid and liquid, resulting from the production, preparation, and consumption of food. These waste products pose potentially severe pollution problems and represent a loss of valuable biomass and nutrients. In this regard, it is interesting to consider not only the potential nutritional quality of the by-product, but also its distribution, cost and other additional benefits. One useful approach to adding value to by-products is to use them as sources of DF, and also as natural antioxidant compounds.

There is estimated to be around 800 000 tons per year of fresh fruit and vegetable matter globally, not counting wastage during processing (Ayala-Zavala et al. 2010). These by-products could account for as much as 60 % of harvested plants. They represent more than 40 % of total plant food in cases such as artichoke, asparagus, cactus pear fruit, tiger nuts, orange, and others.

Many agri-food by-products are good sources of DF and bioactive compounds, and they may even contain more than the edible portion of the food. Table 1 shows the total DF content of some by-products from widely-consumed plant foods. Note the large fiber fraction present in by-products, ranging from 38 up to >80 % and comprising both soluble and insoluble fiber compounds.

Table 1. Total dietary fiber (TDF) content in processing by-products of fruits and vegetables

	TDF (%dm)	Reference
Pea hulls	82.30	Verma et al. 2011
Asparagus	62-77	Fuentes-Alventosa et al. 2009
Grape pomace	64.6	Saura-Calixto, 1998
Artichoke	58.8	Grigelmo-Miguel & Martín-Belloso, 1999
Orange peel	37.8	Grigelmo-Miguel & Martín-Belloso, 1999
Pineapple shell	70.6	Larrauri et al. 1997
Apple pomace	63.3	Goñi et al. 1989
Cladodes (Opuntia ficus-indica)	63.0	Bensadón et al. 2010
Tuna green peel (Opuntia ficus-indica)	42.8	Bensadón et al. 2010

Table 2 shows polyphenol contents of some by-products generated by industrial plant food processers.

As noted above, DF in plant foods transports a significant amount of polyphenols and carotenoids linked to the fiber matrix. Likewise, waste products derived from them are also sources of phytochemicals associated with the fiber matrix; and for the same reason a significant proportion of the antioxidant capacity in plant foods is also associated with DF and may contribute to a healthy antioxidant environment and help counteract the effects of dietary pro-oxidants.

Table 2. Polyphenol content in processing by-products of fruits and vegetables

	Polyphenol content[1] (mg/g dry matter)	Reference
Blanched artichoke	3.6 - 4.4[2]	Llorach et al. 2002
Cauliflower	1.1 - 1.8[2]	Llorach et al. 2002
Cladodes (Opuntia ficus-indica)	3.2	Bensadón et al. 2010
Tuna green peel (Opuntia ficus-indica)	2.7	Bensadón et al. 2010
Orange peel	1.6	Larrauri et al. 1996
Grape pomace	2.0	Saura-Calixto, 1998
Pineapple shell	2.7	Larrauri et al. 1997

[1] extractable polyphenols; [2] fresh weight.

Use of Antioxidant Dietary Fibers As Functional Ingredients

DF and natural antioxidants possess the requisite characteristics for consideration as important ingredients in the formulation of functional foods, owing to their proven beneficial effects. Natural antioxidants have the capacity to act as powerful antioxidants by scavenging free radicals and terminating oxidative reactions. These properties have prompted proposals for their use as natural food preservatives. Then again, the inclusion of DF in food products improves physicochemical and sensory properties in processed foods. Both DF and antioxidants are used as food additives and as health-promoting agents.

Antioxidant additives are used in processed meats to prevent oxidative damage and to prolong the shelf life of meat products. Synthetic antioxidants have been used to control lipid oxidation in meat. However, the use of synthetic antioxidants is restricted because of their toxic and carcinogenic effects. The use of natural preservatives to prolong the shelf life of meat products is a promising technology since many vegetable substances have antioxidant and antimicrobial properties.

One example of this type of material is grape antioxidant dietary fiber (GADF). GADF is a concentrate rich in phenolic compounds, which has been developed at our laboratory from wine by-products.

GADF is a natural product that combines large amounts of DF and phenolic antioxidants obtained from grape pomace. GADF contains around 78 % of DF, 5 % of extractable polyphenols and 18 % of non-extractable polyphenols on a dry matter basis. It presents a high level of antioxidant activity (124 μmol trolox equivalent/g dm, ABTS method; 214 μmol trolox equivalent/g dm, ORAC method). GADF meets the definition of antioxidant dietary fiber since it combines the properties of both DF and antioxidants in a single material.

GADF has been used successfully as a food ingredient in meat products (Sáyago-Ayerdi, 2009) and restructured fish products (Sánchez-Alonso, 2007) with maintenance of nutritional quality and prolongation of shelf life.

In recent years DF has been commonly added to several foodstuffs as a functional ingredient and has also been included in several dietary supplements. Similarly, dietary antioxidants may be critical mediators in the lower mortality associated with healthy diets such as the Mediterranean dietary pattern, and this has prompted more research into natural antioxidants with possible health effects.

GADF has been tested as a possible dietary supplement in studies in both animals and humans. Studies in rats have found a significant reduction in total cholesterol, antiproliferative capacity in their colonic epithelium through a decrease in the total number of crypts, higher caecal antioxidant capacity and a more antioxidant status in the colon (López-Oliva et al. 2012). In addition, a prebiotic effect stimulating the growth of *Lactobacillus* and *Bifidobacterium* has been demonstrated when GADF is added to the rat diet as a source of DF (Pozuelo et al. 2012). Numerous beneficial effects have been demonstrated experimentally when GADF is used as a supplement in humans (Pérez-Jimenez et al. 2008). In short, GADF as a functional ingredient may prevent lipid oxidation in food products, and as a dietary supplement is a health-promoting agent.

Experience in the development of GADF may serve as a basis for development of other materials that meet the definition of antioxidant dietary fiber. Several plant products, especially Mediterranean and tropical fruits and seaweeds, appear to be suitable materials for antioxidant dietary fiber.

Conclusion

Most of the phenolic antioxidants in the diet are carried through the gastrointestinal tract by other non-digestible compounds (DF). A substantial proportion of dietary polyphenols are polymeric or polyphenols trapped in cores of the fiber matrix, which can become fermentable substrates for the microbiota. Therefore, dietary polyphenols may be bioavailable in the small intestine (a small proportion due to the action of digestive enzymes) and in the large intestine (due to the enzymatic activity of the human microbiota), where they may exert a twofold healthy effect: on the host by enhancing the antioxidant status at a systemic and a local level, and on the microbiota by inhibiting pathogenic bacteria and stimulating beneficial bacteria.

Materials rich in DF and antioxidants (antioxidant dietary fiber) may be obtained from agri-food by-products for use as functional ingredients to prevent dietary lipid oxidation, and as dietary supplements to promote health.

References

Bäckhed, F; Ley, RE; Sonnenburg, JL; Peterson, DA; Gordon, JI. Host-bacterial mutualism in the human intestine. *Science*. 2005 307, 1915-1920.

Bauer, E; Williams, BA; Smidt, H; Mosenthin, R; Verstegen, MW. Influence of Dietary Components on Development of the Microbiota in Single-Stomached Species. *Nutr. Res. Rev*. 2006, *19*, 1, 63-78.

Bensadón, S; Hervert-Hernández, D; Sáyago-Ayerdi, S; Goñi, I. By-products of opuntia ficus-indica as a source of antioxidant dietary fiber. *Plant Food Hum. Nutr.*, 2010 65, 210-216.

Buttriss, JL; Stokes, CS. Dietary fiber and health: an overview. *Nutrition Bulletin*, 2008 33, 3, 186-200.

Chong, MF-F; Macdonald, R; Lovegrove, JA. Fruit polyphenols and CVD risk: a review of human intervention studies. *Br. J. Nutr.*, 2010 104, S28-S39.

Choy, YY; Jaggers, GK; Oteiza, PI; Waterhouse, AL. Bioavailability of intact proanthocyanidins in the rat colon after ingestion of grape seed extract. *J. Agric. Food Chem.*, 2012 61, 121-127.

Chuang, SC; Norat, T; Murphy, N; Olsen, A; Tjønneland, A; et al. Fiber intake and total and cause-specific mortality in the European Prospective Investigation into Cancer and Nutrition Cohort. *Am. J. Clin. Nutr.*. 2012 96, 1, 164-174.

Clifford, MN. Diet-derived phenols in plasma and tissues and their implications for helath. *Planta Medica*, 2004 70, 1103-1114.

Cummings, JH; Macfarlane, GT. The control and consequences of bacterial fermentation in the human colon. *J. Appl. Bacteriol.* 1991 70, 443-459.

Del Rio, D; Borges, G; Croizer, A. Berry flavonoids and phenolics: bioavailability and evidence of protective effects. *Br. J. Nutr*, 2010 104, S67-S90.

Del Rio, D; Costa, LG; Lean, MEJ; Crozier, A. Polyphenols and health: what compounds are envolved?. *Nutr. Metab. Cardiovasc. Dis.* 2009 20, 1, 1-6.

Deprez, S; Brezillon, C; Rabot, S; Philippe, C; Mila, I; Lapierre, C; Scalbert, A. Polymeric proanthocyanidins are catabolized by human colonic microflora into low-molecular-weight phenolic acids. *J. Nutr.* 2000, 130, 2733-2738.

EFSA, European Food Safety Authority, 2007. Statement of the Scientific Panel on Dietetic products, Nutrition and allergies on a request from the Commission related to dietary fiber, Nº EFSA-Q-2007-121.

Elmadfa, I editor. European nutrition and health report 2009. Forum Nutrition. Basel, Karger, 2009 62, 43-59.

FAO/WHO. Carbohydrates in human nutrition. FAO Food and Nutrition paper-66. Report of a joint FAO/WHO Expert Consultation. Rome. 1998.

Fuentes-Alventosa, JM; Jaramillo-Carmona, S; Rodriguez-Gutierrez, G; Rodriguez-Arcos, R; Fernández-Bolaños, J; Guillén-Bejarano, R; Espejo-Calvo, JÁ; Jimenez-Araujo, A. Effect of the extraction method on phytochemical composition and antioxidant acrivity of high dietary fiber powders obtained from asparagus by-products. *Food Chem.*, 2009 116, 484-490.

Goñi, I; Brenes, A, Centeno, C; Viveros, A; Saura-Calixto, F; Rebolé, A; Arija, I; Esteve, R. Effect of dietary grape pomace and vitamin e on growth performance, nutrient digestibility and susceptibility to meat lipid oxidation in chickens. *Poultry Science*, 2007 86, 508-516.

Goñi, I; Hervert-Hernández, D. By-products from plant foods are sources of dietary fiber and antioxidants. In: Rasooli I, editor. Phytochemicals – Bioactivities and impact on health. Rijeta, Croatia: INTECH Publisher, 2011; 95-116.

Goñi, I; Serrano, J. The intake of dietary fiber from grape seeds modifies the antioxidant status in rat. *J. Sci. Food Agric.*, 2005 85, 1877-1881.

Goñi, I; Serrano, J; Saura-Calixto, F. Bioaccessibility of beta-carotene, lutein, and lycopene from fruits and vegetables. *J. Agric. Food Chem.*. 2006 54, 15, 5382-5387.

Goñi, I; Torre, M; Saura-Calixto, F. Determination of dietary fiber in cider wastes. Comparison of methods. Food Chem, 1989 3, 2, 151-159.

Hervert-Hernández, D: Pintado, C; Rotger, R; Goñi, I. Stimulatory role of grape pomace polyphenols on Lactobacillus acidophilus growth. *Int. J. Food Microbiol.* 2009 136, 119-122.

Hervert-Hernández, D; Goñi, I. Dietary poluphenols and human gut microbiota: a review. *Food Rev. Int.*, 2011, 27, 154-169.

Laparra, JM; Sanz, Y. Interactions of gut microbiota with functional food components and nutraceuticals. *Pharm Res.*, 2010 61, 3, 219-225.

Larrauri, JA; Ruperez, P; Borroto, B; Saura-Calixto, S. Mango peels as a new tropical fiber: Preparation and characterization. *Lebensm Wiss Technol.*, 1996 29, 729-733.

Larrauri, JA; Ruperez, P; Bravo, L; Saura-Calixto, F. High dietary fiber powders from orange and lime peels: associated polyphenols and antioxidant capacity. *Food Res. Int.*, 1996 29, 8, 757-762.

Larrauri, JA; Ruperez, P; Saura-Calixto, F. Pineapple shell as a source of dietary fiber with associated polyphenols. *J. Agric. Food Chem.*, 1997 45, 4028-4031.

Larrauri, JA; Ruperez, P; Saura-Calixto, F. Pineapple shell as a source of dietary fiber with associated polyphenols. *J. Agric. Food Chem.*, 1997 45, 4028-4031.

Lee, HC; Jenner, AM; Lowa, CS; Lee, YK. Effect of tea phenolics and their aromatic fecal bacterial metabolites on intestinal microbiota. *Res. Microbiol.*, 2006 157, 876-884.

Llorach, R; Espín, JC; Tomás-Barberán, FA; Ferreres, F. Artichoke (Cynara scolymus L) byproducts as a potencial source of Elath-promoting antioxidante phenolics. *J. Agric. Food Chem.*, 2002 50, 3458-3464.

López-Oliva, ME; Pozuelo, MJ; Rotger, R; Muñoz-Martinez, E; Goñi, I. Grape antioxidant dietary fiber prevents mitochondrial apoptotic pathways by enhancing Bcl-2 and Bcl-x_L expression and minimizing oxidative stress in rat distal colonic mucosa. *Br. J. Nutr.*, 2012 19, 1-13.

MacDonald, RS; Wagner, K. Influence of dietary phytochemicals and microbiota on colon cancer risk. *J. Agric. Food Chem.*, 2012 60, 6728-6735.

Manach, C; Scalbert, A; Morand, C; Remesy, C; Jimenez, L. Polyphenols: food sources and bioavailability. *Am. J. Clin. Nutr.*, 2004 79, 5, 727-747.

Manach, C; Williamson, G; Morand, C; Scalbert, A; Remesy, C. Bioavailability and bioefficiency of polyphenols in humans. I. Review of 97 bioavailability studies. *Am. J. Clin. Nutr.*, 2005 81, 1, 230S-242S.

Mañas, E; Saura-Calixto, F. dietary fiber análisis: methodological errors sources. *Eur J Clin Nutr*, 1995 49 S3, S158-S162.

Murphy, N; Norat, T; Ferrari, P; Jenab, M; Bueno-de-Mesquita, B. et al. Dietary Fiber Intake and Risks of Cancers of the Colon and Rectum in the European Prospective Investigation into Cancer and Nutrition (EPIC). *PLoS ONE* 2012 7(6): e39361. doi:10.1371/journal.pone.0039361.

Nilnakara, S, Chiewchan, N; Devahastin, S. Production of antioxidant dietary fiber powder from cabbage outer leaves. *Food Bioproducts Processing*, 2009 87, 4, 301-307.

Ottaviani, JI; Kwik-Uribe, C; Keen, CL; Schroeter, H. Intake of dietary procyanidins does not controbute to the pool of circulating flavanols in humans. *Am. J. Clin. Nutr.*, 2012 95, 4, 851-858.

Palafox-Carlos, H; Ayala-Zabala, JF; González-Aguilar, GA. The role of dietary fiber in the bioaccessibility and bioavailability of fruit and vegetable antioxidants. *J. Food Sci.*, 2011 76, 1, R6-R15.

Parkar, SG; Stevenson, DE; Skinner, MA. The potential influence of fruit polyphenols on colonic microflora and human gut health. *Int. J. Food Microbiol.*, 2008 124, 295-298.

Pérez-Jimenez, J; Serrano, J; Tabernero, M; Diaz Rubio, E; Arranz, S; García-Diz, L; Goñi, I; Saura-Calixto, F. Effect of grape Antioxidant Dietary Fiber in Cardiovascular Disease Risk Factors. *Nutrition,* 2008 24, 646-653.

Pozuelo, MJ; Agis-Torres, A; Hervert-Hernández, D; López-Oliva, ME; Muñoz-Martínez, E; Rotger, R; Goñi, I. Grape antioxidant dietary fiber stimulates *Lactobacillus* growth in rat cecum. *J. Food Sci.*, 2012 77, 2, H59-H62.

Rossi, M; Negri, E; Parpinel, M; Lagiou, P; Bosetti, C; et al. Proanthocyanidins and the risk of colorectal cancer in Italy. *Cancer Causes Control*, 2010 21, 243-250.

Salminen, S; Isolauri, E; Salminen, E. Clinical uses of probiotics for stabilizing the gut mucosal barrier: successful strains and future challenges. *Antonie Van Leeuwnhoek.* 1996, 70, 347-358.

Sánchez-Alonso, I; Jiménez-Escrig, A; Saura-Calixto, F; Borderías, AJ. Effect of grape antioxidant dietary fiber on the prevention of lipid oxidation in minced fish: evaluation by different methodologies. *Food Chem.*, 2007 101, 372-378.

Saura–Calixto, F; Goñi, I. The intake of dietary indigestible fraction in the Spanish diet shows the limitations of dietary fiber data for nutritional studies *Eur. J. Clin. Nutr.*, 2004 58, 1078-1082.

Saura-Calixto, F. Antioxidant dietary fiber product: A new concept and a potencial food ingrediente. *J. Agric. Food Chem.*, 1998 46, 4303-4306.

Saura-Calixto, F; García-Alonso, A; Goñi, I; Bravo, L. In vitro determination of the indigestible fraction in foods: an alternative to dietary fiber analysis. *J. Agric. Food Chem.* , 2000 48, 3342-3347.

Saura-Calixto, F; Goñi, I. Definition of the Mediterranean diet based on bioactive compounds. *Crit. Rev. Food Sci. Nutr., 20*09 49, 145-152.

Saura-Calixto, F; Pérez-Jiménez, J; Goñi, I. Dietary fiber and associated antioxidants in fruit and vegetables. In: de la Rosa LA; Álvarez-Parilla, E; González-Aguilar, GA, editors. *Fruit and vegetable phytochemical*s, Iowa: Wiley-Blackwell; 2010 a; 223-234.

Saura-Calixto, F; Pérez-Jiménez, J; Touriño,S; Serrano, J; Fuguet, E; Torres, JL;Goñi, I. Proanthocyanidin metabolites associated with dietary fiber from in vitro colonic fermentation and proanthocyanidin metabolites in human plasma. *Mol. Nutr. Food Res.,* 2010 b 54, 7, 939-946.

Saura-Calixto, F; Serrano, J; Goñi, I.Intake and bioaccessibility of total polyphenols in a whole diet. *Food Chem.,* 2007 101, 492-501.

Savage, DC. Microbial ecology of the gastrointestinal tract. Ann Rev Microbiol. 1977 31, 107-133.

Sáyago-Ayerdi, SG; Brenes, A; Goñi, I. Effect of grape antioxidant dietary fiber on the lipid oxidation of raw and cooked chicken hamburgers. *LWT-Food Sci. Technol.*, 2009 42, 971-976.

Selma, MV; Espín, JC; Tomás-Barberán, FA. Interaction between phenolics and gut microbiota: role in human health. *J. Agric. Food Chem.*. 2009 57, 6485-6501.

Serrano, J; Goñi, I; Saura-Calixto, F. Determination of β-carotene and lutein available from green leafy vegetables by an in vitro digestion and colonic fermentation method. *J. Agric. Food Chem.*, 2005 53, 8, 2936-2940.

Tapiero, H; Townsend, DM; Tew, KD. The role of carotenoids in the prevention of human pathologies. *Biomed. Pharmacother*, 2004 58, 2, 100-110.

Theodoratou, E; Kyle, J; Cetnarskyi, R; Farrington, SM; Tenesa, A; et al. Dietary flavonoids and the risk of colorectal cancer. *Cancer Epidemiol. Biomarkers Prevention*, 2007 16, 684-693.

Trichopoulou, A; Costacou, T; Bamia, Ch; Trichopoulou, D. Adherence to a Mediterranean diet and survival in a Greek population. *N. Engl. J. Med.*, 2003 348, 26, 2599-2608.

Tulipani, S; Urpi-Sarda, M; García-Villalba, R; Rabassa, M; López-Uriarte, P; et al. Urolithins are the main urinary microbial-derived phenolic metabolites discriminating a moderate consumption of nuts in free-living subjects with diagnosed metabolic syndrome. *J. Agric. Food Chem.*, 2012 60, 8930-8940.

Tuohy, KM; Conterno, L; Gasperotti, M; Viola, R. Up-regulating the human intestinal microbiome using whole plant foods, polyphenols, and/or fiber. *J. Agric. Food Chem.*, 2012 60, 8776-8782.

USDA. Department of Agriculture, Agricultural Research Service, 2010. Nutrient intakes from food: mean amounts consumed per indiv idual, by gender and age. What we eat in America?. NHANES 2007-2008. wwww.ars.usda.gov/ba/bhnrc/fsrg.

Verma, N; Mukesh, C; Vivek, K. Pea Peel waste: a lignocellulosic waste and its utility in cellulase production by *Trichoderma reesei* under solid state cultivation. *BioResources*, 2011 6, 2, 1505-1519.

Williamson, G; Clifford, MN. Colonic metabolites of berry polyphenols: the missing link to biological activity?. *Br. J. Nutr.*, 2010 104, S48-S66.

Williamson, G; Manach, C. Bioavailability and Bioefficacy of Polyphenols in Humans. II. Review of 93 Intervention Studies. *Am. J. Clin. Nutr* 2005 81, 243S-55S.

In: Dietary Fiber
Editors: D. Betancur-Ancona, L. Chel-Guerrero et al.
ISBN: 978-1-62808-931-8

Chapter 6

Antioxidant Dietary Fiber from Tropical Fruits

Manuel Viuda-Martos, Juana Fernández-López and José A. Pérez-Alvarez*
IPOA Research Group (UMH-1 and REVIV-Generalitat Valenciana),
AgroFood Technology Department. Escuela Politécnica Superior de Orihuela,
Universidad Miguel Hernández, Orihuela Alicante (Spain)

Abstract

It is widely accepted that a plant-based diet with a high intake of fruits, vegetables, and other nutrient-rich plant foods may reduce the risk of oxidative stress-related diseases. Epidemiologic data have shown that persons with a high consumption of fruit and vegetables are at a lower risk of several types of cancer, cardiovascular disease and stroke than are persons with a low consumption.

Tropical fruit production, trade and consumption have increased significantly on the domestic and international markets due to their attractive sensory properties and a growing recognition of its nutritional and therapeutic value. In addition, there has been increase in the availability of tropical fruit drinks. Nutrient-rich beverages are gaining popularity due to the desire of consumers for healthy eating and drinking while experiencing new and exotic flavors, and the same time, due to the focus of industries to produce beverages with health claim as a parameter of differentiation.

It has been demonstrated that both seeds and pericarp of tropical fruits are rich in bioactive compounds, especially phenolic constituents, flavonoids, anthocyanidins, vitamin C and carotenoids that positively influence human health due to their high antioxidant activity. In addition, tropical fruits are rich in dietary fibre. Dietary fibers obtained from fruits and vegetables, in general, and from tropical fruits in particular, contained attached appreciable amount of colorants, antioxidants compounds or other substances with positive health effects, such as protecting against cardiovascular disease, improvements in gastrointestinal health, glucose tolerance and the insulin response; reduction in the risk of developing some cancers; and hence some degree of weight

* Phone: +34 966749739; e-mail address: ja.perez@umh.es.

management. There are two fundamental sources of fiber from tropical fruits. (i) the fiber obtained from the fruit fresh consumption and (ii) the fiber present in the co-products generated by the industrialization of fruit to obtained juice.

Introduction

Dietary fiber as a class of compounds includes a mixture of plant carbohydrate polymers, both oligosaccharides and polysaccharides, e.g., cellulose, hemicelluloses, pectic substances, gums, resistant starch, inulin, that may be associated with lignin and other non-carbohydrate components (e.g., polyphenols, waxes, saponins, cutin, phytates, resistant protein) (Elleuch et al., 2011).

Dietary guidelines advise a diet rich in fruit and vegetables for a healthy lifestyle. Epidemiological studies have revealed that consumption of diets with high amounts of dietary fiber leads to many health-related benefits such as maintaining the functional integrity of the gastrointestinal system, and reducing the risks of colon cancer and coronary heart disease (Peerajit et al., 2012). Additionally, dietary fiber can also impart some functional properties to foods, e.g., increase water holding capacity, oil holding capacity, emulsification and/or gel formation (Ayala-Zavala et al., 2011). Indeed, dietary fiber, incorporated into food products (bakery products, dairy, jams, meats, soups), can modify textural properties, avoid sineresys (the separation of liquid from a gel caused by contraction), stabilize high fat food and emulsions, and improve shelf life (Elleuch et al., 2011).

Cereals have been the traditional source of dietary fiber, although lately are using fruits and vegetables as sources of dietary fiber to fortified foods. The most important characteristics of these sources are its wide availability and low cost, since many of them are co-products that pose an environmental problem. At present up to one third of fruit and vegetables in the form of peels, pips and skins can be discarded during preparation and processing, therefore creating a 'waste', while also decreasing the maximum nutritional potential of the fruit or vegetable.

Researchers are discovering new alternative uses for such 'waste' as potential value added ingredients (O'Shea et al., 2012). However, the use of dietary fiber from new sources is not currently exploited and its ability to modify them by chemical treatments, enzymatic and physical surely expands their uses (Elleuch et al., 2011). Several research groups have been working on the development of multifunctional ingredients from fruits and vegetables residues and its application in different food products. The crude fiber content combined with at least one other property enables them to fulfill several functions in food as depicted by Laufenberg et al., (2003).

Tropical exotic fruit production, trade and consumption have increased significantly on the domestic and international markets. Thus, World production of the major tropical fruits reached 62,000,000 t by 2010, an increase of 15,000,000 t from 1998 to 2000 (FAO, 2010). Brazil, Colombia and Ecuador are considered the main producer and exporter of tropical fresh fruit worldwide. This dynamic exportation of fruits is highly linked to the exotic fruit species, which are within the new preferences in the international markets due to they are innovative and exhibit excellent sensory, nutritional and/or nutraceuticals qualities (Bicas et al., 2011; Jiménez et al., 2011). The exotics fruits represent an opportunity for local growers to gain access to special markets where consumers appreciate the exotic character of such products and the presence of bioactive compounds capable of preventing degenerative diseases (Alves et al., 2008).

In many cases the raw tropical exotic fruit is not consumed directly by humans, but first undergoes processing to separate the desired value product from other constituents of the plant tissue (Ayala-Zavala et al., 2011). In addition, there has been increase in the availability of tropical fruit drinks. Nutrient-rich beverages are gaining popularity due to the desire of consumers for healthy eating and drinking while experiencing new and exotic flavours, and the same time, due to the focus of industries to produce beverages with health claim as a parameter of differentiation (Sabbe, et al., 2009). These processes generated large amount of co-products. From economic and environmental points of view, adding value to these tropical fruit co-products is always desirable. Such co-products are usually used for animal feed; however, the potentially valuable compounds they contain, mainly fiber with high content of bioactive compounds as polyphenols or condensed tannins, could be used to make high-value food products. Depending on the availability of an adequate technology, the co-products can be converted into commercial products either as raw materials for secondary processes (intermediate foods ingredients), as operating supplies, or as ingredients of new products (Sánchez-Zapata et al., 2009).

Thus, this chapter will examine current literature on antioxidant dietary fiber obtained from tropical fruits with a special focus in dietary fiber obtained from tropical fruits co-products.

Bioactive Compounds with Antioxidant Activity

Antioxidant capacity is an important property of dietary fiber (DF) that is given by the presence of different antioxidant linked compounds. Antioxidants associated with the dietary fiber matrix are substances that are not detected in the usual analytical procedures for either dietary antioxidants (targeting antioxidants extracted by aqueous organic solvents) or dietary fiber (targeting carbohydrates and lignin) quantification (Ayala-Zavala et al., 2011). However, these antioxidant compounds make up a substantial portion of the dietary antioxidant capacity; they are not minor constituents of DF, and as such they may contribute significantly to the health effects attributed to DF and dietary antioxidants (Saura-Calixto, 2011).

Phenolic Acids

Phenolic acids are to be found in most plants and, in many cases, they contribute to their color and taste. There are two classes of phenolic acids: derivates of benzoic acid and derivates of cinnamic acid. Hydroxybenzoic acids (Figure 1a) are components of complex structures such as hydrolyzable tannins (gallotannins or ellagitannins) (Manach et al., 2004) while the hydroxycinnamic (Figure 1b) acids are more common than the hydroxybenzoic acids and consist chiefly of *p*-coumaric, caffeic, ferulic, and sinapic acids (El Gharras 2009).

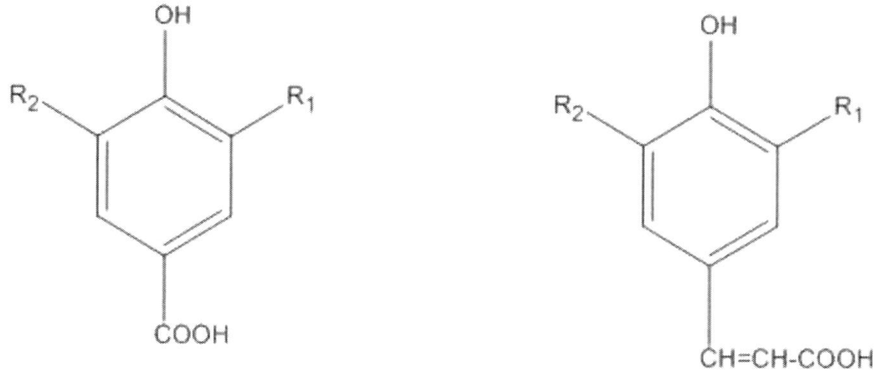

Figure 1. Phenolic acids structures as example of common fruit natural antioxidants.

Flavonoids

Flavonoids are naturally occurring substances in vegetables and fruits and are thought to have positive effects on human health. They are low-molecular-weight compounds consisting of 15 carbon atoms, arranged in a C_6-C_3-C_6 configuration. The flavonoids may themselves be divided into seven subclasses depending the type of heterocycle involved: flavonols, flavones, isoflavones, flavanones, flavanols, anthocyanidins and anthocyanins. They can participate in protection against the harmful action of reactive oxygen species and exhibit a wide range of biological effects, including; antioxidant activity (Sreeramulu and Raghunath 2010). Flavonoids have also been found to inhibit a wide range of enzymes involved in oxidation systems such as 5-lipoxygenase, cyclooxygenase, monooxygenase or xanthine oxidase (Crespo et al., 2008).

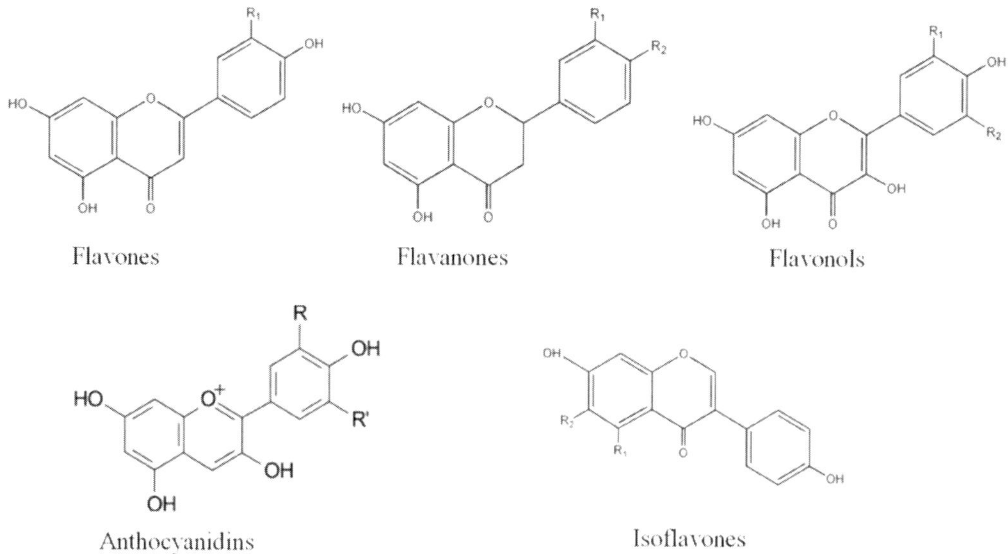

Figure 2. Structure of flavones, flavanones, flavonols, anthocyanidins and isoflavones.

Carotenoids

Carotenoids are a family of more than 600 substances that are synthesized by higher plants and algae. They are a class of natural pigment, familiar to all through the orange-red to yellow colors of many fruits, vegetables, and flowers as well as for the provitamin A activity which some of them possess (Ribaya-Mercado et al., 2000). Of the more than 600 naturally occurring carotenoids identified to date, six (β-carotene, β-cryptoxanthin, α-carotene, lycopene, lutein and zeaxanthin) are commonly found in blood (Figure 3) (>95% total blood carotenoids) (Maiani et al., 2009). Carotenoids have potential antioxidant properties due to their chemical structure consisting of abundant conjugated double bonds that interact with cellular membranes because of their fat-soluble nature (Riccioni 2009).

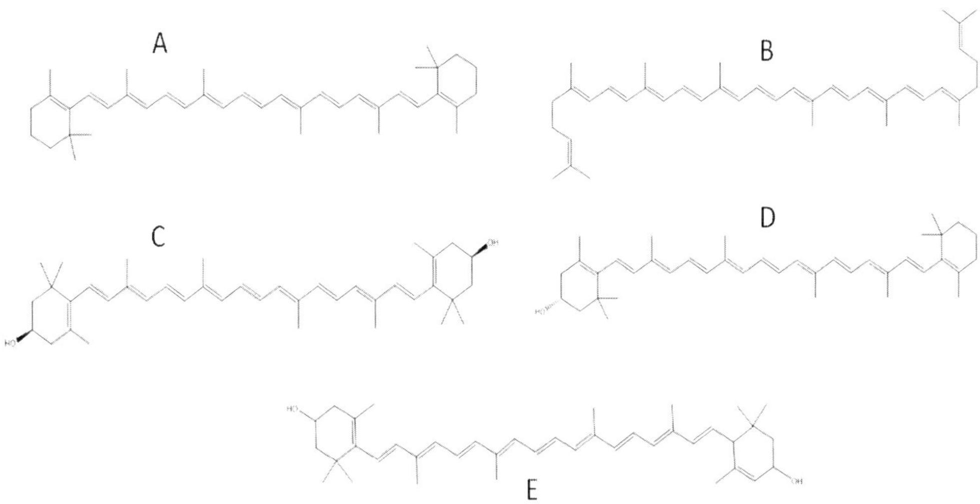

Figure 3. The main carotenes present in blood: A: β-carotene; B: Lycopene; C: Zeaxantin; D: Criptoxantin; E: lutein.

Dietary Fiber Derivated from Tropical Fruits

Mango

Mango (*Mangifera indica* L.), which belongs to family Anacardiaceae, is one of the most cultivated fruit in the world. Several million tons of mango co-products are produced annually from factories. Because mango is a seasonal fruit, about 20% of fruits are processed products such as puree, nectar, leather, pickles and canned slices, among others, which have worldwide. During processing of mango, peel is a major co-product. Peel contributes about 15-20% of the fruit and it has been found to be a good source of phytochemicals (González-Aguilar et al., 2008). The main polyphenols in mango in terms of antioxidative capacity and/or quantity are: mangiferin, catechins, quercetin, kaempferol, rhamnetin, anthocyanins, gallic and ellagic acids, propyl and methyl gallate, benzoic acid, and protocatechuic acid carotenoids, and vitamin C (Vijaya Kumar Reddy et al., 2010; Dembitsky et al., 2011). Some studies have recently analyzed the composition of mango co-products as a potential functional ingredient. Thus, Martínez et al., (2012a) informed that the total dietary fiber of Mango co-products composed mainly by peel and pulp were 69.98 g/100 g dry matter (d.m.). This comprised 28.15 g/100 g d.m. soluble fiber and 41.48 g/100 g d.m. insoluble fiber. Ajila et al., (2008) and Ajila et al., (2009) reported levels of 51.2% d.m. total dietary fiber. This comprised 19% d.m. soluble fiber and 32% d.m. insoluble fiber. In more recently studies Ajila and Prasada Rao (2013) reported that the total dietary fiber content in mango peel was in the range of 40.6-72.5%. Bound polyphenolic and flavonoid contents were in the range of 8.1-29.5 and 0.10-0.39 mg/g, respectively, and were found to be more in ripe peel than in raw peel. Vergara-Valencia et al., (2007) also investigated the dietary fiber content of the mango fruit ('Tommy Atkins' cultivar) and found it to contain 28.05% d.m. dietary fiber (13.80% d.m. insoluble fiber and 14.25% d.m. soluble). The bioactive compounds content and the antioxidant activity of the fiber obtained from mango are widely demonstrated. Therefore, Ayala-Zabala et al., (2010) informed that the peel of mango showed the high values of bioactive compounds and antioxidant capacity. The peel presented values of 5.997mg of gallic acid/g of fresh weight (fw), 4.455 mg of quercetin/g fw and 47.97% DPPH radical scavenging activity at the concentration of 322 mg/mL. Ajila et al., (2007) studied the bioactive compounds and antioxidant activities of mango peel rich-fiber extracts. These authors reported that ripe peels contained higher amount of anthocyanins and carotenoids compared to raw peels while raw mango peel had high polyphenol content. Antioxidant activity, determined using different antioxidant systems, showed IC_{50} values in the range of 1.39-5.24 μg of gallic acid equivalents. In a similar study, Martínez et al., (2012a) reported an antioxidant activity of mango ('Tommy Atkins' cultivar) co-products, measured with different tests systems, comprise between 19.1 and 38.0 μM Trolox equivalents/g of fiber.

Dietary fiber from mango has been included in different functional food to improve their antioxidant and "healthy" properties. Thus, Vergara-Valencia et al., (2007) reported that bakery products prepared with mango dietary fiber conserved the balance of soluble dietary fiber and insoluble dietary fiber and most of its anti-radical efficiency. *In vitro* starch digestibility tests of mango dietary fiber bakery products indicated a low predicted glycemic index. Ajila et al., (2010) incorporated mango peel into macaroni at three different levels (2.5, 5.0 and 7.5%). The total dietary fiber content in macaroni increased from 8.6 to 17.8%. The content of polyphenols increased from 0.46 to 1.80 mg/g and carotenoid content increased from 5 to 84 μg/g of macaroni with 7.5% incorporation of mango peel powder. The macaroni products incorporated with mango peel exhibited improved antioxidant properties. Similarly, Ajila et al., (2008) incorporated mango peel into biscuits. These authors informed that the total dietary fiber content increased from 6.5 to 20.7% with a high proportion of soluble dietary fiber with incorporation of 20% mango peel. The content of polyphenols increased from 0.54 to 4.50 mg/g and carotenoid content increased from 17 to 247 μg/g of biscuit with 20% incorporation of mango peel. Additionally, the biscuits incorporated with mango peel exhibited improved antioxidant properties.

Guava

Guava (*Psidium guajava* L.), which belongs to the Myrtaceae family, is a native of tropical America and is widespread throughout the tropical and subtropical areas (Chopda and Barrett, 2001). Guava is consumed fresh or made into processed products such as juice, nectar, puree, jam and jelly (Kashyap et al., 2001). These processes generated large amount of co-products such as peel, pulp and seeds. These co-products are rich in fiber and bioactive compounds. Therefore, Martínez et al., (2012a) analyzed the dietary fiber powder obtained from guava co-products. These authors reported that the total dietary fiber of guava was 69.10 g/100g d.m. with an insoluble dietary fiber content of 57.70 g/100g d.m. and soluble dietary fiber content of 11.10 g/100g d.m. Jiménez-Escrig et al., (2001) analyzed the dietary fiber powder obtained from guava peel and pulp co-products. These authors reported that the total dietary fiber of peel guava was 48.55 g/100g d.m. with an insoluble dietary fiber content of 46.72 g/100g d.m. and soluble dietary fiber content of 1.83 g/100g d.m; whilst the total dietary fiber of guava pulp was 49.42 g/100g d.m. with an insoluble dietary fiber content of 47.65 g/100g d.m; and soluble dietary fiber content of 1.77 g/100 g d.m. Marquina et al., (2008) informed that the pulp and peel fractions of guava had high content of dietary fiber (48.55-49.42 g/100g d.m.) and extractable polyphenols (2.62-7.79%) methoxylated pectin, which can be a suitable source of natural antioxidants. However, Ramulu and Rao (2003) reported that the total dietary fiber, insoluble dietary fiber and soluble dietary fiber content of guava fruits cultivated in India were 8.5, 7.1 and 1.4 g/100g d.m, respectively. In this way, Li et al., (2002) reported that the total dietary fiber, insoluble dietary fiber and soluble dietary fiber content of guava fruits were 12.72, 11.81 and 1.54 g/100g d.m. respectively.

Diverse studies analyzed the antioxidant activity of guava fiber. Thus, Martínez et al., (2012a) reported a total phenol content of 243 mg gallic acid equivalents/100 g sample with a remarkable antioxidant activity. These authors reported an antioxidant activity of guava co-products, measured with different tests systems, comprise between 19.1 and 38.0 µM Trolox equivalents/g of fiber. Guava fruits were analyzed by Lim et al., (2007) for total phenol contents, ascorbic acid contents and antioxidant activities. These authors reported that these fruits had a total phenol content of 138 mg/100 g and ascorbic acid content of 144 mg/100 g. The antioxidant activity showed an IC_{50} of 1.71 mg/mL. Jiménez-Escrig et al., (2001) informed that all fractions of guava peel and pulp tested showed a remarkable antioxidant capacity, and this activity was correlated with the corresponding total phenolic content. These authors reported that one-gram (dry matter) portion of peel contained DPPH· activity, FRAP activity, and inhibition of copper-induced *in vitro* LDL oxidation, equivalent to 43 mg, 116 mg, and 176 mg of Trolox, respectively.

Passion Fruit

Passion fruit (*Passiflora edulis*) a tropical fruit belonging to the family of *Passifloraceae*. There are several types of this fruit: purple passion fruit (*Passiflora edulis* Sims), granadilla (*Passiflora ligularis*), gulupa (*Passiflora edulis* Sims. fo *edulis*) and yellow passion fruit (*Passiflora edulis* var. *flavicarpa* Degenerer) (Chen & Lu, 1994). These fruits are considered as vitamin A, thiamine, riboflavin, niacin, calcium, phosphorus, and ascorbic acid source (Wenkam, 1990). Previous studies have described the presence of flavonoids as the major constituents of *P. edulis*, mainly C-glycosylflavones (Pereira and Vilegas 2000). The flavonoids schaftoside, isoschaftoside, isoorientin, orientin, isovitexin, luteolin-6-C-chinovoside and luteolin-6-C-fucoside have been identified in the fruit (Mareck et al., 1990).

Most of the fruit is intended for the production of juices and soft drinks. However, the juice industry alone generates several thousand tons of seeds, pulp and peels as agricultural co-products. There are several researches to analyze the composition of passion fruit co-products as a potential functional ingredient. Thus, Salgado et al., (2010) reported that the total dietary fibre content of passion fruit peel was 57.76 g/100 g with an insoluble dietary fibre content of 54.27 g/100 g and soluble dietary fibre content of 3.49 g/100 g. Martínez et al., (2012a) informed that the total dietary fiber of passion fruit co-products composed mainly by peel, pulp and seeds were 81.49 g/100 g d.m.; this comprised 35.45 g/100 g d.m. soluble fiber and 45.99 g/100 g d.m. insoluble fiber. In a similar study, Lopez-Vargas et al., (2013) analyzed the dietary fiber powder obtained from yellow passion fruit (*Passiflora edulis* var. flavicarpa) co-products (pulp and seeds or albedo). These authors reported that the total dietary fiber of passion fruit albedo was 71.79 g/100g d.m. with an insoluble dietary fiber content of 52.34 g/100g d.m. and soluble dietary fiber content of 19.45 g/100g d.m. While the total dietary fiber of passion fruit peel and seeds was 53.51 g/100g d.m. with an insoluble dietary fiber content of 48.25 g/100g d.m. and soluble dietary fiber content of 5.26 g/100 g d.m. Chau and Huang (2004) reported that raw passion fruit (Passiflora edulis) seed is rich in crude lipid (24.5 g/100 g) and insoluble dietary fiber (64.1 g/100 g). After defatting, the insoluble fibre-rich fractions including insoluble dietary fiber, alcohol-insoluble solids and water-insoluble solids (84.9-93.3 g/100 g) became the predominant component in the (defatted) seed, and were mainly composed of cellulose, pectic substances and hemicellulose.

The antioxidant activity of dietary fiber obtained from passion fruit has been determined. Martínez et al., (2012a) reported an antioxidant activity of guava co-products, measured with different tests systems (ABTS, DPPH and FRAP), were 5.50, 5.10 and 6.90 μM Trolox equivalents/g of fiber respectively. Vasco et al., (2008) reported that the antioxidant activity of passion fruit measured with the DPPH assay was 0.5 μM TE/g (fresh weight). Contreras-Calderón et al., (2011) reported that the antioxidant activity of *Passiflora mollissima*, measured with the ABTS and FRAP assays, was 34.4 and 42.2 μM TE/g (fresh weight), respectively, while the antioxidant activity of *Passiflora tarminiana* was 36.7 and 48.9 μM TE/g (fresh weight), respectively. Lopez-Vargas et al., (2013) reported that the IC_{50} values of passion fruits peel and seeds extracted with dimethylsulfoxide, methanol or water and measured with DPPH assay were 12.73, 252.68 and 25.16 mg/mL; whilst, the IC_{50} values of passion fruits albedo extracted with dimethylsulfoxide or methanol and measured with DPPH assay were 89.06 and 289.74 mg/mL. Kuskoski et al., (2006) reported total phenol content in passion fruit co-products of 20.0 mg acid gallic equivalent/g. In a similar study Cabral de Oliveira et al., (2009) reported total phenol content in passion fruit (*Passiflora alata*) co-products of 41.20 mg acid gallic equivalent/g with a high antioxidant activity.

Cocoa

Cocoa-derived foods such as cocoa powders, chocolate, and other cocoa-related products are polyphenol-rich foods derived from the fermented, roasted, and industrially processed seeds of *Theobroma cacao* L. (Sterculiaceae). Once the cocoa dry bean has been obtained, the co-products that remain are composed mainly by three fractions (i) cocoa pod husk, (ii) cocoa bean shells and (iii) cocoa mucilage. In most cases, these co-products are underexploited and considered an undesirable "waste" of the cocoa/chocolate industry (Martinez et al., 2012b). However, their composition gives them the potential to be used for other end, for example to obtain bioactive compounds and dietary fiber that could be used as ingredient in food processing. The polyphenol content in cocoa-derived products is lower than that found in the raw material used in their production. The major flavan-3-ol enantiomer identified in unfermented, dried, unroasted cocoa beans is the (-)-epicatechin compound. However, during the processing of cocoa, a significant degradation of (-)-epicatechin and (+)-catechin compounds takes place (Schinella et al., 2010). There are several researches to analyze the composition of cocoa co-products as a potential functional ingredient. Serra-Bonvehí & Aragay-Benería, (1998) informed that cocoa hull might be a good source of dietary fiber, with reported values of total dietary fibre ranging from 38 to 44 g/100 g sample as non-starch polysaccharides plus Klason lignin. Martinez et al., (2012b) analyzed the total, insoluble and soluble dietary fiber of cocoa co-products such as cocoa pod husks, cocoa bean shell and cocoa mucilage obtained from two lactations (Cone and Taura) in Ecuador. As regards cocoa mucilage, the total dietary fibre content range between 16.75 and 16.86 g/100 g d.m.; soluble dietary fiber values ranged between 16.06 and 16.11 g/100 g d.m., while the small amount of insoluble dietary fiber ranged between 0.69 and 0.78 g/100 g d.m.; total dietary fiber content of cocoa pod husks was 55.99 and 56.10 g/100 g d.m. for Taura and Cone respectively. While, cocoa bean shell, the total dietary fiber content ranged between 52.23 and 56.98 g/100 g d.m. Dietary fiber content of a fiber-rich product obtained from cocoa was studied by Lecumberri et al., (2007). This product contained 60.54 g/100 g (dry matter basis) of dietary fiber, made of mainly insoluble fiber although with appreciable amounts of soluble dietary fiber (10.09 g/100 g d.m.). Chung et al., (2003) reported values of total dietary fiber of 32 g/100 g in cocoa hulls. Ramos et al., (2008) informed that the enzymatic treatment of cocoa husks yielded a product with only minor amounts of insoluble fiber (2.6 g/100 g dry matter) and rich in soluble dietary fiber (48.6 g/100 g dry matter). The analysis of neutral sugars in the soluble dietary fiber fraction showed appreciable amounts of galactose and mannose residues, suggestive of the presence of hemicellulosic galactomannans, yet the major constituents of the soluble dietary fiber were pectic polysaccharides as shown by the high uronic acid content, accounting for 49% of the SDF.

The antioxidant activity of cocoa fiber has been widely investigated. Martinez et al., (2012b) analyzed the antioxidant properties of several cocoa co-products. All samples analyzed showed a good antioxidant capacity in the three different methods used with values ranging between from 2.48 to 22.93 μM Trolox Equivalents (TEs)/g in ABTS assay; 1.57-33.93 μM TEs/g in DPPH assay and 0.67 and 4.69 μM TEs/g sample in FRAP assay. Ramos et al., (2008) reported that the antioxidant activity of cocoa husks measured with the TEAC, ORAC and FRAP assays, were 83.30, 569.0 and 112.6 μM Trolox equivalent/g, respectively. Lecumberri et al., (2007) informed that the presence of associated polyphenolic compounds (1.32% and 4.46% of soluble polyphenols and condensed tannins, respectively) provides to dietary fibre rich cocoa product material with intrinsic antioxidant capacity as determined by the FRAP and TEAC methods with values of 72.32 and 7.73 μM Trolox Equivalents/g

Others

There are a large number of exploited and underexploited native and exotic fruit species that are of potential interest to the agro-industry and constitute a possible future source of income for the local population. In recent years, a wide variety of fruit products with beneficial health effects have been developed and marketed. However, only limited information on the nutritional value and bioactive compounds of tropical fruits, especially the more exotic species, is currently available (Botero et al., 2007). Glorio et al., (2008) informed that papaya (*Carica papaya*) a fruit of great acceptance among consumers shows a total dietary fiber value of 18.51 g/100 g with an insoluble dietary fiber content of 8.92 g/100g d.m. and soluble dietary fiber content of 9.59 g/100g d.m; this value were higher than reported by Ramulu and Rao (2003) who informed that de total dietary fiber obtained from papaya cultivated in India was 11.40 g/100 g., Similarly, Ittimongkol et al., (2002) reported a total dietary fiber content in ripe papaya fruits cultivated in Thailand was 66.12 g/100 g; the insoluble and soluble dietary fiber contents were 62.60 and 3.61 g/100 g. respectively. Other important tropical fruit is banana (*Musa sapientum*). Emaga et al., (2008) informed that banana peel accounts for 30-40% of the total fruit weight and is rich in hemicellulose, pectin and minerals. Glorio et al., (2008) reported that the total dietary fiber values of banana cv. palillo cultivated in Peru, shows a total dietary fiber value of 9.24 g/100 g with an insoluble dietary fiber content of 4.99 g/100g d.m. and soluble dietary fiber content of 4.25 g/100g d.m; this values a were close to those reported by Pak (2001) (total dietary fiber 11.03 g/100 g 11,03) for Chilean varieties of banana. Gonzalez-Montelongo et al., (2010) reported that banana peels contain large amounts of dopamine and L-dopa, catecholamines, which have substantial antioxidant activity. The physical and chemical characteristics and nutritional coconut (*Cocos nucifera*). Dietary fiber has been studied by Gunathilake et al., (2009), reporting dietary fiber content of 38 g/100g. The large amount of dietary fiber present in coconut is directly associated with its formation. In a mature coconut, white meat corresponds to 28% of the weight, surrounded by a hard shell protection, equivalent to 12% of the weight, and the outer shell of 35% of the weight. The shell is formed by 30 g/100 g dietary fiber (Rodriguez et al., 2011). This has been confirmed by Raghavendra et al., (2004), defatted coconut residue, as dietary fiber source. Trinidad et al., (2006) evaluated the addition of coconut flour as a source of dietary fiber to different types of foods: granola bars (5%), cinnamon bread (5%), multigrain bread (10%), chocolate chip cookies (15 %), hotcake (15%), chocolate cakes (20%), carrot cake (20%), macaroni (25%) and brownies (25%). The results identified that coconut flour is a rich source of dietary fiber and that an addition of 15 to 25% in food generates a release of short chain fatty acids with little or no effect on the availability of minerals; along with a reduction of the glycemic index and a reduction in total cholesterol, LDL cholesterol and triglycerides in persons with moderate levels of cholesterol.

Conclusion

Exotic fruit co-product are available in large quantities as a co-product of juice production, it could be used as an intermediate foods ingredient (IFI) in the development of functional foods. Dietary fibre obtained from exotic fruit co-products represents a potential material to be used as an ingredient in the food industry due to the high content in total dietary fibre with a good balanced ratio between insoluble dietary fibre and soluble dietary fibre which is important for the nutritional effects of fibre. In addition, these fibre-rich co-products have potential applications as ingredients in products requiring hydration, viscosity development and freshness preservation, such as baked foods or cooked meat products, due to their high total dietary fibre content and good technological properties, especially their water holding and swelling capacities.

These co-products show considerable levels of polyphenolic compounds with a remarkable antioxidants capacity. Due to the low cost of fruit co-products, which otherwise would be discharged as waste in the environment, they should be regarded as potential nutraceutic resources, capable of offering significant low-cost, nutritional dietary supplements for low-income communities. In addition, it could be also used in the pharmaceutical sector as a nutritional supplement, due to the health-related properties of dietary fibre and associated bioactive compounds.

References

Ajila, C. M., Naidu, K. A., Bhat, S. G. & Prasada Rao, U. J. S. (2007). Bioactive compounds and antioxidant potential of mango peel extract. *Food Chemistry, 105,* 982-988.

Ajila, C. M., Leelavathi, K. & Prasada Rao, U. J. S. (2008). Improvement of dietary fiber content and antioxidant properties in soft dough biscuits with the incorporation of mango peel powder. *Journal of Cereal Science, 48(2),* 319-326.

Ajila, C. M., Aalami, M. & Prasada Rao, U. J. S. (2009). Mango peel powder: A potential source of antioxidant and dietary fiber in macaroni preparations. *Innovative Food Science & Emerging Technologies, 11(1),* 219-224.

Ajila, C. M., Aalami, M., Leelavathi, K. & Prasada Rao, U. J. S. (2010). Mango peel powder: A potential source of antioxidant and dietary fiber in macaroni preparations. *Innovative Food Science & Emerging Technologies, 11,* 219-224.

Ajila, C. M. & Prasada Rao, U. J. S. (2013). Mango peel dietary fibre: Composition and associated bound phenolics. *Journal of Functional Foods, 5,* 444-450.

Alves, R. E., Brito, E. A., Rufino, M. S. M., & Sampaio, C. G. (2008). Antioxidant activity measurement in tropical fruits: A case study with acerola. *Acta Horticulturae, 773,* 299-305.

Ayala-Zavala, J. F., Rosas-Domínguez, C., Vega-Vega, V., & González-Aguilar, G. A. (2010). Antioxidant enrichment and antimicrobial protection of fresh-cut fruits using their own byproducts: Looking for integral exploitation. *Journal of Food Science, 25,* 175-181.

Ayala-Zavala, J. F., Vega-Vega, V., Rosas-Domínguez, C., Palafox-Carlos, H., Villa-Rodriguez, J. A., Siddiqui, W., Dávila-Aviña, J. E. & González-Aguilar, G. A. (2011). Agro-industrial potential of exotic fruit byproducts as a source of food additives. *Food Research International, 44*(7), 1866-1874.

Bicas, J., Molina, G., Dionisio, A., Cavalcante Barros, F., Wagner, R., Marostica, M. & Pastore, G. (2011). Volatile constituents of exotic fruits from Brazil. *Food Research International, 44(7),* 1843-1855.

Botero, M., Ricaute, S., Monsalve, C. & Rojano, B. (2007). Capacidad reductora de 15 frutas tropicales. *Scientia et Thechnica, 33,* 295-296.

Cabral de Oliveira, A., Barros Valentim, I., Silva, C. A., Bechara, E. J. H., Paes de Barros, M., Mano, C. M. & Fonseca Goulart, M. O. (2009). Total phenolic content and free radical scavenging activities of methanolic extract powders of tropical fruit residues. *Food Chemistry, 115,* 469-475.

Chau, C. F. & Huang, Y. L. (2004). Characterization of passion fruit seed fibres—a potential fibre source. *Food Chemistry, 85,* 189-194.

Chen, X. J., & Lu, L. X. (1994). Karyotype analysis of two major cultivated forms of *Passiflora* L. *Journal of Fujian Agricultural University, 23,* 24-25.

Chopda, C. A. & Barrett, D. M. (2001). Optimization of guava juice and powder production. *Journal of Food Processing and Preservation, 25,* 411-417.

Contreras-Calderón, J., Calderón-Jaimes, L., Guerra-Hernández, E. & García-Villanova, B. (2011). Antioxidant capacity, phenolic content and vitamin C in pulp, peel and seed from 24 exotic fruits from Colombia. *Food Research International, 44,* 2047-2053.

Crespo, I., García-Mediavilla, M. V., Almar, M., González, P., Tuñón, M. J., Sánchez-Campos, S., González-Gallego, J. (2008). Differential effects of dietary flavonoids on reactive oxygen and nitrogen species generation and changes in antioxidant enzyme expression induced by pro-inflammatory cytokines in Chang Liver cells. *Food and Chemical Toxicology, 46(5),* 1555-1569.

Dembitsky, V. M., Poovarodom, S., Leontowicz, H., Leontowicz, M., Vearasilp, S., Trakhtenberg, S. & Gorinstein, S. (2011). The multiple nutrition properties of some exotic fruits: Biological activity and active metabolites. *Food Research International, 44(7),* 1671-1701.

El Gharras, H. (2009). Polyphenols: food sources, properties and applications-a review. *International Journal of Food Science and Technology, 44,* 2512-2518.

Elleuch, M., Bedigian, D., Roiseux, O., Besbes, S., Blecker, C. & Attia, H. (2011). Dietary fibre and fibre-rich by-products of food processing: Characterisation, technological functionality and commercial applications: A review. *Food Chemistry, 124,* 411-421.

Emaga, T. H., Robert, C., Ronkart, S. N., Wathelet, B. & Paquot, M. (2008). Dietary fibre component and pectin chemical features of peels during ripening in banana and plantain varieties. *Bioresource Technology, 99,* 4346-4354.

FAO (2010). Tropical fruits. http://www.fao.org/docrep/006/y5143e/y5143e1a.htm. Accessed [25/03/2013].

Glorio, P. Repo-Carrasco, R., Velezmoro, C., Anticona, S., Huaranga, R., Martínez, P., Melgarejo, S., Astuhuaman, L., Huamán, N. E., Icochea, J. C., Peña, J. C. (2008). Fibra dietaria en variedades peruanas de frutas, tubérculos, cereales y leguminosas. *Revista de la Sociedad Quimica Peruana, 74,* 46-56.

González-Aguilar, G. A., Celis, J., Sotelo-Mundo, R. R., De La Rosa, L. A., Rodrigo-Garcia, J. & Alvarez-Parrilla, E. (2008). Physiological and biochemical changes of different fresh-cut mango cultivars stored at 5 °C. *International Journal of Food Science & Technology, 43(1),* 91-101.

González-Montelongo, R., Gloria Lobo, M. & González, M. (2010). Antioxidant activity in banana peel extracts: Testing extraction conditions and related bioactive compounds. *Food Chemistry, 119,* 1030-1039.

Gunathilake, K., Yalegam, C. & Kumara. A. (2009). Use of coconut flour as a source of protein and dietary fibre in wheat bread. *Journal Asian of Food and Agro-Industry, 2(3),* 382-391.

Ittimongkol, B., Srisukh, V., Tungrugsasut, E., Sukkhow, B., Chinganjanarod, P. & Jaicharoenl P. (2002). Instant dietary fiber-supplemented beverage mixes from papaya. *Thai Journal of Phytopharmacy, 9(1),* 13-21.

Jiménez-Escrig, A., Rincón, M., Pulido, R. & Saura-Calixto, F. (2001). Guava fruit (*Psidium guajava* L.) as a new source of antioxidant dietary fiber. Journal of Agricultural and Food Chemistry, *49,* 5489-5493.

Jiménez, A. M., Sierra, C. A., Rodríguez-Pulido, F. J., González-Miret, M. L., Heredia, F., & Osorio, C. (2011). Physicochemical characterisation of gulupa (*Passiflora edulis* Sims. Fo *edulis*) fruit from Colombia during the ripening. *Food Research International, 44, 7,* 1912-1918.

Kashyap, D. R., Vohra, P. K., Chopra, S. & Tewari, R. (2001). Application of pectinase in the commercial sector: a review. *Bioresource Technology, 77,* 215-227.

Kuskoski, E. M., Asuero, A., Morales, M. & Fett, R. (2006). Wild fruits and pulps of frozen fruits: antioxidant activity, polyphenols, and anthocyanines. *Ciência Rural Santa Maria, 36(4),* 1283-1287.

Laufenberg, G., Kunz, B., and Nystroem, M. (2003). Transformation of vegetable waste into value added products: (A) the upgrading concept; (B) practical implementations. *Bioresource Technology, 87,* 167-198.

Lecumberri, E., Mateos, R., Izquierdo-Pulido, M., Rupérez, P., Goya, L. & Bravo, L. (2007). Dietary fibre composition, antioxidant capacity and physico-chemical properties of a fibre-rich product from cocoa (*Theobroma cacao* L.). *Food Chemistry, 104,* 948-954.

Li, B. W., Andrewsw, K. W. & Pehrssonw, P. R. (2002). Individual sugars, soluble, and insoluble dietary fiber contents of 70 high consumption foods. *Journal of Food Composition and Analysis, 15,* 715-723.

Lim, Y. Y., Lim, T. T. & Tee, J. J. (2007). Antioxidant properties of several tropical fruits: A comparative study. *Food Chemistry, 103,* 1003-1008.

López-Vargas, J. H., Fernández-López, J., Pérez-Álvarez, J. A. & Viuda-Martos, M. (2013). Chemical, physico-chemical, technological, antibacterial and antioxidant properties of dietary fiber powder obtained from yellow passion fruit (*Passiflora edulis* var. *flavicarpa*) co-products. *Food Research International, 51,* 756-763.

Manach, C., Scalbert, A., Morand, C., Rémésy, C. & Jiménez, L. (2004). Polyphenols: food sources and bioavailability. *American Journal of Clinical Nutrition, 79,* 727-747.

Mareck, U. Galensa, R. & Herrmann, K. (1990). Identizierung von passionsfruchtsaft in fruchtprodukten mitels HPLC. Zeitschrift für Lebensmittel-Untersuchung und Forschung, 191, 269-274.

Marquina, V., Araujo, L., Ruíz, J., Rodríguez-Malaver A. & P. Vit, P. (2008). Composition and antioxidant capacity of the guava (*Psidium guajava* L.) fruit, pulp and jam. Archive Latinoam of Nutrition, 58, 98-102.

Martínez, R., Torres, P., A. Meneses, M. A., Figueroa, J. G., Pérez-Álvarez, J. A. & Viuda-Martos, M. (2012a). Chemical, technological and *in vitro* antioxidant properties of mango, guava, pineapple and passion fruit dietary fibre concentrate. *Food Chemistry, 135, Issue 3,* 1520-1526.

Martínez, R., Torres, P., A. Meneses, M. A., Figueroa, J. G., Pérez-Álvarez, J. A. & Viuda-Martos, M. (2012b). Chemical, technological and in vitro antioxidant properties of cocoa (*Theobroma cacao* L.) co-products. *Food Research International 49,* 39-45.

O'Shea, N., Arendt, E. K. & Gallagher, E. (2012). Dietary fibre and phytochemical characteristics of fruit and vegetable by-products and their recent applications as novel ingredients in food products. *Innovative Food Science and Emerging Technologies, 16,* 1-10.

Pak, N. (2001). Fibra dietética en alimentos Chilenos. In: Layolo, F.M., Saura-Calixto, F., Witting de Penna, E., and Menezes, E.W. eds. "Fibra Dietetica en Iberoamerica: Tecnología y Salúd". Editorial Valera. Brazil. p.p. 179-185.

Peerajit, P., Chiewchan, N. & Devahastin, S. (2012). Effects of pretreatment methods on health-related functional properties of high dietary fibre powder from lime residues. *Food Chemistry, 132,* 1891-1898.

Pereira, C. A. M. & Vilegas, J. H. Y. (2000). Constituintes químicos e farmacologia do gênero Passiflora com ênfase a *P. alata* Dryander, *P. edulis* Sims e *P. incarnata* L. *Revista Brasilera de Medicina, 3,* 1-12.

Raghavendra, S., Rastogi, N., Raghavarao, K. & R. Tharanathan, R. (2004). Dietary fiber from coconut residue: effects of different treatments and particle size on the hydration properties. *European Food Research and Technology, 218(6),* 563-567.

Ramos, S., Moulay, L., Granado-Serrano, A. B., Vilanova, O., Muguerza, B., Goya, L. & Bravo, L. (2008). Hypolipidemic effect in cholesterol-fed rats of a soluble fiber-rich product obtained from cocoa husks. *Journal of Agricultural and Food Chemistry, 56,* 6985-6993.

Ramulu, P. & Rao, P. U. (2003). Total, insoluble and soluble dietary fiber contents of Indian fruits. *Journal of Food Composition and Analysis, 16,* 677-685.

Ribaya-Mercado, J. D., Solon, S. F., Tang, G., Solon, J. A., Fjeld, C. R. & Russell, R. M. (2000). Bioconversion of plant carotenoids to vit-A in Filipino school-aged children varies inversely with vit-A status. *American Journal of Clinical Nutrition, 72,* 455-465.

Riccioni G. (2009). Carotenoids and cardiovascular disease. *Current Atherosclerosis Report* 11, 434-439.

Rodríguez N., Yáñez, M., Gutiérrez, F., Gomez, O., Matadamas, T., Lagunez, L. & J. Vazquez, J. (2011). Assessment of coconut fibre insulation characteristics and its use to modulate temperatures in concrete slabs with the aid of a finite element methodology. *Energy and Buildings, 43(6),* 1264-1272.

Sabbe, S., Verbeke, W., Deliza, R., & Van Damme, P. (2009). Effect of a health claim and personal characteristics on consumer acceptance of fruit juices with different concentration of açai (*Euterpe oleracea* Mart.). *Appetite, 53,* 84-92.

Salgado, J. M., Bombarde, T. A. D., Mansi, D. N., Piedade, M. S. & Meletti, L. M. M. (2010). Effects of different concentrations of passion fruit peel (*Passiflora edulis*) on the glicemic control in diabetic rat. *Ciência e Tecnologia de Alimentos, 30(3),* 784-789.

Sánchez-Zapata, E., Fuentes-Zaragoza, E., Fernández-López, J., Sendra, E., Sayas, E., Navarro, C., & Pérez-Alvarez, J. A. (2009). Preparation of dietary fibre powder from tiger nut (*Cyperus esculentus*) milk ("horchata") byproducts and its physicochemical properties. *Journal of Agricultural and Food Chemistry*, 57, 7719-7725.

Saura-Calixto, F. (2011). Dietary fiber as a carrier of dietary antioxidants: An essential physiological function. *Journal of Agricultural and Food Chemistry, 59(1),* 43-49.

Schinella, G., Mosca, S., Cienfuegos-Jovellanos, E., Pasamar, M. A., Muguerza, B., Ramón, D. & Ríos, J. L. (2010). Antioxidant properties of polyphenol-rich cocoa products industrially processed. *Food Research International, 43,* 1614-23.

Serra-Bonvehí, J. & Aragay-Benería, M. (1998). Composition of dietary fibre in cocoa husk. *Zeitschrift für Lebensmittel-Untersuchung und -Forschung A, 207,* 105-109.

Sreeramulu, D. & Raghunath, M. (2010). Antioxidant activity and phenolic content of roots, tubers and vegetables commonly consumed in India. *Food Research International, 43,* 1017-1020.

Trinidad, T., Mallillin, A. Valdez, D. Loyola, A. Askali, F. Castillo, J. Encabo, R. Masa, D. Maglaya, A. &Chua, M. (2006). Dietary fiber from coconut flour: a functional food. *Innovative Food Science and Emerging Technologies, 7(4),* 309-317.

Vasco, C., Ruales, J. & Kamal-Eldin, A. (2008). Total phenolic compounds and antioxidant capacities of major fruits from Ecuador. *Food Chemistry, 111,* 816-823.

Vergara-Valencia, N., Granados-Pérez, E., Agama-Acevedo, E., Tovar, J., Ruales, J., & Bello-Pérez, L. A. (2007). Fibre concentrate from mango fruit: Characterization, associated antioxidant capacity and application as a bakery product ingredient. *LWT-Food Science and Technology, 40(4)*, 722-729.

Vijaya Kumar Reddy, C., Sreeramulu, D., Raghunath, M. (2010). Antioxidant activity of fresh and dry fruits commonly consumed in India. *Food Research International, 43*, 285-288.

Wenkam, N. S. (1990). Food of Hawaii and the pacific basin, fruit and fruit products. Raw, processed and prepared, Vol 4, Honolulu: University of Hawaii.

In: Dietary Fiber
Editors: D. Betancur-Ancona, L. Chel-Guerrero et al.
ISBN: 978-1-62808-931-8

Chapter 7

Pomegranate: A Potential Source of Antioxidant Dietary Fiber

***Manuel Viuda-Martos*[1], *Juana Fernández-López*[1] *and José A. Pérez-Alvarez*[1,*]**
[1]IPOA Research Group (UMH-1 and REVIV-Generalitat Valenciana),
AgroFood Technology Department, Escuela Politécnica Superior de Orihuela,
Universidad Miguel Hernández, Crta, Beniel
Orihuela Alicante, Spain

Abstract

Since ancient times, pomegranate (Punica granatum L.) has been regarded as a "healing food" with numerous beneficial effects on several diseases. Indeed, pomegranate was usually used in folk medicine for eliminating parasites as an anti-helmintic and vermifuge and to treat and cure aphtae, ulcers, diarrhea, acidosis, dysentery, hemorrhage, microbial infections, respiratory pathologies and as an antipyretic. All these beneficial properties are due to pomegranate as an important source of minerals; and complex polysaccharides. Additionally, in their composition, pomegranate presents high levels of a diverse range of bioactive compounds such as phenolics, flavonoids and fiber.

At present, pomegranate is consumed fresh, as juice, jam, wine or oil, and in extract supplements. There is growing interest in this fruit because it is considered to be a functional product of great potential benefit in the human diet as it contains several groups of substances that are useful in several diseases.

In the process used to obtain juice from pomegranate fruit several co-products are obtained: (i) pulp and bagasse and (ii) peel. Uses for these co-products are scarce and their disposal presents a problem. One way of avoiding this problem would be to re-use the pomegranate bagasse and peel obtained from the pomegranate industries to take advantage of the large quantity of potentially beneficial compounds such as dietary fiber or bioactive compounds mainly phenolic acids and flavonoids which could be used as ingredient in food processing.

* Phone: +34 966749739; E-mail: ja.perez@umh.es.

Introduction

The pomegranate (*Punica granatum* L.) belongs to the family Punicaceae. It is native from the area of Iran to the Himalayas in northern India, and has been cultivated and naturalized over the entire Mediterranean region since ancient times (Meerts et al. 2009).

The pomegranate are mainly consumed as a raw staple food due to their desirable nutritional properties, the arils contain proteins, crude fibres, vitamins, minerals, pectin, sugars, polyphenols, and so on (Viuda-Martos et al., 2010). The arils are also used to elaborate increasingly popular pomegranate products such as canned beverages, jam, jelly, paste (Mousavinejad et al., 2009) and, especially, fresh juice which can be obtained from the arils or the whole fruit.

In addition, it is widely used in therapeutic formulas, cosmetics, and food seasonings. Since ancient times, the pomegranate has been regarded as a "healing food" with numerous beneficial effects in several diseases (Vidal et al. 2003).

The pomegranate fruit has valuable compounds in different parts of the fruit. These can be divided into several anatomical origins: peel, seeds, and arils (Figure 1). Another important product obtained from pomegranate fruit is the juice that can be obtained from arils or from whole fruit. The chemical composition of the fruits differs depending on the cultivar, growing region, climate, maturity, cultivation practice, and storage conditions (Poyrazoglu et al. 2002). About 50% of the total fruit weight corresponds to the peel which is an important source of minerals, mainly potassium, nitrogen, calcium, phosphorus, magnesium, and sodium (Mirdehghan and Rahemi 2007), complex polysaccharides (Jahfar et al. 2003) and bioactive compounds such as phenolics, flavonoids compounds (Li et al. 2006) and ellagitannins, such as punicalagin and its isomers, as well as lesser amounts of punicalin, gallagic acid, ellagic acid and ellagic acid-glycosides (hexoside, pentoside, rhamnoside, etc.) (Devatkal et al. 2010). The edible part of the pomegranate fruit (50%) consists of 40% arils and 10% seeds. Arils contain 85% water, 10% total sugars, mainly fructose and glucose, and 1.5% pectin, organic acid such as ascorbic acid, citric acid, and malic acid, and bioactive compounds such as phenolics and flavonoids, principally anthocyanins such as cyanidin-3-glucoside, cyanidin-3,5-diglucoside and delphindin-3-glucoside (Aviram et al. 2000; Tezcan et al. 2009).

As mentioned above, the pomegranate fruits are either consumed fresh or used commercially in the juice industries. Once the pomegranate juice has been extracted, the wastes that remain are composed mainly by two fractions (i) pulp and bagasse and (ii) peel. Uses for these co-products are scarce and their disposal represents a problem. One way of avoiding this problem would be to re-use the pomegranate bagasse obtained from the pomegranate industries to take advantage of the large quantity of potentially beneficial compounds such as dietary fiber or bioactive compounds mainly phenolic acids, flavonoids and tannins, which could be used as ingredient in food processing. Thus, new aspects concerning the use of these co-products for further exploitation as food additives or supplements with high nutritional value have gained increasing interest because these are high-value products and their recovery may be economically attractive (Murthy and Naidu, 2012). This chapter examines the antioxidant properties of the dietary fiber obtained from pomegranate or pomegranate co-products.

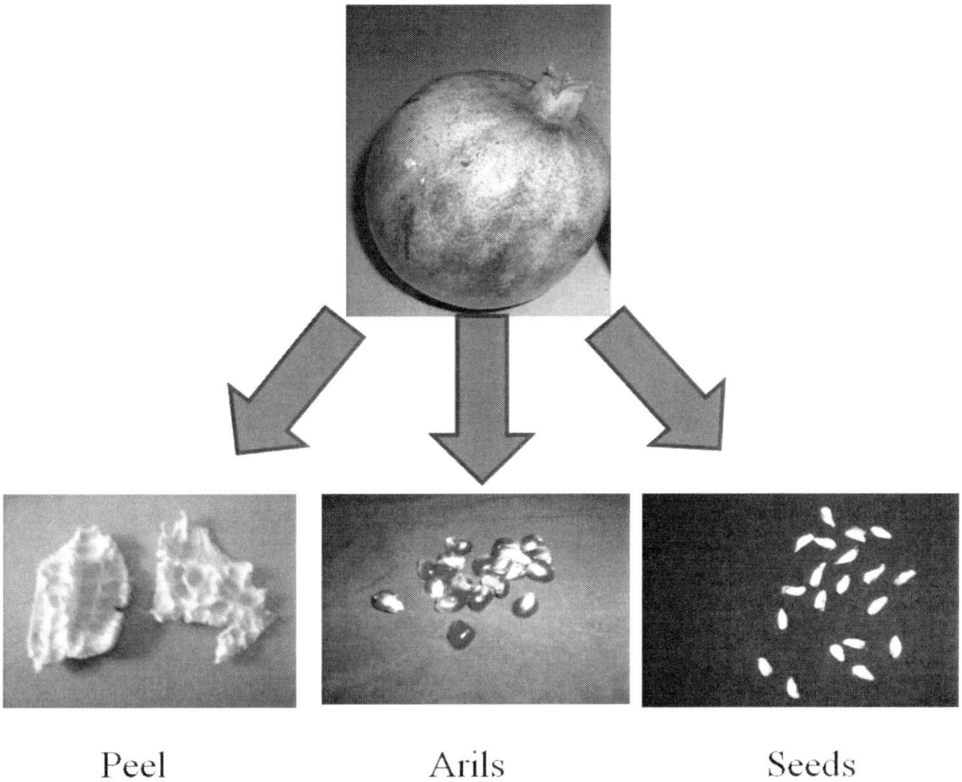

Figure 1. Different parts of the pomegranate fruit.

Total Dietary Fiber in Pomegranate Co-Product

The industrial transformation of vegetables and fruits generates large quantities of co-products rich in bioactive compounds that may well be suitable for other purposes (Viuda-Martos et al., 2009). Public institutions are supporting the food industry in the implementation of new technologies to recover valued-added ingredients from co-products. The importance of natural food additives or food ingredients are increasing due to a more extensive use of natural compounds in food, cosmetics and pharmaceuticals industries, following EU directives in favor of natural rather than synthetic compounds. Indeed, the recycling or re-usage of these co-products that are accumulated during processing and available in high amounts can reduce the treatment costs (Vági et al., 2007).

There are not many studies that reported the total dietary fibre content of pomegranate bagasse and/or peel. Thus, Viuda-Martos et al. (2012a) analyzed the total dietary fiber content and functional properties of pomegranate juice extraction bagasse, which were obtained in two different ways (Figure 2): (i) direct extraction that involved arils and peel (WFB) and (ii) only from arils (AB). The total dietary fiber, insoluble dietary fiber and soluble dietary fiber content was higher in WFB samples (50.3, 30.4 and 19.9 g/100 g d.m. respectively) than AB samples (45.6, 29.0 and 16.6 g/100 g d.m.). AB showed a pH of 4.40 while WFB showed a pH of 4.5. AB and WFB exhibited a water holding capacity of 4.5 and 4.9 g water/g d.m.

respectively while the oil holding capacity was 5.9 g oil/g d.m. for AB sample and 5.9 g oil/g d.m. for WFB.

Viuda-Martos et al. (2012b) informed that the pomegranate peel powder co-product showed good functional properties. These extract contains a high proportion of total dietary fiber (72.68 g/100 g), composed mainly of insoluble dietary fiber (42.53 g/100 g). It has a high water-holding capacity (5.03 g/g) and oil-holding capacity (6.60 g/g) and low water absorption (0.76 g/g) and water adsorption (0.29 g/g) capacities. The emulsifying ability was 20.33 mL/100 mL, and the emulsifying stability was 95 mL/100 mL. The total dietary fiber content of these extractg was found to be higher than that of some other fruit peels such as dietary preparations from mango dietary fiber (28.1 g/100 g dry sample), coconut fiber (60.9 g/100 g dry sample) apple (60.1 g/100 g dry sample) and cocoa fiber (60.54 g/100 g dry sample) (Trinidad et al. 2006; Vergara-Valencia et al. 2007; Lecumberri et al. 2007).

Total Polyphenol Content in Pomegranate

The phenolic compounds content could be used as an important indicator of the antioxidant capacity which may be used as a preliminarily screen for fruit co-products when intended as natural sources of antioxidants in functional foods (Liu et al. 2008).

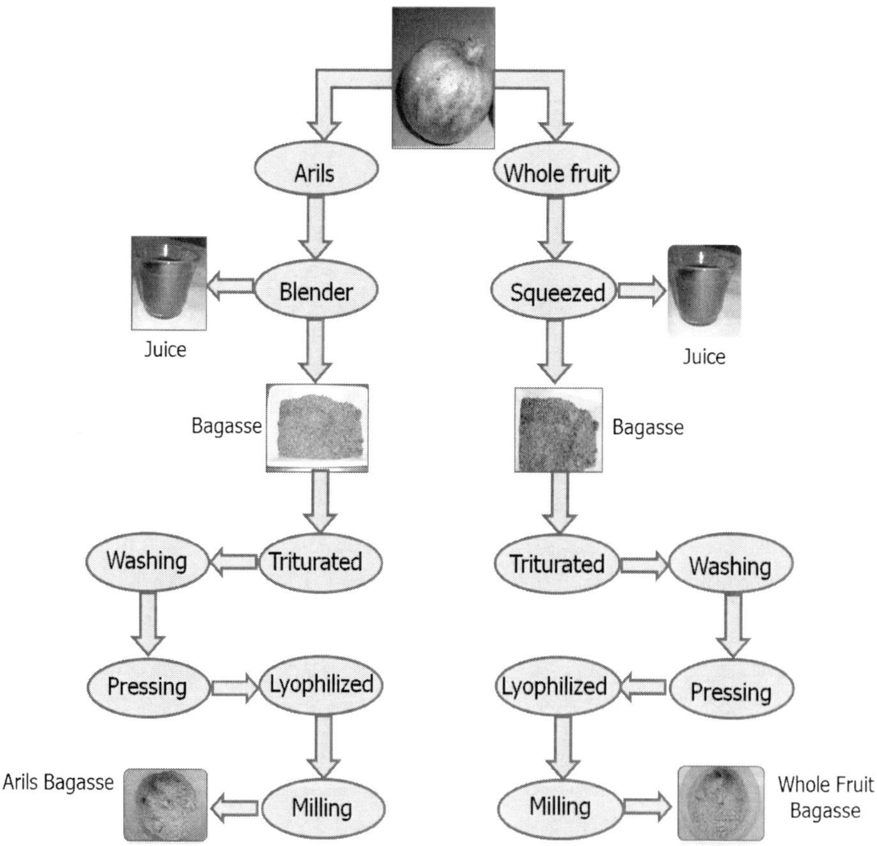

Figure 2. Process to obtain pomegranate juice arils bagasse and pomegranate juice whole fruit bagasse.

Many authors (Gomez-Estaca et al. 2009; Hernández-Hernández et al. 2009) have described the potential antioxidant properties of polyphenols. These compounds act as antioxidants by donating of a hydrogen atom, as an acceptor of free radicals, by interrupting chain oxidation reactions, or by chelating metals (Gramza et al. 2004). The phenolic and flavonoids contents in pomegranate extracts depend on the cultivar, growing region, climate, maturity, cultivation practice, storage conditions (Poyrazoglu et al., 2002) and method used to obtain the juice.

The total phenolic contents of pomegranate peel and bagasse are widely demonstrated. In the case of peel, Çam and Hişil (2010) reported that the total phenolic contents of pomegranate peels obtained by pressurized water extraction at optimized conditions and conventional solid–liquid methanol extraction were determined as 264.3 and 258.2 mg/g tannic acid equivalents, respectively. In a similar study, Li et al. (2006) analyzed the total phenol content and total flavonoid content of pomegranate peel co-products. These authors reported that the peel had a total phenolic content values of 249.4 mg tannic acid equivalents /g sample; whilst the total flavonoid content was of 59.1 mg rutin equivalent /g sample. Viuda-Martos et al. (2012c) informed that the pomegranate peel powder co-product showed total phenolic content values of 54.84 mg gallic acid equivalents/g sample; whilst the total flavonoid content was of 42.36 mg rutin equivalent /g sample. These values were similar than reported Hayrapetyan et al. (2012) in pomegranate peels (46.58-54.84 mg gallic acid equivalent/g). However, Cuccioloni et al. (2009) observed lower phenolic contents 16.90-27.10 mg gallic acid equivalents/g dry-peel solids (depending on the variety). However, there are several reports that shown a higher total phenolic content in pomegranate peel. Therefore, the total polyphenols was analyzed by Saad et al. (2012) for 4 Tunisian pomegranate cultivars (Mekki, Chelfi, Gabsi, Jbeli). They reported that the total polyphenolic content ranged from 134.3 mg gallic acid equivalents/g d.m. to 181.0 mg gallic acid equivalents/g d.m; the content was minimum for ‘Mekki’ and maximum for ‘Jbeli’. Similarly Ramadan et al., (2009) found phenolic contents in pomegranate peel as 667 mg gallic acid equivalents/g dry-peel solids (i.e. 175 mg GAE/100 g fresh peel). As regards the total phenolic content in the bagasse, Viuda-Martos et al. (2011) analyzed the total phenol and total flavonoid content pomegranate juice extraction bagasses, which were obtained in two different ways (i) direct extraction that involved arils and peel and (ii) only from arils. In the first case, the total phenolic content value was 10.05 mg gallic acid equivalents/g sample; whilst the total flavonoid content was of 7.19 mg rutin equivalent /g sample. In the second case, the total phenolic content value was 4.62 mg gallic acid equivalents/g sample; while the total flavonoid content was of 5.71 mg rutin equivalent /g sample. Li et al. (2006) analyzed the total phenol content and total flavonoid content of pomegranate pulp co-products. These authors reported that pulp had a total phenolic content value of 24.4 mg tannic acid equivalents /g sample; whilst the total flavonoid content was of 17.20 mg rutin equivalent /g sample.

Antioxidant Properties of Pomegranate Extracts

The determination of the antioxidant capacity of pomegranate components and their derivatives is being given greater importance by researchers and those involved in the agrofood industry for use as natural additives to replace synthetic antioxidants, whose use is increasingly restricted due to the secondary effects they may produce (Table 1).

Table 1. Overview of antioxidant pomegranate studies

Part of the plant	Assays	Effect	Reference
Peels	FRAP and DPPH	FRAP and DPPH values varied from 24.30 to 63.37 mM $^{Fe2+}$/100 g d.m and 60.12-83.52% inhibition	Tabaraki et al. (2012)
Peels	Phosphomolybdenum complex	Ethyl acetate, acetone, methanol exhibited marked antioxidant capacity, but the water extract was the lowest	Negi and Jayaprakasha (2003)
Pith and carpellary membrane	DPPH free radical and superoxide radicals	Strong lipid peroxidation inhibitory activity in a liposome model system	Kulkarni et al. (2004)
Peels	DPPH	Scavenging activity of 5.8 g/g	Pan et al. (2012)
Peels	DPPH	Scavenging activity 96.24 %	Ashoush et al. (2013)
Arils, peels and Ellagic acid extracts	DPPH	Good antioxidant activity. Extrongest from ellagic acid extracts of arils	Ricci et al. (2006)
Peel, Pulp and seeds	FRAP	High antioxidant activity and might be rich sources of natural antioxidants	Guo et al. (2003)
Peel	TEAC	Prodelphinidin potent antioxidants in aqueous phase. Gallocatechin-(4,8)-catechin more effective than prodelphinidin in lipid phase	Plumb et al. (2002)
Peel	DPPH and ABTS	Strong antioxidant activity	Rout and Banerjee (2007)
Peel	DPPH and ABTS	High free radical-scavenging power	Okonogi et al. (2007)
Arils	FRAP and TEAC	Variability among cultivars was great	Ozgen et al. (2008)
Peel, pulp and seeds	FRAP	Peel of the fruit have a greater antioxidant activity than pulp and seed	Hajimahmoodi et al. (2009)
Seeds	FRAP	The extracts obtained using various solvents exhibited various degrees of antioxidant activity.	Sadeghi et al. (2009)
Peels and seeds	FRAP	Peels showed very high total antioxidant but seed had lower capacity	Surveswaran et al. (2007)
Juice and sour concentrate	Linoleic acid system	Sour concentrate present higher antioxidant activity that juice	Orak (2009)

The antioxidant and sensory qualities of pomegranates depend on several factors, such as cultivar and climatic conditions during fruit maturation and ripening and the part of the fruit used (Borochov-Neori et al. 2009). Thus, Tzulker et al. (2007) reported that the homogenates prepared from the whole fruit exhibited an approximately 20-fold higher antioxidant activity than the level found in the aril juice. Singh et al. (2002) reported that a methanol extract of pomegranate peel had much higher antioxidant capacity than that of seeds. Li et al. (2006) reported that pomegranate peel had the highest antioxidant activity among the peel, pulp and seed fractions of 28 kinds of fruits commonly consumed in China. The antioxidant activity of pomegranate components has been the subject of many studies (Naveena et al. 2008; Çam et al. 2009; Mousavinejad et al. 2009; Tezcan et al. 2009), most conducted *in vitro* and *in vivo*. Viuda-Martos et al. (2011) analyzed the antioxidant activity of pomegranate juice extraction bagasses, which were obtained in two different ways (i) direct extraction that involved arils and peel (WFB) and (ii) only from arils (AB) using different methods. The AB and WFB samples were examined for their ability to act as radical scavenging agents in the TBARs assay. A concentration-dependent lipid peroxidation inhibitory potency was found in both samples. The EC_{50} achieved was 4.87% for AB and 1.82% for WFB. As regards the 2,2'-diphenyl-1-picrylhydrazyl radical scavenging assay (DPPH), AB samples showed IC_{50} value of 37.8%; while IC_{50} value for WFB sample was 11.6%. Fischer et al. (2011) analyzed the antioxidant activity of peel obtained from Peruvian pomegranate.

These authors reported that the pomegranate peel extracts had antioxidant capacity measure with Trolox-Equivalent Antioxidant Capacity (TEAC) assay of 1361.9 mMol/kg whilst when the Ferric Reducing Antioxidant Power (FRAP) assay was used the values obtained were 589.1 mMol/kg.

To study the antioxidant effects of extracts from the peel, leaf, seed and flower of pomegranate, their ethanolic extracts were added to soy bean oil determining the peroxide value (POV) and malondialdehyde (MDA) (Zhang et al., 2010). Experimental results indicated that the peel was the strongest one, and the petal, the stamen and the receptacle were of about a same level, but the leaf was weaker than them. The polyphenol content was significantly correlative to the antioxidant effect and antibacterial activity, which indicated that polyphenols were the main active compounds of pomegranate. Sagdic et al. (2010) studied the antioxidant and antiradical potential of pomegranate seeds extracted by methanol, ethanol and water. The highest phenolic content was found in the methanol extracts and the lowest in aqueous extracts of pomegranate seeds and hulls. The values of IC_{50} in methanol extracts of the pomegranate seeds and hulls were founded as 39.40 and 7.02, respectively. The *in vitro* antioxidant activities of the whole fruits and leaves of pomegranate was studied by Zhang et al. (2008) which presented the radical scavenging activities of water soluble extracts of leaves, fruit peel, seeds and juice of pomegranate were measured by DPPH assay and 2,2'-azino-bis(3-ethylbenzothiazoline-6-sulphonic acid) (ABTS) assay. In both methods, both leaf and peel exhibited very strong antioxidant activity and high polyphenol content when compared to seeds and juice and they had the same IC_{50} values of 0.14 mg/mL in the DPPH method. Kanatt et al. (2010) analyzed the antioxidant activity of pomegranate peel extract. They reported that the iron chelation capacity of pomegranate peel extract was found to be relatively high (45.5% chelation at a concentration of 1 mg/mL); while, in the DPPH assay pomegranate peel extract showed a concentration dependent radical scavenging activity with an IC_{50} of 4.9 μg/mL. The sequentially extracted pomegranate peel fractions were tested for their antioxidant activity by DPPH free radical scavenging, phospho-molybdenum, FRAP

(Fe^{3+} reducing power) and CUPRAC (cupricions (Cu^{2+}) reducing ability) assays by Zahin et al. (2010). The methanol fraction showed highest antioxidant activity by all the four *in vitro* assays comparable to ascorbic acid and butylated hydroxytoluene (BHT) followed by activity in ethanol, acetone, and ethyl acetate fractions.

In vivo, animal, and human trials have examined the effects of various pomegranate constituents on the prevention and attenuation of atherosclerosis and Low-density Lipoprotein (LDL) oxidation. Rosenblat et al. (2006) investigated the anti-atherosclerotic effects of a pomegranate co-product extract after the juice was removed. Mice with significant atherosclerosis were given pomegranate co-product extract (containing 51.5 μg gallic acid equiv / kg / day) with a 8-fold higher polyphenol concentration than pomegranate juice for 3 months. This resulted in a significant reduction in oxidative status as evidenced by a 27% decrease in total macrophage peroxide levels, a 42% decrease in cellular lipid peroxide levels, and a 19% decrease in peritoneal macrophage uptake of oxidized LDL.

Murthy et al. (2002) evaluated the effect of administration of methanolic peel extracts (50 mg/kg/day) during 28 days to healthy albino Wistar rats. These authors informed that methanolic peel extracts had a protective effect of antioxidant enzymes catalase, peroxidase and superoxide dismutase. Hossin (2009) conducted a study where hyperlipidemic Albino Sprague Dawley rats were supplemented with pomegranate peel extracts (5, 10, 15%) for 28 days. the author reported a Reduction of total cholesterol, LDL-cholesterol, triglycerides and VLDL-cholesterol. Althunibat et al. (2010) carried out a study whether daily consumption of pomegranate Methanolic peel extracts (20 mg/kg/day) during 28 days in diabetic Albino Wistar rats. These authors reported an increase the activities of antioxidant enzymes catalase, superoxide dismutase, glutathione peroxidase, glutathione-S-transferase, and glutathione reductase, in liver and kidney. All these activities may be related to the diverse phenolic compounds present in pomegranate, including punicalagin isomers, ellagic acid derivatives, and anthocyanins (delphinidin, cyanidin and pelargonidin 3-glucosides, and 3,5-diglucosides). These compounds are known for their properties to scavenge free radicals and to inhibit lipid oxidation *in vitro* (Gil et al. 2000; Noda et al. 2002). However, Tzulker et al. (2007) suggested that punicalagin originating from the peels is one of the major phytochemicals contributing to the total antioxidant capacity of pomegranate juice, whilst anthocyanins play only a minor role in this activity. The action mechanism set in motion by the antioxidant activity of these compounds is still not clearly understood, although it is a known fact that antioxidant mechanisms involved in biological matrixes are quite complex and several different factors may play a role (Çam et al. 2009). Madrigal-Carballo et al. (2009) suggested that pomegranate polyphenolic molecules undergo redox reactions because phenolic hydroxyl groups readily donate hydrogen to reducing agents. Negi and Jayaprakasha (2003) have also reported a significant increase in the reducing power of pomegranate peel extracts with increases in concentration from 50 to 400 ppm. Reducing properties are generally associated with the presence of reductones (Pin-Der 1998). Gordon (1990) reported that the antioxidative action of reductones is based on the breaking of the free radical chain by the donation of a hydrogen atom. Reductones also react with certain precursors of peroxides, thus preventing peroxide formation (Naveena et al. 2008). However, Amarowicz et al. (2004) suggested that the antioxidant activity of phenolic compounds is due to their ability to scavenge free radicals or chelate metal cations. The next step, in further research, is to try to identify the exactly mechanism or mechanisms by which antioxidant effect occurs, identifying too, the compounds responsible for antioxidant activity.

Pomegranate Extracts and Meat Products

In response to recent demand for natural products and consumers' willingness to pay significant premiums for natural foods (Sebranek and Bacus 2007), the meat industry is actively seeking natural solutions to minimize oxidative rancidity and increase products' shelf life (Naveena et al. 2008). Recent investigation has focused towards identification of novel antioxidants from natural sources. Due to their high content of phenolic compounds, fruits and other plant materials are a good source of natural antioxidants and provide an alternative to currently used conventional antioxidants (Karre et al. 2013).

Pomegranate fruit parts contain a high concentration of antioxidants. The peel and rind are good sources of tannins, anthocyanins, and flavonoids (Naveena et al. 2008). These co-products could be used as potential ingredients in meat and meat products although their nutritional and functional properties make them suitable for other purposes, such as the enhancement of functional foods. Thus, Devatkal and Naveena (2010) studied effect of salt, kinnow and pomegranate peel in raw ground goat meat. Samples treated with fruit powders showed lower TBARS values compared with control and salted samples. Pomegranate peel-treated patties showed greater reduction in TBARS (134% and 443% compared with control and salted samples, respectively). In a similar study, Devatkal et al. (2010) used pomegranate rind powder in raw goat meat patties stored for 12 days at 4 °C. These authors informed that incorporation of pomegranate rind powder was effective in reducing TBARS formation up to 67%. The effect of addition of pomegranate peel extract on the oxidative stability of chicken chilly and lollipop stored under chilled condition was analyzed by Kanatt et al. (2010). In all the samples there was an increase in TBARS during chilled storage. However, oxidative rancidity was less in chicken chilly and lollipop containing pomegranate peel extract throughout the storage period as compared to untreated control samples. Naveena et al. (2008) evaluated the addition of pomegranate rind powder into cooked chicken patties. These authors reported that total phenolic content (as tannic acid equivalent) significantly increased from 308 in control to 441 μg/g in patties added with pomegranate rind powder. The values of thiobarbituric acid reactive substances were significantly reduced from 1.530 in control patties to 0.135 mg malonaldehyde/kg samples in pomegranate rind powder patties. Pomegranate rind powder extract treatment substantially inhibited lipid oxidation in cooked chicken patties to a much greater extent than Vitamin C treatment. Additionally pomegranate rind powder to chicken patties did not affect any of the sensory attributes. The addition of pomegranate fiber to bologna-type products have been studied by Ruiz-Navajas et al. (2011). The addition of pomegranate peel to pork product increased fiber content and decreased fat, TBA values of control samples were higher than samples with 0.25% pomegranate peel extracts.

Conclusion

The consumption of pomegranate has grown tremendously due to its reported health benefits. The rich bioactive profile of pomegranate makes it a highly nutritious and desirable fruit crop. Pomegranate and derivates, such as peel and seeds, are rich sources of several high-value compounds with potential beneficial physiological activities.

Pomegranate co-products mainly peel and bagasse may be considered good sources of natural compounds with significant antioxidant activity which can be attributed to the high percentages of the main constituents or to synergy among their different components, especially phenolic acids, flavonoids and tannins. Due to these characteristics pomegranate peel or bagasse could be suitable for applications in the food industry as potential ingredient for food products. These important sources of bioactive compounds with antioxidant properties could be very appreciated in avoiding oxidation in a wide number of food processes during processing, and also during their storage period. Another important reason for their suitability as a food ingredient is their natural origin, which consumers find comforting and which is beneficial for the environment.

References

Althunibat, O. Y., Al-Mustafa, A. H., Tarawneh, K., Khleifat, K. M., Ridzwan, B. H. and Qaralleh, H. N. (2010). Protective role of Punica granatum L. peel extract against oxidative damage in experimental diabetic rats. *Processing Biochemistry,* 45(4), 581-585.

Amarowicz, R., Pegg, R. B., Rahimi-Moghaddam, P., Barl, B. and Weil, J. A. (2004). Free-radical scavenging capacity and antioxidant activity of selected plant species from the Canadian prairies. *Food Chemistry,* 84, 551-562.

Ashoush, I. S., El-Batawy, O. I. and El-Shourbagy, G. H. (2013). Antioxidant activity and hepatoprotective effect of pomegranate peel and whey powders in rats. *Annals of Agricultural Sciences, In Press,* http://dx.doi.org/10.1016/j.aoas.2013.01.005.

Aviram, M., Dornfeld, L., Rosenblat, M., Volkova, N., Kaplan, M., Coleman, R., Hayek, T., Presser, D. and Fuhrman B. (2000). Pomegranate juice consumption reduces oxidative stress, atherogenic modifications to LDL, and platelet aggregation: studies in humans and in atherosclerotic apolipoprotein E-deficient mice. *American Journal of Clinical Nutrition,* 71, 1062-1076.

Borochov-Neori, H., Judeinstein, S., Tripler, S., Harari, M., Greenberg, A., Shomer, I. and Holland, D. (2009). Seasonal and cultivar variations in antioxidant and sensory quality of pomegranate (Punica granatum L.) fruit. *Journal of Food Composition and Analysys,* 22(3), 189-195.

Çam, M., Hısıl Y. and Durmaz, G. (2009). Classification of eight pomegranate juices based on antioxidant capacity measured by four methods. *Food Chemistry,* 112, 721-726.

Çam, M. and Hişil, Y. (2010). Pressurised water extraction of polyphenols from pomegranate peels. *Food Chemistry*, 123, 878-885.

Cuccioloni, M., Mozzicafreddo, M. and Sparapani, L. (2009). Pomegranate fruit components modulate human thrombin. *Fitoterapia*, 80, 301-305.

Devatkal, S. K. and Naveena, B. M. (2010). Effect of salt, kinnow and pomegranate fruit by-product powders on color and oxidative stability of raw ground meat during refrigerated storage. *Meat Science,* 85, 306-311.

Devatkal, S.K., Narsaiah, K. and Borah, A. (2010). Anti-oxidant effect of extracts of kinnow rind, pomegranate rind and seed extracts in cooked goat meat patties. *Meat Science,* 85(1), 155-159.

Fischer, U. A., Carle, R. and Kammerer, D. R. (2011). Identification and quantification of phenolic compounds from pomegranate (Punica granatum L.) peel, mesocarp, aril and differently produced juices by HPLC-DAD–ESI/MSn. *Food Chemistry,* 127, 807-821.

Gómez-Estaca, J., Bravo, L., Gómez-Guillén, M. C. Alemán, A., and Montero P. (2009). Antioxidant properties of tuna-skin and bovine-hide gelatin films induced by the addition of oregano and rosemary extracts. *Food Chemistry,* 112(1), 18-25.

Gordon, M. F. (1990). The mechanisam of antioxidant action in vitro. In: Food Antioxidants. pp 1-18. Hudson, B. J. F. ed. London: Elsevier applied Science.

Gramza, A., Khokhar, S., Hes, M., and Jedrusek-Golinska, A. (2004). Tea extracts influence on catalytical properties of Fe^{2+} in lipids. *Polish Journal of Environment Studies*, 13, 143-146.

Guo, C., Yang, J., Wei, J., Li, Y., Xu, J. and Jiang, Y. (2003). Antioxidant activities of peel, pulp and seed fractions of common fruits as determined by FRAP assay. *Nutrition Research,* 23(12), 1719-1726.

Hajimahmoodi, M., Oveisi, M. R., Sadeghi, N., Jannat, B. and Nateghi, M. (2009). Antioxidant capacity of plasma after pomegranate intake in human volunteers. *Acta Medical of Iran,* 47(2), 125-132.

Hayrapetyan, H., Hazeleger, W. C. and Beumer, R. R. (2012). Inhibition of Listeria monocytogenes by pomegranate (Punica granatum) peel extract in meat paté at different temperatures. *Food Control,* 23, 66-72.

Hernández-Hernández, E., Ponce-Alquicira, E., Jaramillo-Flores, M. E., and Guerrero-Legarreta, I. (2009). Antioxidant effect rosemary (Rosmarinus officinalis L.) and oregano (*Origanum vulgare* L.) extracts on TBARS and colour of model raw pork batters. *Meat Science,* 81(2), 410-417.

Hossin, F. L. A. (2009). Effect of pomegranate (Punica granatum) peels and its extract on obese hypercholesterolemic rats. *Pakistan Journal of Nutrition,* 8, 1251-1257.

Jahfar, M., Vijayan, K. K. and Azadi, P. (2003). Studies on a polysaccharide from the fruit rind of Punica granatum. *Research Journal of Chemistry and Environment,* 7, 43-50.

Kanatt, S. R., Chander, R. and Sharma, A. (2010), Antioxidant and antimicrobial activity of pomegranate peel extract improves the shelf life of chicken products. *International Journal of Food Science and Technology,* 45, 216-222.

Karre, L. Keyla Lopez, K. and Getty, K. J. K. (2013). Natural antioxidants in meat and poultry products. *Meat Science,* 94, 220-227.

Kulkarni, A. P., Aradhya, S. M. and Divakar, S. (2003). Isolation and identification of a radical scavenging antioxidant-punicalagin from pith and carpellary membrane of pomegranate fruit. *Food Chemistry,* 87(4), 551-557.

Lecumberri, E., Mateos, R., Izquierdo-Pulido, M., Rupérez, P., Goya, L. and Bravo, L. (2007). Dietary fibre composition, antioxidant capacity and physico-chemical properties of a fibre-rich product from cocoa (Theobroma cacao L.). *Food Chemistry,* 104, 948-954.

Li, Y., Guo, C., Yang, J., Wei, J., Xu, J. and Cheng, S. (2006). Evaluation of antioxidant properties of pomegranate peel extract in comparison with pomegranate pulp extract. *Food Chemistry,* 96(2), 254-260.

Liu, H., Qiu, N., Ding, H., and Yao, R. (2008). Polyphenols contents and antioxidant capacity of 68 Chinese herbals suitable for medical or food uses. *Food Research International*, 41, 363-370.

Madrigal-Carballo, S., Rodriguez, G., Krueger, C. G., Dreher, M. and Reed, J. D. (2009). Pomegranate (Punica granatum L.) supplements: Authenticity, antioxidant and polyphenol composition. *Journal of Functional Foods,* 1, 324-329.

Meerts, I. A. T. M., Verspeek-Rip, C. M., Buskens, C. A. F., Keizer, H. G., Bassaganya-Riera, J., Jouni, Z. E., van Huygevoort, A. H. B. M., van Otterdijk, F. M. and van de Waart, E. J. (2009). Toxicological evaluation of pomegranate seed oil. *Food Chemistry and Toxicololy,* 47(6), 1085-1092.

Mirdehghan, S. H. and Rahemi, M. (2007). Seasonal changes of mineral nutrients and phenolics in pomegranate (Punica granatum L.) fruit. *Scientia Horticulturae,* 111(2), 120-127.

Mousavinejad, G., Emam-Djomeh, Z., Rezaei, K. and Khodaparast, M. H. H. (2009). Identification and quantification of phenolic compounds and their effects on antioxidant activity in pomegranate juices of eight Iranian cultivars. *Food Chemistry,* 115, 1274-1278.

Murthy, K. N. C., Jayaprakasha, G. K. and Singh, R. P. (2002). Studies on antioxidant activity of pomegranate (*Punica granatum*) peel extract using in vivo models. *Journal of Agricultural and Food Chemistry,* 50(17), 4791-4795.

Murthy, P. S. and Naidu, M. M. (2012). Recovery of Phenolic Antioxidants and Functional Compounds from Coffee Industry By-Products. *Food and Bioprocess Technology,* 5(3), 897-903.

Naveena, B. M., Sen, A. R., Kingsly, R. P., Singh, D. B. and Kondaiah, N. (2008). Antioxidant activity of pomegranate rind powder extract in cooked chicken patties. *International Journal of Food Science and Technology,* 43, 1807-1812.

Negi, P. S. and Jayaprakasha, G. K. (2003). Antioxidant and antibacterial activities of Punica granatum peel extracts. *Journal of Food Science,* 68, 1473-1477.

Okonogi, S., Duangrat, C., Anuchpreeda, S., Tachakittirungrod, S. and Chowwanapoonpohn, S. (2007). Comparison of antioxidant capacities and cytotoxicities of certain fruit peels. *Food Chemistry,* 103(3), 839-846.

Orak, H. H. (2009). Evaluation of antioxidant activity, colour and some nutritional characteristics of pomegranate (Punica granatum L.) juice and its sour concentrate processed by conventional evaporation. *International Journal of Food Science and Nutrition,* 60, 1-11.

Ozgen, M., Durgaç, C., Serçe, S. and Kaya, C. (2008). Chemical and antioxidant properties of pomegranate cultivars grown in the Mediterranean region of Turkey. *Food Chemistry,* 11(3), 703-706.

Pan, Z., Qu, W., Haile Ma, H., Atungulu, G. G. and McHugh, T. H. (2012). Continuous and pulsed ultrasound-assisted extractions of antioxidants from pomegranate peel. *Ultrasonics Sonochemistry,* 19, 365-372.

Pin-Der, D. (1998). Antioxidant activity of Budrock (Arctium lappa L.): its scavenging effects on free radical and active oxygen. *Journal of American Oil Chemistry Society,* 75, 455-461.

Plumb, G. W., de Pascual-Teresa, S., Santos-Buelga, C., Rivas-Gonzalo, J. C. and Williamson, G. (2002). Antioxidant properties of gallocatechin and prodelphinidins from pomegranate peel. *Redox Report,* 7, 41-46.

Poyrazoglu, E., Gökmen, V. and Artık, N. (2002). Organic acids and phenolic compounds in pomegranates (Punica granatum L.) grown in Turkey. *Journal of Food Composition and Analysis, 15*, 567-575.

Ramadan, A., El-Badrawey, S., Abd El-Ghany, M., *et al.* (2009). Rind and juice of pomegranate as natural antioxidants in cotton seed oil. The 5th Arab Annual Scientific Conference, Egypt, 8-9 April.

Ricci, D., Giamperi, L., Bucchini, A. and Fraternale D. (2006). Antioxidant activity of Punica granatum fruits. *Fitoterapia, 77*, 310-312.

Rosenblat, M., Volkova, N., Coleman, R., Aviram, M. (2006). Pomegranate by-product administration to apolipoprotein e-deficient mice attenuates atherosclerosis development as a result of decreased macrophage oxidative stress and reduced cellular uptake of oxidized low-density lipoprotein. *Journal of Agricultural and Food Chemistry*, 54, 1928-1935.

Rout, S. and Banerjee, R. (2007). Free radical scavenging, anti-glycation and tyrosinase inhibition properties of a polysaccharide fraction isolated from the rind from Punica granatum. *Bioresource Technology*, 98, 3159-3163.

Ruiz-Navajas, Y., Viuda-Martos, M., Pérez-Álvarez J. A., Sayas, E., Sendra, E. and Fernández-López, J. (2011). Effect of added pomegranate peel extract on the chemical and physic-chemical characteristics of a bologna sausage. In: Proceedings of 2011 EFFoST Annual Metting. Process-Structure-Function Relationships. pp: 3.49.

Saad, H., Charrier-El Bouhtoury, F., Pizzi, A., Rode, K., Charrier, B. and Ayed, N. (2012). Characterization of pomegranate peels tannin extractives. *Industrial Crops and Products*, 40, 239-246.

Sadeghi, N., Jannat, B., Oveisi, M. R., Hajimahmoodi, M. and Photovat, M. (2009). Antioxidant activity of Iranian pomegranate (Punica granatum L.) seed extracts. *Journal of Agricultural Science and Technology*, 11, 633-638.

Sagdic, O., Ozturk, I., Ekici, L., Simsek, H. and Yetim, H. (2010). Antioxidant, antiradical and antimicrobial potential of pomegranate seed and hull extracts. *Ernaehrung*, 34, 376-380.

Sebranek, J., and Bacus, J. (2007). Natural and organic cured meat products: Regulatory, manufacturing, marketing, quality and safety issues. American Meat Science Association. White Paper Series 1 (Retrieved March 24, 2009, from http://www.meatscience.org /pubs/White%20Papers/wp_001_2007_Natural_Organic_Cured_Meat.pdf).

Singh, R. P., Murthy, K. N. C. and Jayaprakasha, G. K. (2002). Studies on the antioxidant activity of pomegranate peel and seed extracts using in vitro models. *Journal of Agricultural and Food Chemistry*, 50, 81-86.

Surveswaran, S., Cai, Y. Z., Corke, H. and Sun, M. (2007). Systematic evaluation of natural phenolic antioxidants from 133 Indian medicinal plants. *Food Chemistry*, 102, 938-953.

Tabaraki, R., Heidarizadi, E. and Benvidi, A. (2012). Optimization of ultrasonic-assisted extraction of pomegranate (Punica granatum L.) peel antioxidants by response surface methodology. *Separation and Purification Technology*, 98, 16-23.

Tezcan, F., Gültekin-Özgüven, M., Diken, T., Özçelik, B. and Erim, F. B. (2009). Antioxidant activity and total phenolic, organic acid and sugar content in commercial pomegranate juices. *Food Chemistry*, 115(3), 873-877.

Trinidad, T., Mallillin, A. Valdez, D. Loyola, A. Askali, F. Castillo, J. Encabo, R. Masa, D. Maglaya, A. andChua, M. (2006). Dietary fiber from coconut flour: a functional food. *Innovative Food Science and Emerging Technologies,* 7(4), 309-317.

Tzulker, R., Glazer, I., Bar-Ilan, I., Holland, D., Aviram, M. and Amir, R. (2007). Antioxidant activity, polyphenol content, and related compounds in different fruit juices and homogenates prepared from 29 different pomegranate accessions. *Journal of Agricultural and Food Chemistry,* 55, 9559-9570.

Vági, E., Simándi, B., Vásárhelyiné, K. P., Daood, H., Kéry, A., Doleschall, F. and Nagya, B. (2007). Supercritical carbon dioxide extraction of carotenoids, tocopherols and sitosterols from industrial tomato by-products. *Journal of Supercritical Fluid,* 40, 218-226.

Vergara-Valencia, N., Granados-Pérez, E., Agama-Acevedo, E., Tovar, J., Ruales, J., and Bello-Pérez, L. A. (2007). Fibre concentrate from mango fruit: Characterization, associated antioxidant capacity and application as a bakery product ingredient. *LWT-Food Science and Technology,* 40(4), 722-729.

Vidal, A., Fallarero, A., Pena, B. R., Medina, M. E., Gra, B., Rivera, F., Gutierrez, Y. and Vuorela, P. M. (2003). Studies on the toxicity of Punica granatum L. (Punicaceae) whole fruit extracts. *Journal of Ethnopharmacology,* 89, 295-300.

Viuda-Martos, M., Ruiz-Navajas, Y., Fernández-López, J., Pérez-Álvarez, J. A. (2009). Effect of adding citrus waste water, thyme and oregano essential oil on the chemical, physical and sensory characteristics of a bologna sausage. *Innovative Food Science and Emerging Technology,* 10, 655-660.

Viuda-Martos, M., Fernández-López, J. and Pérez-Alvarez, J. A. (2010). Pomegranate and its many functional components as related to human health: a review. *Comprehensive Reviews in Food Science and Food Safety,* 9, 635-654.

Viuda-Martos, M., Ruiz-Navajas, Y., Fernández-López, J., Sendra, E., Sayas-Barberá, E. and Pérez-Álvarez, J. A. (2011). Antioxidant properties of pomegranate (*Punica granatum* L.) bagasses obtained as co-product in the juice extraction. *Food Research International,* 44, 1217-1223.

Viuda-Martos, M., Ruiz-Navajas, Y., Martin-Sánchez, A., Sánchez-Zapata, E., Fernández-López, J., Sendra, E., Sayas-Barberá, E., Navarro, C. and Pérez-Álvarez, J. A. (2012a). Chemical, physico-chemical and functional properties of pomegranate (Punica granatum L.) bagasses powder co-product. *Journal of Food Engineering,* 110, 220-224.

Viuda-Martos, M., Sánchez-Zapata, E., Martin-Sánchez, A. M., Ruiz-Navajas, Y. Fernández-López, J., Sendra. E., Sayas-Barberá E., Navarro C. and Pérez Álvarez J.A. (2012b). Technological properties of pomegranate (Punica granatum L.) peel extract obtained as co-product in the juice processing. In: Dietary Fiber and Health. CRC Press; Taylor and Francis Inc. Boca Ratón, USA. pp. 433-442.

Viuda-Martos, M., Pérez-Álvarez, J. A., Sendra, E. and Fernández-López, J. (2012c), In vitro antioxidant properties of pomegranate (Punica granatum) peel powder extract obtained as coproduct in the juice extraction process. *Journal of Food Processing and Preservation.* doi: 10.1111/j.1745-4549.2012.00715.x.

Zahin, M., Aqil, F. and Ahmad, I. (2010). Broad spectrum antimutagenicactivity of antioxidant active fraction of *Punica granatum* L. peel extracts. *Mutation Research/Genetic Toxicology and Environmental Mutagenesis,* 703, 99-107.

Zhang, L., Zhang, Y. and Yang X. (2010). Antioxidant effects on oil and antibacterial activities of extracts from different parts of pomegranate. *Zhongguo Liangyou Xuebao,* 25, 38-42.

Zhang L., Li L., Li Y., Zhang Y. (2008). In vitro antioxidant activities of fruits and leaves of pomegranate. *Acta Horticulturae,* 765, 31-36 (2008).

In: Dietary Fiber
Editors: D. Betancur-Ancona, L. Chel-Guerrero et al.
ISBN: 978-1-62808-931-8

Chapter 8

Characterization and Functionality of By-Products from Chia (*Salvia hispanica* L.) Seeds of Argentina

Marianela I. Capitani[1,2]***, Susana M. Nolasco***[2]
and Mabel C. Tomás[1,*]
[1]Centro de Investigación y Desarrollo en Criotecnología de Alimentos (CIDCA) (UNLP-CCT-CONICET), La Plata, Buenos Aires, Argentina;
[2]TECSE, Facultad de Ingeniería, Departamento de Ing. Química, (UNCPBA), Olavarría, Buenos Aires, Argentina

Abstract

The aim of this chapter was to characterize the physicochemical and functional properties of meals (M) and fibrous and protein fractions (FRF and PRF, respectively) of chia seeds, and to compare the effect of oil extraction methods (cold pressing -p- and solvent -s- extraction) and sieving processes on these properties. Both methods affected the properties of meals and their corresponding residual fractions. Mp, FRFp and PRFp showed a significantly higher residual oil content than Ms, FRFs and PRFs (11.39, 10.85, 13.40, 0.21, 0.21 and 0.31% dry basis, respectively).

After sieving both meals, two fractions were obtained: one retained on the sieve mesh, with an increase in fiber content, and the other one with an increase in protein content.

Total dietary fiber and its respective components (soluble and insoluble dietary fiber) were significantly higher in FRF than in the other samples. All samples exhibited a high antioxidant activity. By-products of the solvent extraction process exhibited better functional properties than those corresponding to cold-pressing extraction. The physicochemical and functional properties of chia by-products make them important ingredients for the food industry (formulation and development of various products) and,

[*] E-mail: mabtom@hotmail.com.

from the physiological standpoint, for the prevention of diseases such as cholesterol, diabetes and constipation.

Introduction

Chia (*Salvia hispanica* L.) is an annual herbaceous plant that belongs to the Lamiaceae family, which is native to southern Mexico and northern Guatemala. Chia seed, as well as corn, amaranth and beans were the basis of the diet of many pre-Columbian civilizations in America (Ayerza and Coates, 2005). With time its use was abandoned, but by the end of last century research on chia became more relevant due to its content and quality of oil (25-38%), mainly of α-linolenic acid (~60%), dietary fiber (~40%, with 5% of soluble dietary fiber), proteins (15-25%), minerals and vitamins (Bushway and Belya, 1981; Weber et al. 1991; Ixtaina et al. 2011). Today, chia is grown commercially in Mexico, Bolivia, Argentina, Ecuador and Guatemala.

In Argentina, it is a summer-autumn crop that could be grown commercially instead of as a non-profitable traditional crop in the north-western region. After oil extraction from the chia seeds, a by-product is obtained (residue meal) with an important content of fiber, proteins and other compounds with antioxidant activity, such as flavonols (myricetin, quercetin, kaempferol) and cinnamic acids (caffeic and chlorogenic acids) (Taga et al. 1984). It also exhibits some interesting functional properties for its use in the food industry (Capitani et al. 2012). Functional properties are generally associated with the presence of proteins (Badui, 1999) and also of dietary fiber (Chau and Huang, 2003; Wong and Cheung, 2005; Raghavendra et al. 2006).

The functional properties of food components can be defined as any physicochemical property that affects some of its characteristics and that contributes to the quality of the final product. Knowledge on functional properties such as water-holding, absorption and adsorption capacity, as well as those linked to the affinity for lipid components is useful for the food industry because during the food processing some modifications can occur that must be taken into account according to the end use of the product and marketing conditions (Zambrano et al. 2001). Thus, fibers are added to cooked meat products in order to increase the cooking yield due to their water and lipid retention properties. On the other hand, in fried food products, the addition of fiber reduces lipid retention and increases moisture content (Raghavendra et al. 2006). The *in vitro* determination of these properties could provide information on its potential use, and complementary *in vivo* tests would enable to study its possible positive correlation with the intestinal functionality from a physiological viewpoint (Zambrano et al. 2001).

The need to find new sources of high-fiber or protein products lies in the health benefits associated with them. For example, supplements with high fiber content are recommended in the treatment of irritable bowel syndrome to improve intestinal transit (Singh et al. 2008). It has also been found that rich-fiber and rich-protein products help reduce by 12.8% the plasma levels of low-density lipoproteins (LDL) cholesterol, and by 12.3% glucose levels (Aller et al. 2004). For obtaining products with a high content of certain component various methods and processes exist, which can affect the properties of the raw material. One disadvantage of wet separation treatments is the loss of soluble proteins (Bergthaller et al. 2001), as well as the structural changes of some components, for example the loss of phenolic compounds. On the other hand, dry fractionation has been used to obtain starches and proteins from legumes (Otto et al. 1997). The main advantage of this type of fractionation is the simplicity of the process, along with the lower or no use of water or other solvents, generating no effluents or residues. The search for protein-rich sources has led to the development of protein concentrates (≈ 70% dry basis, d.b.), protein isolates (> 90%) and protein-rich fractions (with a higher content than whole-wheat flower) (Endres, 1989). In general, proteins are separated based on differences in some properties, such as relative molecular mass, relative charge, affinity for other molecules, degrees of solubility and particle size (Mathews and Van Holde, 1990). Based on the latter characteristic, it is possible to use a method of physical separation to obtain a protein-rich fraction by fluidization or sieving the meal (Endres, 1989).

Dietary fiber (DF) consists of a heterogeneous mixture of compounds that are classified according to their physical properties and effects of their intake into soluble dietary fiber (SDF) and insoluble dietary fiber (IDF) (Gorinstein et al., 2001), referring to the solubility of fibers in water. Plant secretions (pectins and gums), components such as mucilage, and chelating agents such as phytates are sources of SDF, whereas cellulose, lignin, some fractions of hemicellulose, phenolic compounds such as tannins and lipid structures such as waxes, suberins and cutins constitute IDF. Given the capacity of SDF to form gels, it increases the viscosity of the bolus in the gastrointestinal tract, slowing the intestinal transit, thus making digestion and the absorption of nutrients more efficient, providing more of a feeling of satiety. Soluble fibers are fermentable fibers that can be microbiologically decomposed in the colon, producing gases such as carbon dioxide, hydrogen and methane, and short-chain fatty acids (acetic, propionic and butyric acid) which are absorbed and used as energy sources, being one of the most important beneficial effects of SDF that it regulates blood sugar and lowers cholesterol levels. On the other hand, IDF is responsible for adding bulk to the stool, speeding the passage of stool through the intestine by promoting peristalsis, alleviating constipation and other gastrointestinal disorders (McDougall et al. 1996). In addition, both types of fiber may reduce the risk of obesity, hypertension, appendicitis, and other disorders (Rehinan et al. 2004). The beneficial effects noted above show the important role that DF plays in human diet. That is why a daily intake of 25-30 g is recommended, with a good SDF/IDF balance (a minimum of 30% SDF and 70% IDF, optimum 50/50 ratio) in order to benefit from both fractions of fiber (Saura-Calixto et al. 2002).

The aim of this study was to characterize the physicochemical and functional properties of meals (M) and fibrous and protein fractions (FRF and PRF, respectively) of chia seeds, and to compare the effect of oil extraction methods (cold pressing -p- and solvent -s- extraction) and sieving processes on these properties.

Materials and Methods

Seeds

Commercial chia seeds used in this work were obtained in Salta (25° south and 65.5° west), Argentina (10 kg). Seeds were packed in hermetic plastic containers and stored at 5° C until further use.

Meals

Meals were obtained as by-products of two oil extraction methods:

Solvent Extraction

Meal (Ms) was obtained after oil solvent extraction (n-hexane) in a Soxhlet apparatus (Buenos Aires, Argentina) by thermal cycles at 80 °C for 8 h, following the IUPAC standard method (1992), from chia seeds previously ground in a laboratory grinding mill (Moulinex, horizontal blade grinder, Buenos Aires Argentina) at 424 μm.

Pressing Extraction

Seeds were pressed at 25-30 °C using a Komet screw press (Model CA 59 G, IBG Monforts, Mönchengladbach, Germany) with a 5-mm restriction dye and a screw speed of 20 rpm. The screw press was first run for 15 min without seed material, but with heating via an electrical resistance-heating ring attached around the press barrel to raise the screw press barrel temperature to the desired temperature (25 ± 2 °C). Running temperature was checked with a digital thermometer inserted in the restriction dye. The meal obtained by pressing (Mp) was ground with a laboratory grinding mill (Moulinex, horizontal blade grinder, Buenos Aires, Argentina) at 498 μm.

Meals from both extraction methods (Ms and Mp) were homogenized and stored in plastic containers at 5 °C until further use.

Fibrous and Protein Fractions of Chia

The fibrous and protein fractions were obtained by dry fractionation of defatted meals (Vázquez-Ovando et al. 2010). The meals (Ms and Mp) were sieved in a Zonitest agitator (Buenos Aires, Argentina) using a 100 ASTM mesh (149 μm) for 20 min. The material retained by the sieve was considered rich in fiber (FRFs and FRFp, respectively), while the fraction passing through the sieve was considered rich in protein (PRFs and PRFp, respectively).

Characterization of Meals and Fibrous and Protein Fractions

Proximate Composition

Moisture, crude fiber and ash content were determined according to AOCS recommended practices Ba 2^a-38, Ba 6-84 and Ba 5^a-49, respectively (AOCS, 1998). Oil and nitrogen content (N) were determined following IUPAC standard method (1992) and AOAC method (1997), respectively. Protein content was calculated as nitrogen x 6.25. Carbohydrate content was estimated by calculating the nitrogen-free extract (NFE) by difference using Eq. (1).

$$NFE : 100 - (oil + protein + crude\ fiber + ash) \quad (Eq.\ 1)$$

Total, Soluble and Insoluble Dietary fiber

Total dietary fiber (TDF), soluble dietary fiber (SDF) and insoluble dietary fiber (IDF) were determined according the enzymatic gravimetric method (Prosky et al. 1988).

Neutral Detergent Fiber (NDF), Acid Detergent Fiber (ADF), Lignin, Cellulose and Hemicelluloses

The vegetable cell was separated into two parts (Van Soest method): cell content (highly digestible) and cell wall (partially digestible). The cell wall was analyzed and its components (cellulose, hemicelluloses and lignin) were determined. The technique uses acidic and neutral detergent (AOAC, 1997, method 973.18; Guiragossian et al. 1979).

Minerals

Calcium, magnesium, iron, copper and zinc were measured by flame atomic absorption spectrophotometry using a GBC 902 atomic absorption spectrometer (GBC Scientific Equipment, Victoria, Australia). Samples were mineralized (550 °C 2 h) to obtain carbon free white ashes. Ashes were dissolved in chlorhydric acid, filtered and analyzed. Results were expressed as mg/kg meals or fibrous and protein fractions.

Phosphorus content was determined following AOCS method Ca 12-55 (1998). This method determines phosphorus or equivalent phosphatide content by ashing the sample in the presence of zinc oxide, followed by the spectrometric measurement of phosphorus as a blue phosphomolybdic acid complex.

Antioxidant Activity

The extraction of phenolic compounds was carried out according to the method of Re et al. (1999). Ten mL ethanol were added to 1 g sample, then it was homogenized in Vortex for 2 min, decanted and filtered (0.45 μm nylon paper). The supernatant was transferred into a flask and evaporated using a rotavapor apparatus (BUCHI R124, Germany) to concentrate the sample. It was then redissolved in 1000 μL ethanol.

A spectrophotometric method was used to determine the antioxidant activity using a Hitachi U-1900 UVeVIS spectrophotometer (Japan). The antioxidant activity was quantified by a dying assay of the radical cation $ABTS^+$ measuring $ABTS^+$ reduction as the percentage of absorption inhibition at 734 nm, just 6 min later. The radical cation ABTS and potassium persulfate were obtained from Sigma Aldrich. Chlorogenic acid was used as standard antioxidant. Results were expressed as μmol/L Trolox g/sample, considering that chlorogenic acid diminishes twice the amount of absorption than Trolox (Walker and Everette, 2009).

Functional Properties

Water-Holding (WHC) and Oil-Holding Capacity (OHC)

Water and oil holding capacities were determined according to the method of Chau et al. (1997). Briefly, 1 g sample (dry basis (d.b.)) was weighed and then stirred into 10 mL distilled water or corn oil (density 0.92 g/mL, Arcor). These suspensions were centrifuged at

2200 x g for 30 min (Rolco Centrifuge Refrigerate, Model CR-5850, 22 cm radius, Buenos Aires, Argentina) and the supernatant volumes were measured. Water-holding capacity was expressed as gram water held per gram sample, and oil-holding capacity as gram oil held per gram sample.

Water Adsorption Capacity (WAdC)

This property was determined according to the method of Chen et al. (1984). Briefly, 1 g (d.b.) sample was placed in an equilibrium micro-environment at 98% relative humidity, generated by placing 20 mL saturated potassium sulfate saline solution and placing these in oven at 25 °C until constant weight. Water adsorption capacity was expressed as g water per g sample.

Water Absorption Capacity (WAbC)

This property was determined according to the AACC method 88-04 (1984). Approximate water absorption capacity was first determined by weighing out 2 g sample (d.b.), adding water until saturation (approx. 35 mL) and centrifuging at 2000 x g for 10 min in a Rolco centrifuge Model CR-5850. Approximate water absorption capacity was calculated by dividing the increase in sample weight (g) by the initial weight, quantifying the water needed to complete the original sample weight (2 g d.b.) to 15 g. Water absorption capacity (WAbC) was then determined by placing samples in four tubes, adding different amounts of water (1.5 and 0.5 mL water above original weight, and 1.5 and 0.5 mL water below; one in each tube), agitating vigorously, and centrifuging the samples at 2000 x g for 10 min in a Rolco centrifuge model CR 5850. The supernatant was discarded and the residue weighed. Average water absorbed was calculated, and WAbC was determined and expressed as gram water absorbed per gram sample.

Organic Molecule Absorption Capacity (OMAC)

This capacity was determined according to the method of Zambrano et al. (2001). A three gram (d b.) sample was placed in excess corn oil (approx. 25 mL) for 24 h at room temperature, and then centrifuged at 2000 x g for 15 min in a Rolco centrifuge model CR-5850. OMAC was expressed as the absorbed hydrophobic component and calculated in terms of sample weight gain (g oil/sample g).

Emulsifying Activity (EA) and Emulsion Stability (ES)

These properties were evaluated according to the method of Chau et al. (1997). Briefly, 100 mL 2 g/100 mL suspension was homogenized using an Ultra-Turrax T25 disperser (Janke & Kunkel, IKA-Labortechnik, Germany) at 7800 rpm for 2 min. Then, 100 mL corn oil (density 0.92 g/mL, Arcor) were added and homogenized at 15,000 rpm for 2 min. Emulsions were centrifuged in a 15 mL graduated centrifuge tube at 455 x g for 10 min, and then the emulsion volume was measured. The EA was expressed as the remaining volume of the centrifuged emulsion corresponding to 100 mL of initial emulsion. The emulsion stability was determined by heating the emulsions to 80 °C for 30 min, cooling them to room temperature and then centrifuging the samples at 455 g for 10 min. ES was expressed as the remaining volume of the centrifuged emulsion corresponding to 100 mL of initial emulsion. On the other hand, all emulsions were evaluated by optical characterization using a Vertical Scan

Analyzer (QuickSCAN, Beckman Coulter, Fullerton, USA). The QuickSCAN head scans the entire length of the sample (approximately 65 mm), collecting backscattering (BS) data every 40μm. Thus, it is possible to obtain curves showing the percentage of backscattering light flux, relative to external standards, as a function of the sample height in mm (Pan et al. 2002). Coalescence kinetics was determined by measuring the mean values of BS as a function of time in the 25-30 mm zone (Backscattering % 25-30 mm).

Statistical Analysis

The obtained results were analyzed with ANOVA and Tukey's test ($p \leq 0.05$), using Infostat software (2004).

Results and Discussion

The process of oil extraction from chia seeds generated 75.2±0.5% (d.b.) residual meal by cold-pressing (Mp) and 80.8±0.3% (d.b.) residual meal by solvent extraction (Ms). The sieving procedure yielded 79.9±0.8 and 85.8±0.5% of fibrous fractions (FRFs and FRFp, respectively) with a particle size > 149 μm, and 20.1±0.7 and 14.2±0.5% of protein-rich fractions (PRFs and PRFp, respectively), with a particle size < 149 μm.

The proximate composition of the chia by-products from both extraction methods (pressing and solvent) is shown in Figure 1.

Both meals (Mp and Ms) exhibited a high percentage of protein and crude fiber, with significantly higher levels in Ms ($p<0.05$). Ms presented a higher crude fiber content that that reported for sesame, soybean, linseed and canola meals, but similar to that of Mexican chia meal, in all the cases obtained by the same method. The protein content for Ms was higher than that reported for sunflower meals, and similar to that of canola and linseed meals (Table 1). As regards the meals obtained by cold-pressing extraction, Mp exhibited a higher protein content than that observed for canola meal, and similar to that of linseed meal (Table 1).

The lipid content in the studied chia meals was significantly higher ($p<0.05$) in Mp (Figure 1), indicating that the oil extraction method affected the level of residual oil in the meals. Similar results were observed in meals obtained following cold-pressing and solvent extraction from a range of linseed varieties (Table 1).

The fractions obtained from the meals presented significant differences ($p<0.05$) among their main components, except for lipid content in the Ms fractions and nitrogen-free extracts in the Mp fractions. In the coarse fractions (FRFp and FRFs), the crude fiber content increased by 6 and 19%, respectively, with respect to that of the meals, at the expense of a decrease, in protein content. In contrast, in the fine fractions the protein content increased by 53 and 30% (PRFs and PRFp, respectively) with respect to that of the meals. Coarse fractions are rich in fiber, and fine fractions are rich in protein (Figure 1).

Thus, the sieving of the meals allowed to retain structural carbohydrates present in the cell wall of the vegetables, as well as the transfer of components of the cell content (Pérez, 2001). A similar behavior was observed following the dry fractionation of defatted meal of Mexican chia, by which two fractions were obtained: a fiber-rich fraction with a level of crude fiber similar to FRFs, and a protein-rich fraction with a lower content than PRFs (Table 1).

It must be noted that the oil extraction method used to obtain the chia meals affected the residual lipid content in both the fiber-rich and protein-rich fractions, but the fractions corresponding to cold-pressing extraction exhibited a higher level of residual lipids (Figure 1).

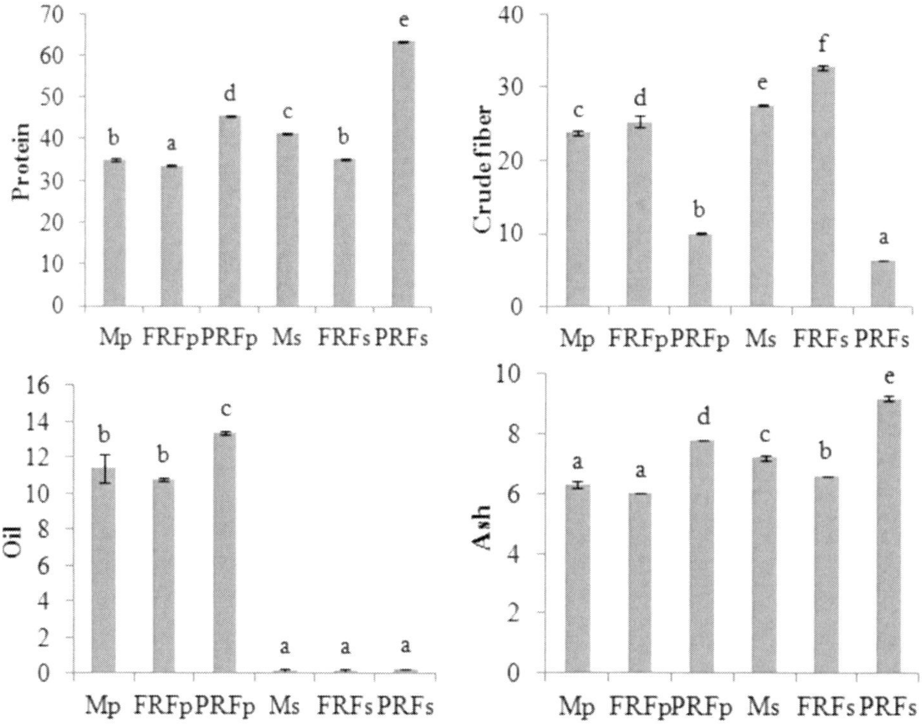

Figure 1. Proximate composition of chia (*Salvia hispanica* L.) by-products. Values followed by different letters indicate significant differences among the samples ($p<0.05$).

Table 1. Chemical composition (g/100 g) of meals of different seed varieties

Species	Protein	Crude fiber	Oil	References
Canola meal -p	30.5		26.4	Sun et al. (2008)
Linseed meal -p	36.9 – 40.9		7.5 - 12.4	Mueller et al. (2010)
Beniseed meal -s	48.8	5.8	10.9	Egbekun and Ehieze (1997)
Canola meal -s	36.1 - 40	11.5	1.1–2.8	Sun et al. (2008); Khattab and Arntfiel (2009)
Chia meal -s	32.2	26.5	0.45	Vázquez-Ovando et al. (2010)
Linseed meal -s	38.9 –43.3	5.3	1.1–2.2	Khattab and Arntfiel (2009); Mueller et al. (2010)
Soybean meal -s	48.3	3.5	1.6	Khattab and Arntfiel (2009)
Sunflower meal -s	37.8		0.8	Pacheco de Delahaye et al. (1994)
Mexican FRF -s	28.1	29.6	0.5	Vázquez-Ovando et al. (2010)
Mexican PRF -s	44.6	11.5	0.5	Vázquez-Ovando et al. (2010)

-p: oil extraction by cold-pressing; -s: solvent extraction.

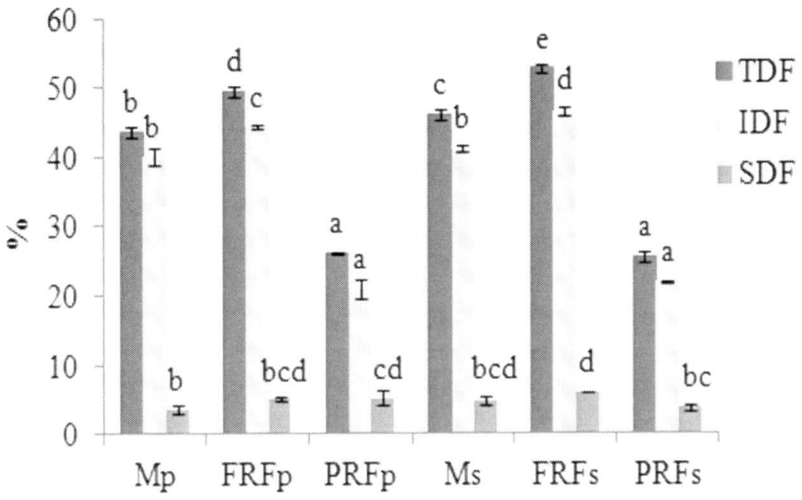

Figure 2. Total dietary fiber (TDF), insoluble dietary fiber (IDF) and soluble dietary fiber (SDF) content in chia by-products (g/100g d.b.). Values followed by different letters indicate significant differences among the samples for each type of fiber ($p<0.05$).

The analysis of the total (TDF), insoluble (IDF) and soluble (SDF) dietary fiber of the chia by-products showed that all the samples presented a high content of TDF, consisting mainly of IDF, compared to a SDF content of 3.5-6% (Figure 2).

The fiber-rich fractions presented a significantly higher ($p<0.05$) TDF and IDF content than the rest of the samples, with the highest values being observed for FRFs. The obtained results reveal that the dry fractionation process using a 100 ASTM mesh could efficiently concentrate the TDF content. In contrast, in the protein-rich fractions the TDF and IDF content was significantly lower than in the rest of the samples. These results are in agreement with the data obtained by the method proposed by Van Soest regarding NDF, consisting mainly of cellulose, hemicellulose and lignin (structural polysaccharides that contribute to the IDF fraction), which were significantly higher in the meals and fiber-rich fractions (Table 2). The ADF content (a less digestible portion of DF, made of cellulose, lignin and acid-insoluble ash) was significantly higher in the meals and FRF, with similar values to those reported for Jack bean residues (30.72%, Betancur-Ancona et al. 2004). Regarding lignin content, significant differences ($p<0.05$) were observed between the fibrous fractions, with a higher level in FRFp. The content of cellulose and hemicellulose in the meals and FRF could indicate that the cell walls were made mainly of cellulose-hemicellulose complexes, and therefore had a low pectin content, as is usually the case with the cell walls of most monocotyledons (Vázquez-Ovando et al. 2010). The FRFs exhibited significantly lower levels of cellulose compared to Ms.

The insoluble and soluble dietary fiber composition presented by the fibrous fractions were in the range of those reported for a fibrous residue of Mexican chia and a fibrous residue of Jack bean, although they were higher than those reported for oat bran and wheat bran, and lower (mainly in SDF content) than that of various fruits and vegetables (Table 3).

The intake of appropriate amounts of dietary fiber is associated with the prevention of diseases such as hypercholesterolemia, diabetes, colon cancer and obesity, among others (Lecumberri et al. 2007). The relation between IDF and SDF is important due to its nutritional and physiological effects. The American Diabetes Association recommends consuming 25-30 g of dietary fiber per day, with an IDF/SDF balance of 3 to 1 (Borderías et al. 2005). In the studied chia by-products, this ratio varied in the range between 4 and 11, with the lower values corresponding to the protein-rich fractions.

In all the by-products it was possible to detect phosphorus, calcium, magnesium, iron, zinc and copper, with the first three minerals being present in a higher proportion (Figure 3). It was also observed that the protein-rich fractions presented a higher concentration of minerals, except for Ca, which had lower values in those samples. The calcium/phosphorus ratio (Ca:P) was in the range 0.49-.79 for all the studied samples, with the lower value corresponding to FRFp and the higher to Ms. For an effective use in ruminant nutrition and to avoid potential nutritional disorders, the Ca:P ratio should range between 1:1 and 2:1. It is also necessary to consider that normally 20-30% of calcium in the diet is absorbed, and that this absorption is affected by other food components such as proteins, fiber, phytic acid and phosphorus (Mota-Blancas and Perales-Caldera, 1999). In view of the above, the obtained results suggest that the analyzed chia by-products could be used as supplements in meals of other cereals due to the high Ca content. Given that all the cases exhibited high levels of DF, it would be necessary to perform an analysis of dialyzability to obtain further information on the bioavailability of this mineral (Kernefick and Cashman, 2000).

Table 2. Composition of chia by-products according to the Van Soest method, expressed as (g/100 g d.b.)

Sample	NDF	ADF	Lignin	Cellulose	Hemicellulose
Mp	59.3 ± 3.3^{cd}	32.3 ± 2.4^{bc}	7.5 ± 0.1^{d}	22.0 ± 1.8^{b}	30.3 ± 2.0^{c}
FRFp	$62{,}2 \pm 2.1^{d}$	35.0 ± 0.3^{bcd}	8.1 ± 0.2^{d}	25.9 ± 1.4^{bc}	29.9 ± 0.6^{c}
PRFp	30.8 ± 2.0^{b}	12.0 ± 0.2^{a}	3.3 ± 0.1^{a}	9.9 ± 0.3^{a}	18.0 ± 0.2^{b}
Ms	52.9 ± 0.3^{c}	38.1 ± 1.2^{d}	4.5 ± 0.7^{ab}	34.6 ± 1.3^{d}	14.8 ± 1.2^{b}
FRFs	65.0 ± 0.1^{d}	35.5 ± 0.0^{cd}	5.5 ± 0.5^{bc}	28.2 ± 0.4^{c}	31.3 ± 0.0^{c}
PRFs	15.8 ± 0.4^{a}	9.9 ± 0.2^{a}	3.0 ± 0.2^{a}	7.6 ± 0.0^{a}	5.9 ± 0.2^{a}

Values followed by different letters indicate significant differences among the samples ($p<0.05$).

Table 3. Total dietary fiber (TDF), insoluble dietary fiber (IDF) and soluble dietary fiber (SDF) content of different fibrous residues (g/100 g d.b.)

Species	TDF	IDF	SDF	References
Apple fruit	60.1	46.3	13.8	Grigelmo-Miguel and Martín-Belloso (1999)
Artichoke	58.8	44.5	14.3	Grigelmo-Miguel and Martín-Belloso (1999)
Asparagus	49.0	38.6	10.4	Grigelmo-Miguel and Martín-Belloso (1999)
Mexican FRF -s	56.5	53.4	3.0	Vázquez-Ovando et al. (2009)
FRF Jack bean	55.9	52.5	3.4	Betancur-Ancona et al. (2004)
Guava fruit	64.1	55.2	8.9	Chau and Huang (2003)
Oat bran	23.8	20.2	3.6	Grigelmo-Miguel and Martín-Belloso (1999)
Passion fruit	57.0	47.6	9.4	Chau and Huang (2003)
Wheat bran	44.0	41.1	2.9	Grigelmo-Miguel and Martín-Belloso (1999)

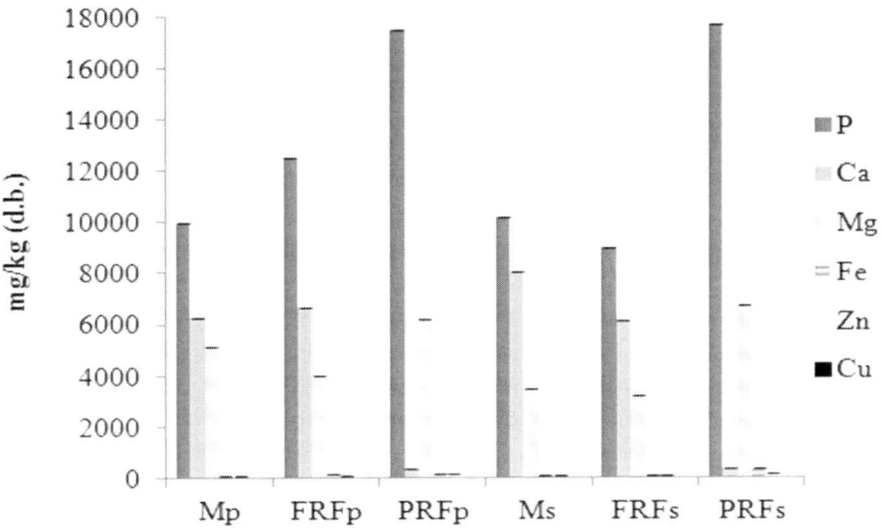

Figure 3. Mineral content in chia (*Salvia hispanica* L.) by-products.

The antioxidant activity of the chia by-products is shown in Figure 4. All the by-products exhibited a high antioxidant activity, a fact that could be associated with the presence of polyphenolic compounds. Capitani et al. (2012) found chlorogenic and caffeic acids, quercetin, myricetin and kaempferol in Ms, FRFs, Mp and FRFp, with a total concentration of polyphenolic components in the range between 3.3 x 10^{-4} and 5.7 x 10^{-4} mol/kg (in Ms and Mp, respectively). In addition, Mp, FRFp and PRFp presented a higher antioxidant activity than Ms, FRFs and PRFs. This behavior could be attributed to the higher residual lipid content present in the samples obtained by cold-pressing extraction, which contain tocopherols (natural substances with antioxidant activity) (Capitani et al. 2012).

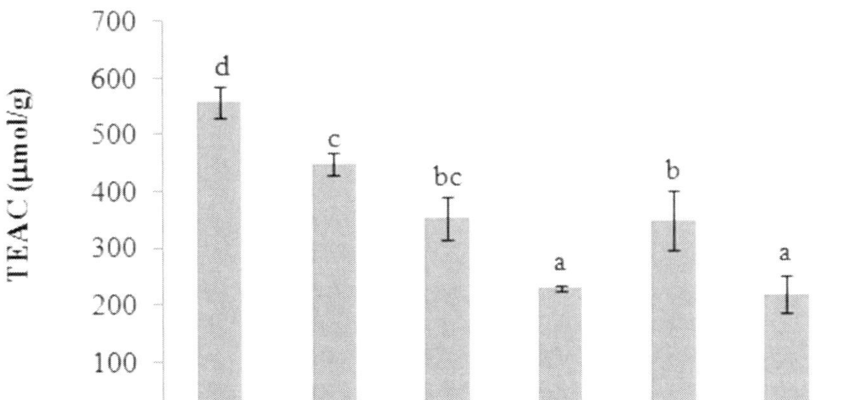

Figure 4. Antioxidant activity of the chia by-products obtained by both oil extractions methods, determined by a dying assay of the radical cation ABTS+ (TEAC, μmol/g). Values followed by different letters indicate significant differences among the samples ($p<0.05$).

Table 4. Antioxidant activity of different species

Species	Trolox equivalent antioxidant activity (TEAC, μmol/g)	References
Mexican FRFs	488.8	Vázquez-Ovando et al. (2009)
Oat meal	14.9	Ragaee et al. (2006)
Sorghum meal	51.7	Ragaee et al. (2006)
Wheat bran	48.5	Iqbal et al. (2005)

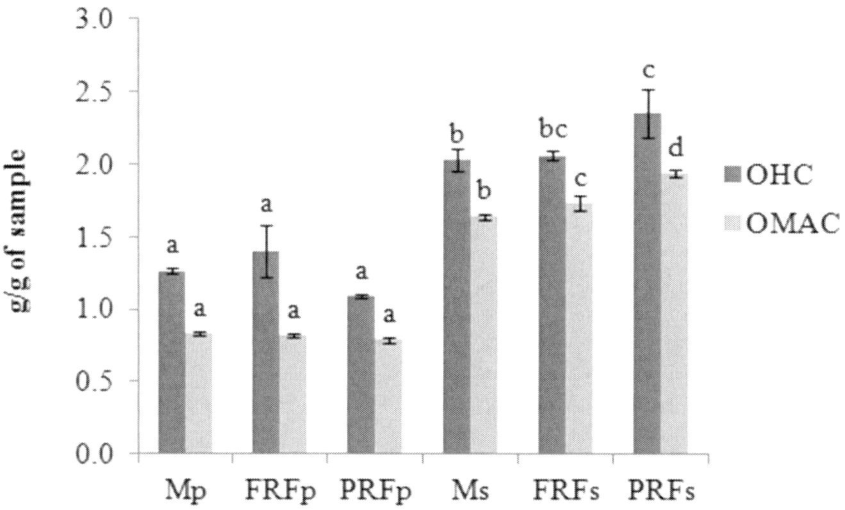

Figure 5. Oil holding (OHC) and organic absorption (OMAC) capacities of chia (*Salvia hispanica* L.) by-products. Values followed by different letters indicate significant differences among the samples, for each property ($p<0.05$).

The antioxidant activity of the studied by-products was higher than that reported for wheat bran and sorghum and barley whole grain meals, and similar to that of a fibrous fraction of Mexican chia (Table 4).

Regarding the functional properties of the studied chia by-products, the main differences between the solvent-extracted samples (Ms, FRFs and PRFs) and the pressing-extracted samples (Mp, FRFp and PRFp) were found for the properties related to the affinity for oil (OHC and OMAC) (Figure 5), which were significantly higher ($p<0.05$) in the samples from solvent extraction. This behavior could be attributed to the higher level of proteins and lipids associated with solvent and pressing extraction, respectively (see Figure 1).

The functional properties relating to water affinity are presented in Figure 6. In general, these properties exhibit high levels, WHC being higher than WAbC, indicating that the material retains almost all the absorbed water (Robertson et al. 1981; Chen et al. 1984). The high capacity of the chia by-products to retain water could be associated with the presence of mucilaginous substances, which act as SDF.

In this sense, chia by-products could be added to various foods given the capacity of SDF to retain water and provide a greater feeling of satiety, as well as to decrease the nutrient absorption time (Scheneeman, 1987).

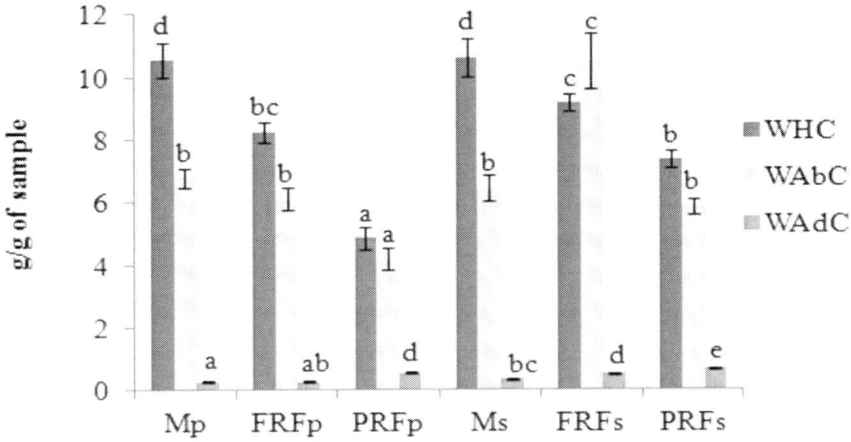

Figure 6. Water holding (WHC), absorption (WAbC) and adsorption (WAdC) capacities of chia (*Salvia hispanica* L.) by-products. Values followed by different letters indicate significant differences among the samples, for each property ($p<0.05$).

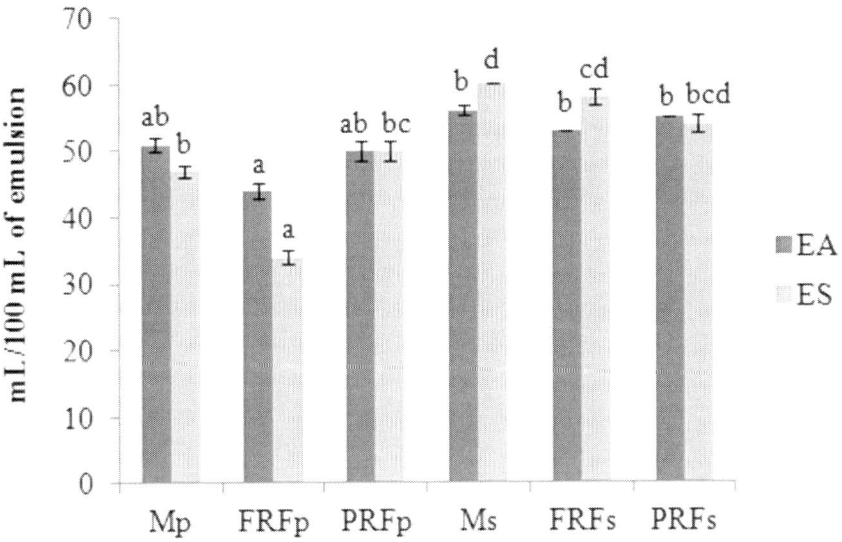

Figure 7. Emulsifying activity (EA) and emulsion stability (ES) of chia (*Salvia hispanica* L.) by-products. Values followed by different letters indicate significant differences among the samples, for each property ($p<0.05$).

Even though differences were observed in general between the functional properties of the meals and those of the corresponding fiber-rich and protein-rich fractions, the sieving process did not generate a clear tendency in those properties, except in the case of WHC. This property was significantly higher in meals than in FRF and PRF, and in turn higher in FRF than in PRF. This could be explained by the particle size of the samples, because as the particle size increases, the water holding capacity also increases (Borroto et al. 1995). On the other hand, it is worth noting that WHC could be affected by certain experimental parameter such as agitation, temperature, soaking time and magnitude of the external force applied, as well as chemical conditions of the medium (pH, ionic force). These factors can alter the physical structure of the fiber source, generating important changes on this property (Sangnark and Noomhorm, 2003). The by-products corresponding to solvent extraction presented a higher capacity to hold water than the pressing-extracted by-products, which could be attributed to the lower residual lipid content and higher protein content of the solvent extraction samples.

The EA and ES were higher in the by-products corresponding to oil solvent extraction (Figure 7). This could be due to the lower percentage of residual lipids and higher protein content present in that by-product, both being substances with emulsifying activity.

The Ms and Mp meals showed a higher WAbC than canola and soybean meals, and similar to linseed meal, whereas the OHC of Ms was similar to that reported for canola and soybean meals. Both Ms and Mp exhibited a higher EA than linseed, canola and soybean meals (Table 5). And the WHC of both fibrous fractions was higher than that reported for soybean fiber, and corn and wheat hull. FRFs presented a higher OHC than that of the fibrous residues of Jack bean and Lima bean, while its WAbC was higher than the values observed for corn, wheat and soybean hull, and similar to those of a fibrous fraction of Mexican chia. Its WAdC and OMAC were higher than that of the Mexican fibrous fraction and soybean fiber, and similar to that of the corn and wheat hull. It was also observed that FRFs presented a similar EA to and a lower ES than a Mexican chia fibrous fraction (Table 5).

O/W emulsions (50:50 p/p) of the studied chia by-products presented high initial backscatter values (BS_0), varying in a range from 57.3 to 69.1% in emulsions prepared with Mp and PRFs, respectively. The emulsions formulated with the solvent-extracted samples (Ms, FRFs and PRFs) showed a greater stability than the emulsions corresponding to the pressing-extracted samples (Mp, FRFp and PRFp) during the tested time. This behavior could be attributed to the higher protein and fiber content, as well as the lower residual lipid content present in the solvent-extracted samples (**Figure 1**). For each extraction method (cold-pressing and solvent), the protein-rich fractions exhibited higher BS values during the analyzed time, with a reduction percentage of 5.5 and 17.2% in PRFs and PRFp, respectively, in contrast with a reduction of 11.2 and 23% in the corresponding meals (Ms and Mp, respectively) and of 9.4 and 29% in FRFs and FRFp, respectively. This could be explained in terms of the high protein content in these fractions with emulsifying properties.

Table 5. Functional properties of different sources of fiber (g/g of sample)

Species	WAbC	WHC	WAdC	OHC	OMAC	EA-ES (%)	References
Canola meal	3.9	2.1		2.1		48.6	Khattab and Arntfield (2009)
Soybean meal	3.3	2.2		2.0		44.1	Khattab and Arntfield (2009)
Linseed meal	6.0	2.0				33.6	Khattab and Arntfield (2009)
Soybean fiber	1.4	1.3	0.4		0.5		Zambrano et al. (2001)
Corn hull	3.2	2.3	0.4		1.7		Zambrano et al. (2001)
Wheal hull	2.9	2.5	0.3		2.1		Zambrano et al. (2001)
Lima bean		0.3		0.2		49.3-28.2	Betancur-Ancona et al. (2004)
Jack bean		0.4		0.2		8.6-100	Betancur-Ancona et al. (2004)
Mexican FRF-s	11.7		0.3		1.1	53.2-94.5	Vázquez-Ovando et al. (2009)

Conclusion

The method of oil extraction (cold-pressing and solid-liquid) from chia seeds affected the physicochemical and functional properties of the residual meals and their corresponding fiber- and protein-rich fractions. This influence is associated with the content of residual lipids of the studied by-products. By sieving the meals (Ms and Mp), two coarse fractions were obtained, with an increase in fiber of 6 and 19%, and two fine fractions, with a 30 and 53% increase in proteins, respectively. In all the cases it was possible to concentrate the compound of interest from the fractions, with respect to the defatted meal. The fiber-rich fractions presented a high content of TDF, consisting mainly of IDF, with a high proportion of cellulose and hemicellulose. These levels of fiber were significantly higher than those observed in the meals and protein-rich fractions. In all the by-products the presence of phosphorus, calcium, magnesium, iron, copper and zinc was detected, with the first three being in a higher proportion. The protein-rich fractions also exhibited a higher concentration of minerals. All the by-products showed high antioxidant activity. In general, the solvent-extracted by-products (Ms, FRFs and PRFs) presented higher levels in their functional properties than the pressing-extracted by-products (Mp, FRFp and PRFp). It is worth noting that the properties relating to oil affinity (OHC and OMAC) were significantly higher in the solvent-extracted by-products. This could be associated with the low residual oil content and high protein content of those samples. The results obtained from the determination of the studied physicochemical and functional properties suggest that chia by-products could have a potential application as functional ingredients in various products.

References

AACC (1984). Official methods of analysis (12th ed.). St. Paul, MN, USA: American Association of Cereal Chemists.

Aller, R., De Luis, D., Izaola O., La Calle, F., Del Olmo, L., Fernández, L., Arranz, T. & Hernández, J. (2004). Effect of soluble fiber intake in lipid and glucose levels in healthy subjects: A randomized clinical trial. *Diabetes Research and Clinical Practice,* 65, 7–11.

AOAC (1997). In W. Horwitz (Ed.), Official methods of analysis (17th ed.), Washington, D.C., USA, Association of Official Analytical Chemists.

AOCS (1998). Official and Recommended Practices of the American Oil Chemists' Society, 5th edn., edited by D. Firestone, AOCS Press, Champaign Illinois.

Ayerza, R. & Coates, W. (2005). Ground chia seed and chia oil effects on plasma lipids and fatty acids in the rat. *Nutrition Reasearch*, 25, 995-1003.

Badui, S. *Química de los Alimentos*. Longman / Alhambra; 1999.

Bergthaller, W., Dijkink, B., Langelaan, H. & Vereijken, J. (2001). Protein from pea mutants as a co-product in starch separation. Isolates from wet and dry separation: Yield, composition and solubility. *Nahrung-Food,* 45, 390-392.

Betancur-Ancona, D., Peraza-Mercado, G., Moguer-Ordoñez, Y. & Fuertes-Blanco, S. (2004). Physicochemical characterization of lima bean (*Phaseolus lunatus*) and jack bean (*Canavalia ensiformis*) fibrous residues. *Journal Food Chemistry,* 84, 287-295.

Borderías, A. J., Sánchez-Alonso, M. & Pérez-Mateos, M. (2005). New applications of fibres in foods: Addition to fishery products. *Food Science Technology,* 16, 458-465.

Borroto, B., Larrauri, J. A. & Cribeiro, A. (1995). Particle size influence on water holding capacity of citrus and pineaple dietary fiber. *Alimentaria,* 268, 89-90.

Bushway, A. & Belya. (1981). Chia seed as a source of oil, polysaccharide and protein. *Journal of Food Science,* 46, 1349-1356.

Capitani, M. I., Spotorno, V., Nolasco, S. M. & Tomás, M.C. (2012). Physicochemical and functional characterization of by-products from chia (*Salvia hispanica* L.) seeds of Argentina. *Lebensmittel Wissenschaft and Technology - Food Science Technology,* 45, 94-102.

Chau, C., Cheung, K & Wong, Y. (1997). Functional properties of protein concentrate from three Chinese indigenous legume seeds. *Journal of Agriculture and Food Chemistry,* 45, 2500-2503.

Chau, C. & Huang, Y. (2003). Comparison of the chemical composition and physicochemical properties of different fibers prepared from the peel of *Citrus sinensis* L. cv. Liucheng. *Journal of Agriculture and Food Chemistry*, 51, 2615-2618.

Chen, J., Piva, M. & Labuza, T.P. (1984). Evaluation of water binding capacity (WBC) of food fiber sources. *Journal of Food Science,* 49 (1), 59-63.

Egbekun, M. K. & Ehieze, M. U. (1997). Proximate composition and functional properties of full fat and defatted beniseed (*Sesamun indicum* L.) flour. *Plant Food Human Nutrition,* 51, 35-41.

Endres, J.G. (1989). Soy protein products characteristics, nutritional aspects, and utilization. Chapter 3. By AOCS Press and the Soy Protein Council. Champaign, Illinois. *Protein Quality and Human Nutrition*, 10-18.

Gorinstein, S., Zachwieja. Z., Folta. M., Barton, H., Piotrowicz, J., Sembré, M., Weisz, M., Trakhtenberg, S. & Martín, O. (2001). Comparative content of dietary fiber, total phenolics, and minerals in persimmons and apples. *Journal of Agriculture and Food Chemistry*, 49, 952-957.

Grigelmo-Miguel, N. & Martín-Belloso, O. (1999). Comparison of dietary fibre from by-products of processing fruits and greens and from cereals. *Lebensmittel Wissenschaft and Technology - Food Science Technology,* 32, 503-508.

Guiragossian, V.Y., Van Scoyoc, S.W. & Auxtell, J.D. (1979). Chemical and Biological Methods for Grain and Forage Sorghum, Departament of Agronomy Internacional Programs in Agricultura, Purdue University, West Lafayette, Indiana, USA.

Infostat Group, Infostat version 2004, Facultad de Ciencias Agrarias, Universidad Nacional de Córdoba, Argentina (2004).

Iqbal, S., Bhanger, M., Anwar, F. (2005). Antioxidant properties and components of some commercially available varieties of rice bran in Pakistan. *Food Chemistry,* 93, 265-272.

IUPAC (1992), International Union of Pure and Aplplied Chemistry – Standard Methods for the Analysis of Oils, Fats and Derivates. 7th edn. Paquot, C. and Hautffene, A., Blackwell Scientific Publications, Inc., Oxford.

Ixtaina, V. Y., Martínez, M. L., Spotorno, V., Mateo, C. M., Maestri, D.M., Diehl, B. W., Nolasco, S. M. & Tomás M. C. (2011). Characterization of chia seed oils obtained by pressing and solvent extraction. *Journal of Food Composition and Analysis*, 24(2), 166-174.

Kernefick, S. & Cashman, K. D. (2000). Investigation of an in vitro model for predicting the effect of food components on calcium availability from meals. *International Journal Food Science Nutrition,* 51, 45-54.

Khattab, R. Y. & Arntfield, S. D. (2009). Functional properties of raw and processed canola meal. *Lebensmittel Wissenschaft and Technology - Food Science Technology,* 42, 1119-1124.

Lecumberri, E., Mateos, R., Izquierdo-Pulido, M., Rupérez, P., Goya, L. & Bravo, L. (2007). Dietary fibre composition, antioxidant capacity and physico-chemical properties of a fibre-rich product from cocoa (*Theobroma cacao* L.). *Food Chemistry,* 104, 948-954.

Mathews, C.K. & Van Holde, K.E. (1990). Biochemistry, Benjamin/ Cummings Pub. Co, (Redwood City, Calif.) 1129 p

McDougall, G.J., Morrison, I.M., Stewart, D. & Hillman, R. J. (1996). Plant cell walls as dietary fibre: range, structure, processing and function. Journal of the Science and Food Agriculture, 70, 133-150.

Mota-Blancas, E. & Perales-Caldera, E. (1999). Los mecanismos de absorción de calcio y los modificadores de absorción como base para la elaboración de una dieta de bajo costo para pacientes osteoporóticas. *Gacetilla Médica de México,* 135 (3), 291-304.

Mueller, K., Eisner, P., Yoshie-Stark, Y., Nakada, R. & Kirchhoff, E. (2010). Functional properties and chemical composition of fractionated brown and yellow linseed meal (*Linum usitatissimum* L.). *Journal of Food Engineering,* 98, 453-460.

Otto, T., Baik, B. & Czuchajowska, Z. (1997). Wet fractionation of garbanzo bean and pea flours. *Cereal Chemistry,* 74, 141-146.

Pacheco de Delahaye, E., Sánchez, M. A., Girlando, R. & Sánchez, E. (1994). Obtención de aislados proteínicos de girasol por hidrólisis con bromelina y papaína, composición química y propiedades funcionales. *Agronomía Tropical,* 44 (2), 299-315.

Pan, L. G., Tomás, M. C. & Añón, M. C. (2002). Effect of sunflower lecithins on the stability of water in oil (W/O) and oil in water (O/W) emulsions. *Journal of Surfactant and Detergents,* 5(2), 135-143.

Pérez, E. E. (2001). Obtención y caracterización de aceites y harinas de girasol silvestre: *Helianthus petiolaris.* Tesis Doctoral. Universidad Nacional del Sur (UNS).

Prosky, L., Asp, N., Schweizer, T., Devries, S. & Furda, I. (1988). Determination of insoluble, soluble and total dietary fiber in food and food products: interlaboratory study. *Journal of the Association of Official Analytical Chemists,* 71, 1017-1023.

Ragaee, S., Abdel-Aal, M. & Norman, M. (2006). Antioxidant activity and nutrient composition of selected cereals for food use. *Food Chemistry,* 98, 32-38.

Raghavendra, S., Ramachandra, S., Rastogi, N., Raghavarao, K., Kumar, S. & Tharanathan, R. (2006). Grinding characteristics and hydration properties of coconut residue: A source of dietary fiber. *Journal of Food Enginering,* 72, 281-286.

Re, R., Pellegrini, N., Proteggente, A., Pannala, A., Yang, M. & Rice-Evans. C. (1999). Antioxidant activity applying an improved ABTS radical cation decolorization assay. *Free Radical Biological Medicine,* 26 (9/10) 1231-1237.

Rehinan, Z., Rashid, M. & Shah, W. (2004). Insoluble dietary fibre components of food legumes as affected by soaking and cooking processes. *Food Chemistry,* 85, 245-249.

Robertson, J. A., Eastwood, M. A. & Yeoman, M. M. (1981). Investigation into the physical properties of prepared from several carrot varieties and different stages of development. *Journal of the Science of Food Agriculture,* 31 (6), 633-638.

Sangnark, A. & Noomhorm, A. (2003). Effect of particle size on functional properties of dietary fibre prepared from sugarcane bagasse. *Food Chemistry,* 80, 221-229.

Saura-Calixto, F. & García-Alonso, A. (2002). Metodología para el análisis de fibra y carbohidratos. Ed. Lajolo, Saura-Calixto, Witting and Wenzel de Menezes, Fibra dietética en Iberoamérica: Tecnología y Salud. Obtención, caracterización, efecto fisiológico y aplicación en alimentos. Brasil: Livraría LTDA. pp. 17-25.

Scheneeman, B. O. (1987). Soluble vs insoluble fibre-different physiological responses. *Food Technology,* 41, 81-82.

Singh, N., Makharia, G. & Joshi, K. (2008). Dietary survey and total dietary fiber intake in patients with irritable bowel syndrome attending a tertiary referral hospital. *Indian Journal Gastronomy,* 27, 66–70.

Sun, M., Xu, L., Saldaña, D. A. (2008). Comparison of canola meals obtained with conventional methods and supercritical CO_2 with and without ethanol. *Journal of the American Oil Chemistry Society,* 85, 667-675.

Taga, M. S., Miller, E.E. & Pratt, D. E. (1984). Chia seeds as a source of natural lipid antioxidants. *Journal of the American Oil Chemists Society*, 61, 928-931.

Vázquez-Ovando, J. A., Rosado-Rubio, J. G., Chel-Guerrero, L. A. & Betancur-Ancona, D. A. (2010). Procesamiento en seco de harina de chía (*Salvia hispanica* L.): caracterización química de fibra y proteína. *CyTA- Journal of Food,* 8 (2), 117-127.

Vázquez-Ovando, J., Rosado-Rubio, G., Chel-Guerrero, L. & Betancur-Ancona, D. (2009). Physicochemical properties of a fibrous fraction from chia (*Salvia hispanica* L.). *Lebensmittel Wissenschaft and Technology - Food Science Technology,* 42, 168-173.

Weber, C. W. (1991). The nutritional and chemical evaluation of Chia seeds. *Ecology of Food and Nutrition*, 26, (2), 119-125.

Wong, K. & Cheung, P. (2005). Dietary fibers from mushroom sclerotia: 1. Preparation and physicochemical and functional properties. *Journal and Agriculture Food Chemistry,* 53, 9395-9400.

Zambrano-Zaragoza, M. L., Meléndez, R. & Gallardo, Y. (2001). Propiedades funcionales y metodología para su evaluación en fibra dietética. Ed/ FM. Lajolo, F Saura-Calixto, E Witting and Wenzel de Menezes/, Fibra dietética en Iberoamérica: *Tecnología y Salud. Obtención, caracterización, efecto fisiológico y aplicación en alimentos*. Brasil: Livraría LTDA. pp. 195-209.

In: Dietary Fiber
Editors: D. Betancur-Ancona, L. Chel-Guerrero et al.
ISBN: 978-1-62808-931-8

Chapter 9

Effect of Drying Treatment on Primary Nutrients and Antioxidant Activities of *Stevia rebaudiana* Bertoni Stems

D. L. Cabrera-Amaro[1,1], *J. C. Ruiz-Ruiz*[2,2], *Y. B. Moguel-Ordóñez*,[1], *M. R. Segura-Campos*[3,3] *and M. L. Murguía-Olmedo*[1]

[1]Instituto Nacional de Investigaciones Forestales, Agrícolas y Pecuarias, Campo Experimental Mocochá. Mocochá, Yucatán, México

[2]Departamento de Ingeniería Química-Bioquímica, Instituto Tecnológico de Mérida, Mérida, Yucatán, México

[3]Facultad de Ingeniería Química, Universidad Autónoma de Yucatán, Mérida, Yucatán, México

Abstract

This study was carried out to evaluate the primary nutrients and antioxidants activity of *Stevia rebaudiana* Bertoni stems. The *S. rebaudiana* (var. Morita II) stems were sourced from Tizimín, Yucatán, México. The stems were obtained fresh, cleaned and washed prior to drying treatments: hot air dried, convection dried, sun dried and shade dried.

The different drying techniques improved the primary nutrient density of the stems. The result also showed that the antioxidant capacities: radical scavenging activity, ferric reducing power, and chelating of metallic ions, were better preserved by both convection dried and shade dried treatments.

[1] Telephone:5299191 6-2215.Email:cabrera.diana@inifap.gob.mx;moguel.yolanda@inifap.gob.mx.

[2] Telephone: 52 999 964-50-00 begin_of_the_skype_highlighting, end_of_the_skype_highlighting Fax: 52 999 944-81-81.

[3] Telephone: 52 999 946-09-56, Fax. 52 999 946-09-94.

The results of the present study suggest the potential use of the processed (convection dried and shade dried) stems of *Stevia rebaudiana* as functional foods for their high fiber content and their multiple antioxidant capacities.

Introduction

Dietary fibre is the edible parts of plants or analogous carbohydrates that are resistant to digestion and absorption in the human small intestine with complete or partial fermentation in the large intestine (Sankhala et al., 2005). Dietary fibre includes polysaccharides, oligosaccharides, lignin and associated plant substances. In addition an analogous carbohydrate is defined as those carbohydrates-based food ingredients that are non-digestible and non-absorbable, and which are similar to plant dietary fibre (Prosky, 2001). The adequate intake of dietary fibre through the high consumption of fruits and vegetables makes possible to achieve a healthy diet, a correct body weight, an acceptable lipoprotein profile, and a normal blood pressure (Sánchez-Muñiz, 2012).

Natural antioxidants have attracted a great deal of public and scientific interest because of their anticarcinogenic potential and other health promoting effects. Plants and vegetables are good source of phenolic components, ascorbic acids, tocopherols, glutathione, vitamins, carotenoids, and flavonoids that may contribute to protection against oxidative damage. This phytochemicals from plants have been shown to possess significant antioxidant capacities that may be associated with lower incidence and lower mortality rates of degenerative diseases in human beings such as ant-allergic, anti-atherogenic, anti-inflammatory, anti-microbial, antioxidant, anti-thrombotic, cardioprotective and vasodilatory effects (Manch et al., 2005).

Fruit and vegetables have been recognized as important sources for a wide array of non-digestible components and phytochemicals that individually, or in combination, may act synergistically to contribute to the nutritional and health benefits. Dietary fibre and antioxidants are generally addressed separately as groups of food constituents in both chemical and nutritional studies (Raghavendra et al., 2006). However, it is a little known fact that a substantial proportion of the antioxidant polyphenols and carotenoids contained in fruit and vegetables are linked to dietary fibre and some of the postulated benefits of the fibre intake can be attributed to these associated compounds. A variety of plant food byproducts are rich in fibre and antioxidants compounds meeting the criteria of antioxidant dietary fibre (Saura-Calixto et al., 2007), Stevia (*Stevia rebaudiana* Bertoni) is a perennial shrub that is indigenous to Paraguay and Brazil, the leaves and its extracts have been studied widely from the sweetener point of view. Nowadays the extraction of sweeteners from stevia leaves is a growing industrial and commercial worldwide sector; more than 750 tons of stevia leaves per year are used as crude extract for consumption and extraction of glycosides. However the stevia stems are less sweet, so are discarded (Atteh et al., 2011). The food industry processing plant foods produces large amounts of waste and residues (leaves, stems, wastewaters, etc.) that are good sources of dietary fibre and phytochemicals. Several of them contain more dietary fibre than their respective edible portion (Raghavendra et al., 2006).

Most of the modern preservation methods require high initial costs for installation of sophisticated machinery and equipment, skilled manpower and large capital investment for modern food processing industries. But the farmers who are producing the perishable food items always expect low cost technology for preserving their produced items (Rahman and

Kumar, 2007). Conventional drying with hot air and convective are commonly encountered in dehydration. However, an alternative way to remove excess water from food is by using traditional methods like shade dried and sun dried which are drying processes based on water evaporation at environment conditions (Verás et al., 2012). The success of drying as a method of food preservation depends on the properties of the dried products like color, nutritive value and biological activities (Bhuiyan et al., 2011). A search through literature shows little information about alternative uses of *S. rebaudiana* stems for human nutrition. Considering that the non-sweetening components make up 80-90% dry weight of this plant, stevia stems would be a potential source of antioxidant dietary fibre. The objective of the present study was to evaluate the effects of different drying treatments on primary nutrients and antioxidant capacities, by several methods, of *Stevia rebaudiana* Bertoni stems.

Materials and Methods

Raw Material and Chemicals

Stevia rebaudiana Bertoni (var. Morita II) was obtained from plots established in Tizimín Yucatan, México. The plantation had a crop management according to the production technology described by Ramirez et al., (2011). Samples were obtained from the first cut of the plot at an age of three months; samples consisted on branches of leaves and stems (Figure 1). All chemicals were reagent grade or better and purchased from Sigma Chemical Co. (St. Louis, MO, USA).

Drying Treatments

Stevia rebaudiana stems were subjected to four treatments of drying: 1) hot air dried, 2) convection dried, 3) shade dried and 4) sun dried. Stoves at 60 °C were used for the first two treatments. For shade and sun dried treatments temperature and relative humidity were monitored during the process. The vegetal material was distributed in aluminum trays, with three replicates for each treatment (Figure 2). To determinate drying kinetics of each treatment vegetal material was weighed at the beginning and every 4 hours for stove treatments, and every 24 hours for drying at environment conditions. Drying was stop until there was no significant weight loss; this is until vegetal material reached equilibrium in moisture content. The stems were milled in a Wiley equipment to obtain a particle size of 1.0 mm (Figure 2). Samples were stored at room temperature in polyethylene bags until analysis.

Proximate Composition

The proximate composition of *S. rebaudiana* stems was determined using AOAC (1998) methods: moisture content (Method 925.09), ash (Method 923.03), crude fat (Method 920.39), crude protein using a 6.25 nitrogen-protein conversion factor (Method 954.01) and crude fiber (Method 962.09). The carbohydrate content was estimated as the nitrogen-free extract (NFE).

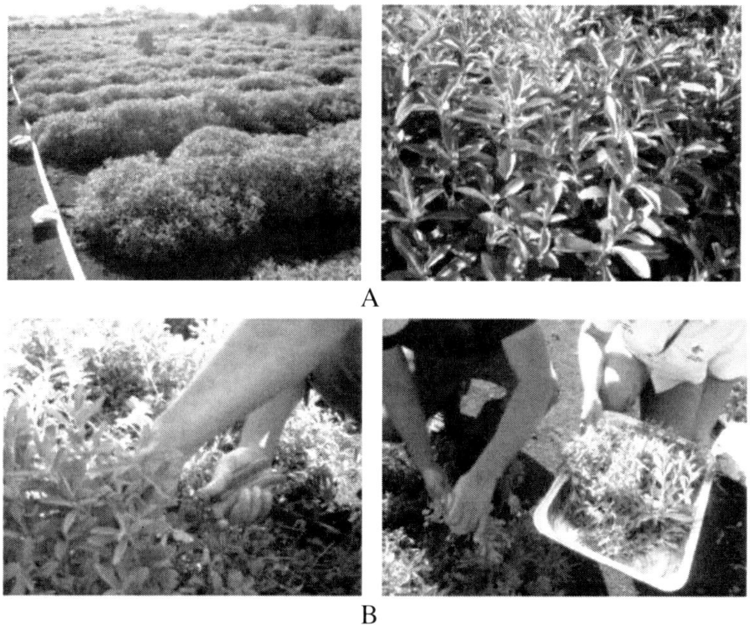

Figure 1. Plots of *Stevia rebaudiana* Bertoni (var. Morita II) established in Tizimín, Yucatán, México. A) Crop management of *Stevia rebaudiana* Bertoni (var. Morita II). B) Samples obtained from the first cut of the plot at an age of three months.

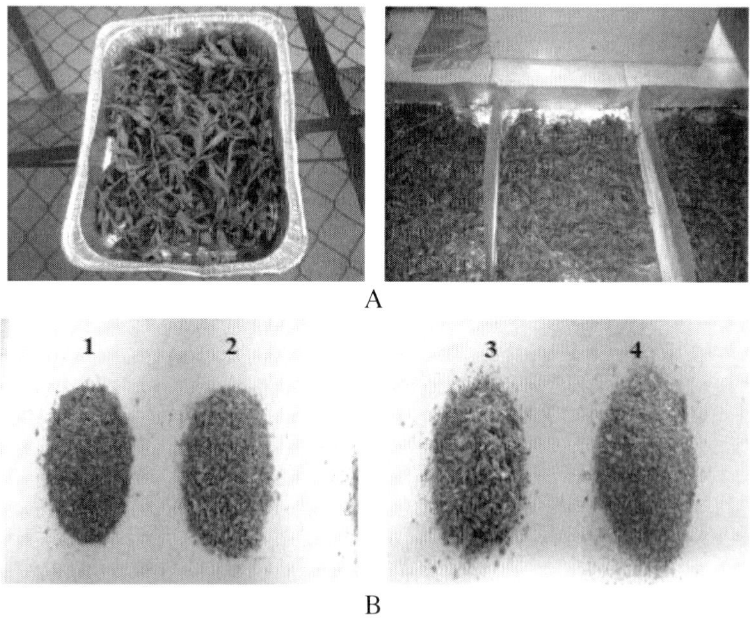

Figure 2. Drying treatments applied to *Stevia rebaudiana* Bertoni (var. Morita II) stems. A) Distribution of vegetal material. B) Dried stems milled (1 = hot air dried, 2 = convection dried, 3 = shade dried, 4 = sun dried).

In Vitro Antioxidant Properties of Stevia Stems

a) 2,2´-Azinobis-(3-Ethylbenzothiazoline-6-Sulfonic Acid, $ABTS^{\bullet+}$) Decolorization Assay

The $ABTS^{\bullet+}$ radical cation was produced by reacting 2,2'-azino-bis(3-ethylbenzthiazoline-6-sulphonic acid (ABTS) with potassium persulfate (Rhee et al. 2004). To prepare the stock solution, ABTS was dissolved at a 2 mM concentration in 50 mL phosphate-buffered saline. The ABTS radical cation was produced by reacting 10 mL ABTS stock solution with 40 μL $K_2S_4O_8$ 70 mM solution and allowing the mixture to stand in darkness at room temperature for 16-17 h before use. The radical was stable in this form for more than 2 days when stored in darkness at room temperature. Antioxidant compound content in the stevia stems was analyzed by diluting the $ABTS^{\bullet+}$ solution with PBS to an absorbance of 0.800 ± 0.030 AU at 734 nm. After adding 990 μL diluted $ABTS^{\bullet+}$ solution (A 734 nm= 0.800 ± 0.030) to 10 μL of 6-hydroxy-2,5,7,8-tetramethylchroman-2-carboxylic acid (TROLOX) standard (final concentration 0.5-3.5 mM) in PBS, absorbance was read at room temperature exactly 6 min after initial mixing. All analyses were run in triplicate. The percentage decrease in absorbance at 734 nm was calculated and plotted as a function of the antioxidant concentration or of Trolox for the standard reference data. To calculate the Trolox equivalent antioxidant coefficient (TEAC), the slope of the absorbance inhibition percentage vs. antioxidant concentration plot was divided by the slope of the Trolox plot. This produces the TEAC at a specific point in time.

b) Ferric Reducing Power Assay

This method is based on the reduction of potassium ferricyanide (Fe^{+3}) to (F^{2+}) in the presence of an antioxidant, KFeIII forming the blue complex [FeII(CN_6)], which absorbing a 700 nm (Sudha et al., 2011). First, 200 μL of sample (containing 1 mg of protein), 500 μL of phosphate buffer (0.2 M, pH 6.6), and 500 μL of potassium ferricyanide (1%) were mixed in a test tube. The test tube was then incubated at 50 ºC for 20 min. Subsequently, 500 mL of trichloroacetic acid (10%) were added, and the tube was centrifuged at 3000 g for 10 min. An aliquot of 500 μL of the supernatant, which is dissolved in an equal amount of distilled water, immediately 500 μL of ferric chloride (0.1%) were added. Absorbance was determined at 700 nm. Samples were tested in a range of concentrations from 200 to 1000 mg/mL. Butylated hydroxytoluene was used as control in the same range of concentrations.

c) Chelating of Metal Ions Cu^{2+} and Fe^{2+}

Cu^{2+}-chelating activity was determined using the pyrocatechol violet reagent according to Saiga et al. (2003). Briefly, 1.0 mL of sodium acetate buffer (100 mM, pH 4.9), 100 mL of Cu (II) standard solution (1.0 mg/mL), and 100 mL of sample (containing 200 mg of sample) were mixed in a test tube. The mixture was allowed to react for 5 min at room temperature and 25 mL of a pyrocatechol violet solution (4.0 mM) was then added. Absorbance was determined at 632 nm. Copper chelating activity was calculated as follows:

Chelating activity (%) = (1 - sample absorbance/control absorbance) x 100.

Fe^{2+}-chelating activity was determined by measuring the formation of the Fe^{2+}-ferrozine complex according to Carter (1971). Briefly, 1.0 mL of sodium acetate buffer (100 mM, pH 4.9), 100 mL of Fe(II) standard solution (1.0 mg/mL), and 100 mL of sample (containing 200 mg of sample) were mixed in a test tube. The mixture was allowed to react for 5 min at room temperature and 50 mL of a ferrozine solution (40 mM) was then added. Absorbance was determined at 562 nm. Iron chelating activity was calculated as follows:

Chelating activity (%) = (1 - sample absorbance/ control absorbance) x 100.

Statistical Analysis

All results were analyzed using descriptive statistics with a central tendency and dispersion measures. One-way ANOVAs were run to evaluate proximate composition and *in vitro* antioxidant activities. The least significant difference (LSD) multiple range test was used to determine differences among drying treatments. All analyses were done according to Montgomery (2004) and processed with the Statgraphics Plus version 5.1 software.

Results and Discussion

Drying Kinetics

Drying curves obtained with hot air and convection treatments are shown in Figure 3. For hot air dried was observed a rapid decrease of the weight difference for the first 8 hours and before the weight difference was stable because the vegetal material reached the equilibrium in moisture content. Instead for convection drying the weight difference gradually decreases until equilibrium in moisture content was reached after 28 hours.

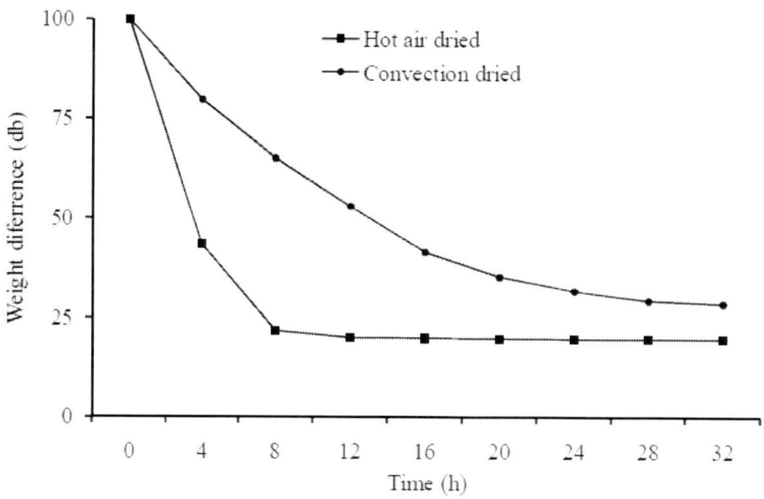

Figure 3. Difference of weight (db) in stems of *Stevia rebaudiana* Bertoni obtained at different conditions of drying (hot air dried and convection dried). Data are presented as means (n = 3).

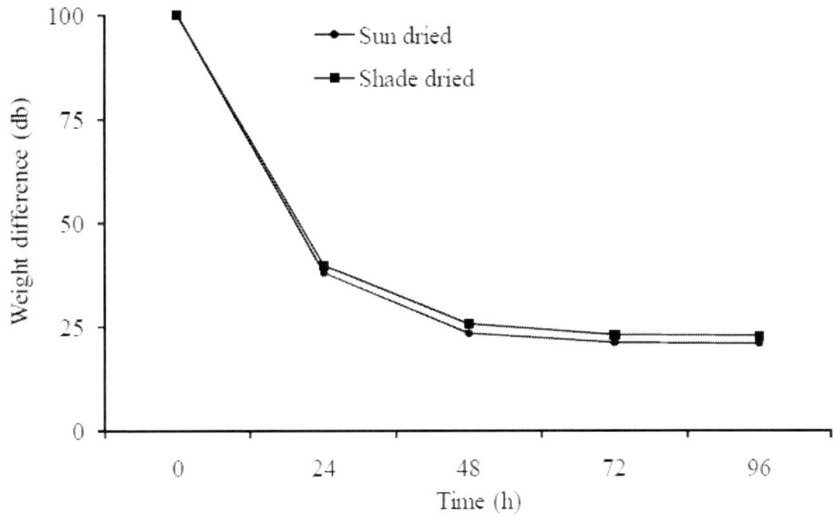

Figure 4. Difference of weight (db) in stems of *Stevia rebaudiana* Bertoni obtained at different conditions of drying (shade dried and sun dried). Data are presented as means (n = 3).

Temperature (60 °C) and time (24 h) were the same for both treatments however hot air dried treatment was more efficient than convection treatment. Thus weight difference is more dependent on both temperature and hot air flow in the process of drying. According to Bhuiyan et al. (2011), one of the most common ways of drying is using air as a drying agent. Heat and mass transfer between air and the solid take place in opposite directions. This would explain the results obtained in this study. Since the hot air dried method better dehydrated the *S. rebaudiana* stems. Dehydration of stems was also evaluated with traditional drying methods (Figure 4). For sun dried was observed a rapid decrease of the weight difference for the first 48 hours and before the weight difference was stable because was reached the equilibrium in moisture content. The shade dried showed the same behavior.

Both treatments were equally effective drying the stems. Sun and shade dried depend on the weather conditions to dehydrate the stems so that reduce costs since do not require equipment and energy. However the dependence of both treatments to weather conditions does not allow establish reproducible conditions to control the drying process.

Proximate Composition

Table 1 summarizes the proximate composition of *S. rebaudiana* stems dehydrated at different drying methods. All methods of drying reduced the moisture content to values less than 10%. The moisture content varied from 7.31% to 8.93%. The convection dried has the highest value followed by hot air dried, shade dried and sun dried. This therefore implied that treatment (different drying techniques) of *S. rebaudiana* stems makes them not to deteriorate faster.

The higher protein content was observed shade dried (4.92%) when correction was made for residual moisture content. This suggests that treatment (different drying techniques) increase the protein content of *S. rebaudiana* stems. The loss in moisture in the processed stems increased nutrient density, a commonly observed phenomenon.

Table 1. Proximate composition of *S. rebaudiana* steams dehydrated at different drying methods

Component (%)	Hot air dried	Convection dried	Shade dried	Sun dried
Moisture	8.38 ± 0.09^{c}	8.93 ± 0.38^{d}	7.89 ± 0.23^{b}	7.31 ± 0.04^{a}
Protein	5.58 ± 0.25^{b}	4.92 ± 0.39^{a}	7.78 ± 0.12^{c}	5.17 ± 0.40^{ab}
Fat	1.13 ± 0.85^{b}	1.13 ± 0.85^{b}	1.32 ± 0.48^{b}	0.68 ± 0.29^{a}
Crude fiber	42.85 ± 1.47^{c}	41.84 ± 1.61^{c}	33.45 ± 2.20^{a}	37.97 ± 1.25^{b}
Ash	7.43 ± 0.72^{a}	9.01 ± 0.41^{b}	11.14 ± 0.42^{c}	9.20 ± 0.34^{b}
NFE	43.14 ± 1.31^{a}	43.09 ± 2.98^{a}	46.30 ± 1.52^{ab}	46.98 ± 1.53^{b}

Data are presented as means (n = 3).
Different letters in the same line indicate significant difference ($p < 0.05$).

The lower fat content of sun-dried stems as compared with the other samples revealed that treatments (hot air dried, convection died and shade dried) did not improve the fat content of the stems. The low fat content of the processed stems (Table 1) suggests that could be used like food for communities that requires low fat diets. The increase in ash content of the processed stems with shade and sun dried treatments (11.4% and 9.20%) as compared with hot air dried and convection dried treatments (7.43% and 9.01%) was again due to the removal of residual moisture and increased nutrient density. The lower fibre content for the shade dried and sun dried stems (33.45% and 37.97%) were attributed to their high nitrogen-free extract content. *S. rebaudiana* stems have high amounts of crude fibre and carbohydrates. Fibre has a useful role in providing roughage that aids digestion and carbohydrates contribute to fat metabolism and spare proteins as energy source for human beings. Considering the primary nutrient composition of the *S. rebaudiana stems*, these could be used as functional foods.

In Vitro Antioxidant Properties of Stevia Stems

Various mechanisms, including radical scavenging, reducing capacity, binding of metal ion catalysts, prevention of chain initiation, decomposition of peroxides, and prevention of continued hydrogen abstraction have been claimed to explain the antioxidant activities (Mao et al., 2006).

The ABTS assay is based on the inhibition by antioxidants of the absorbance of the radical cation $ABTS^{\bullet+}$. The use of Trolox as a standard allows the assay outcome to be called the Trolox equivalent antioxidant capacity (TEAC). The ABTS assay is an excellent tool for determining the antioxidant activity of hydrogen-donating antioxidants and of chain-breaking antioxidants (Leong and Shui, 2007). The result of $ABTS^{\bullet+}$ radical scavenging activity of the stems of *S. rebaudiana* assayed by the $ABTS^{\bullet+}$ decolorization assay system is show in the Figure 5.

TEAC values ranged from 169.54 to 227.87 mM/mg of sample. The ABTS radical scavenging activity of *S. rebaudiana* is comparable to that of other fibrous residues like Oat bran with hulls (7.96 mM/mg of sample), Buckwheat bran (24.24 mM/mg of smaple) and hulls (26.15 mM/mg sample) (Zduńczyk et al., 2006), and Grape antioxidant dietary fibre (375.5 mM/mg of sample) (Pérez-Jiménez and Saura-Calixto, 2008). The radical scavenging activity of the stems was significant related with the conditions of the drying treatment (Figure 5). The lowest value of TEAC was observed in treatment 1 (hot air dried) and the highest value was observed in treatment 3 (shade dried).

The reducing capacity of a sample may serve as a significant indicator of its potential antioxidant activity (Sudha et al., 2011). The Fe^{3+} - Fe^{2+} transformation was determined as the reducing capacity in this study. In ferric reducing power assay, the yellow color of the test solution changes to various shades of green or blue, depending on the reducing power of each sample. The presence of antioxidants could cause the reduction of the Fe3+/ferricyanide complex to the ferrous form.

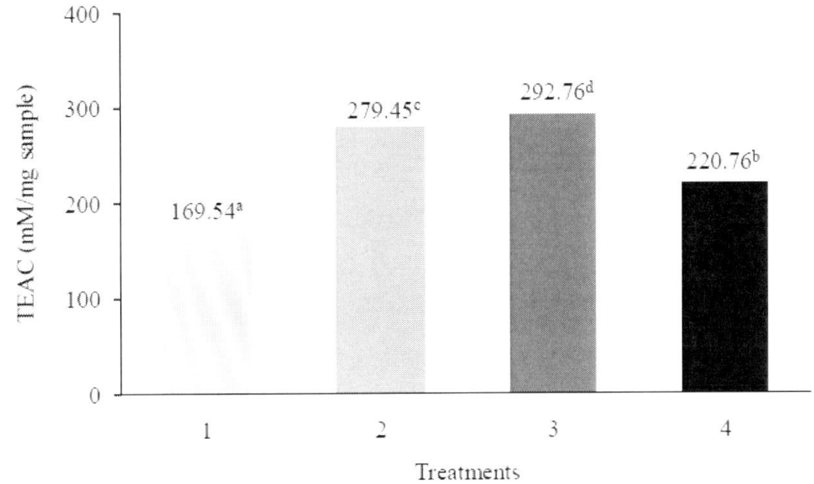

Figure 5. Trolox equivalent antioxidant capacity (TEAC) in stems of *Stevia rebaudiana* Bertoni obtained at different conditions of drying. 1 = hot air dried, 2 = oven dried, 3 = shade dried, 4 = sun-dried. Data are presented as means (n = 3). Different letters indicate significant differences ($p < 0.05$).

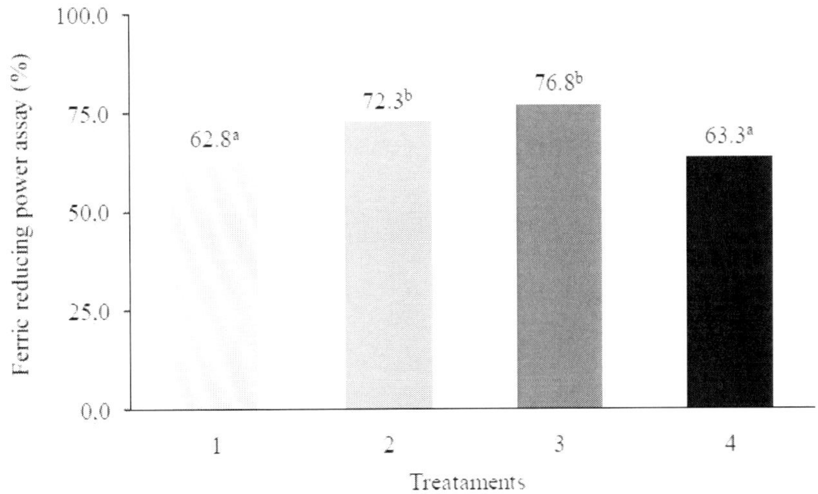

Figure 6. Determination of ferric reducing power of stems of *Stevia rebaudiana* Bertoni obtained at different conditions of drying. 1 = hot air dried, 2 = oven dried, 3 = shade dried, 4 = sun-dried. Data are presented as means (n = 3). Different letters indicate significant differences ($p < 0.05$).

Therefore, measuring the formation of blue complex at 700 nm can monitor the concentration of Fe2+ (Ferreira et al., 2007). The reducing capacity values ranged from 66.3 to 76.8% (Figure 6). This result was consistent with the Trolox equivalent antioxidant capacity (Figure 5), and showed that treatments 2 (convection dried) and 3 (shade dried) preserved most of the reducing power in *S. rebaudiana* stems.

Metal ion chelating activity of an antioxidant molecule prevents oxyradical generation and the consequent oxidative damage. Metal ion chelating capacity plays a significant role in antioxidant mechanisms, since it reduces the concentration of the catalyzing transition metal in lipid peroxidation.

It is reported that chelating agents reduce the redox potential, thereby stabilizing the oxidized form of the metal ions (Duh et al., 1999). Pyrocatechol violet and ferrozine can quantitatively form complexes with Cu^{2+} and Fe^{2+}, respectively. In presence of *S. rebaudiana* stems, the complexes formation are disrupted with the result that the blue (Cu^{2+}) and red (Fe^{2+}) color of the complexes are decreased. Measurement of color reduction therefore allows estimation of the chelating activity of the *S. rebaudiana* stems. The chelating capacities of Cu^{2+} and Fe^{2+} are show in Figure 7.

According to Saura-Calixto et al. (2007), dietary fibre of fruit and vegetables contents a significant amount of polyphenols and carotenoids that exhibit antioxidant capacity. It was confirmed in numerous studies that in addition to direct free radical scavenging, flavonoids exert anti-oxidant activity through interactions with the reduced form of transition metals, primarily Fe(II), Fe(III) and Cu(I), which participate in reactions generating free radicals (Moridani et al., 2003).

The results of the present study suggest that the *S. rebaudiana* stem exhibits chelation activity on cuprous and ferrous ions probably due to their content of flavonoids. Again dried treatment showed significant influence on metal chelating capacity in *S. rebaudiana* stems (Figure 6). Shade dried treatment preserved most metal chelating capacities with a significance difference ($p < 0.05$).

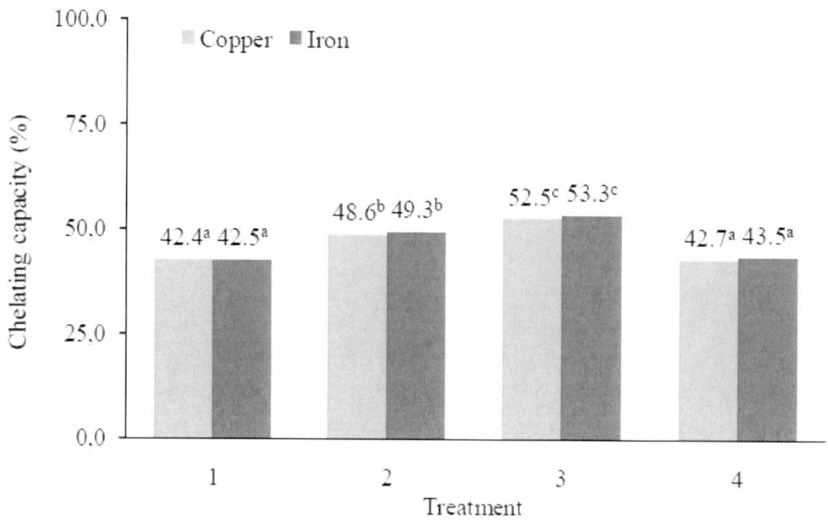

Figure 7. Copper and iron chelating capacity in stems of *Stevia rebaudiana* Bertoni obtained at different conditions of drying. 1 = hot air dried, 2 = oven dried, 3 = shade dried, 4 = sun-dried. Data are presented as means (n = 3). Different letters in same series indicate significant differences ($p < 0.05$).

Conventional drying with hot air and convective are commonly encountered in dehydration (Verás et al., 2012). However, an alternative way to remove excess water from food is by using traditional methods like shade and dried which are drying processes based on water evaporation at environment conditions. When compared to hot air dried stems, those dehydrated by convection, shade and sun dried better preserved the antioxidant activities. The order of antioxidant capacities was shade dried > convection dried > sun dried > hot air dried. According to Howe (2011), the low temperatures and the absence of dry air prevent the degradation of thermolabile substances with antioxidant capacities like vitamins (C and E), carotenoids, and some secondary metabolites (polyphenols, anthocyanins, flavonoids, etc.). This would explain the results obtained in this study. Since the shade drying method better preserves the antioxidant activities of *Stevia rebaudiana* stems. According to Saura-Calixto et al. (2007), part of the total content of antioxidant phytochemicals is linked to dietary fibre and an appreciable proportion of the total antioxidant capacity in fruit and vegetables by products is associated with dietary fibre. This would explain the results obtained in this study. Since *S. rebaudiana* stems which are consider as a byproduct from the extraction of glycosides, exhibit different antioxidant capacities like radical scavenging, reducing capacity, and binding of metal ion catalysts.

Conclusion

The different drying techniques had an effect on the primary nutrients and antioxidant capacities of *S. rebaudiana stems*. For preserving both primary nutrients and antioxidant capacities of stems convection dried was the best conventional treatment while shade dried was the best traditional treatment. Convection dried is suitable for modern food processing industries while shade dried will be a low cost alternative for farmers. The results of the present study suggest the potential use of the processed (convection dried and shade dried) stems of *Stevia rebaudiana* as functional foods for their high fiber content and their multiple antioxidant capacities.

References

AOAC. 1998. *Official Methods of Analysis,* Association of Official Analytical Chemists, Arlington,VA. Secs. 920.39, 923.03, 925.09, 954.01, 962.09, 992.16.

Atteh, J., Onagbesan, O., Tona, K., Buyse, J., Decuypere, E., Geuns, J. (2011). Potential use of *Stevia rebaudiana* in animal feeds. *Archivos de zootecnia*, 60(229): 133-136.

Bhuiyan, M.H.R., Alam, M.M., Islam, N. (2011). The construction and testing of a combined solar and mechanical cabinet dryer. *Journal of Environnemental Science and Natural Resources,* 4(2): 35-40.

Carter, P. (1971). Spectrophotometric determination of serum iron at the submicrogram level with a new reagent (ferrozine). Analytical Biochemistry, 40, 450-458.

Duh, P.D., Tu, Y.Y., Yen, G.C. (1999). Antioxidant activity of water extract of Harng Jyur (*Chrysanthemum morifolium* Ramat). *LWT*, 32: 269-277.

Ferreira, C.F.R., Baptista, P., Vilas-Boas, M. (2007). Free radical scavenging capacity and reducing power of wild edible mushrooms from northeast Portugal: Individual cap and stipe activity. *Food Chemistry*, 100(4): 1511-1516.

Howe, R.M. (2011). Mythology of antioxidant vitamins? *Journal of Evidence-Based complementary and Alternative Medicine,* 16: 149-159.

Leong, L.P. and Shui, G. (2007). An investigation of antioxidant capacity of fruits in Singapore markets. *Food Chemistry*, 76: 69-75.

Manach, C., A. Mazur and A. Scalbert, 2005. Polyphenols and prevention of cardiovascular diseases. *Current Opinion in Lipidology*, 16(1): 77-84.

Mao, L-C., Pan, X., Que, F., Fang, X-H. (2006). Antioxidant properties of water and ethanol extracts from hot air-dried and freeze dried daylily flowers. *European Food Research and Technology*, 222. 236-241.

Montgomery, D. (2004). *Diseño y análisis de experimentos*. México, D.F., México: Limusa-Wiley.

Moridani, M.Y., Pourahmad, J., Bui, H., Siraki, A., O'Brien, P.J. (2003). Dietary flavonoid iron complexes as cytoprotective superoxide radical scavengers. *Free Radical Biology and Medicine*, 34(2): 243-253.

Pérez-Jiménez, J. and Saura-Calixto, F. (2008). Grape products and cardiovascular disease risk factors. *Nutrition Research Reviews*, 21(2): 158-173.

Prosky, L. (2001). What is dietary fibre? A new look at the definition. En: *Advanced dietary fibre technology*. Cleary, B.V., Prosky, L. Blackwell Science Oxford, UK. 2001; pp. 63-88.

Raghavendra, S.N., Ramachandra-Swamy, S.R., Rastogi, N.K., Raghavarao, K.S.M.S., Kumar, S., Tharanathan, R.N. (2006). Grinding characteristics and hydration properties of coconut residue: A source of dietary fiber. *Journal of Food Engineering*, 72(3): 281-286.

Rahman, N. and Kumar, S. (2007). Influence of sample size and shape on transport parameters during drying of shrinking bodies. *Journal of Food Process Engineering*, 30(2):186-203.

Ramírez, J.G., Avilés, B.W., Moguel, O.Y., Góngora, G.S., May, L.C. (2011). Estevia (Stevia rebaudiana, Bertoni), un cultivo con potencial productivo en México. Instituto Nacional de Investigaciones Forestales, Agrícolas y Pecuarias. *Centro de Investigación Regional sureste.*

Rhee, S.J., Lee, C-Y.J., Kim, M-R., Lee C-H. (2004). Potential antioxidant peptides in rice wine. *Journal of Microbiology and Biotechnology*, 14(4): 715-721.

Saiga, A., Tanabe, S., & Nishimura, T. (2003).Antioxidant activity of peptides obtained from porcine myofibrillar proteins by protease treatment. *Journal of Agricultural and Food Chemistry*, 51, 3661-3667.

Saura-Calixto, F., Serrano, J., Goñi, I. (2007). Intake and bioaccessibility of total polyphenols in a whole diet. *Food Chemistry*, 101(2): 492-501.

Sudha, G., Sangeetha, Priya, M.S., Shree, R.I., Vadivukkarasi, S. (2011). *In vitro* free radical scavenging activity of raw pepino fruit (*Solanum muricatum* A.). *International Journal of Current Pharmaceutical Research*, 3(2): 137-140.

Sánchez-Muñiz, F.J. (2012). Dietary fibre and cardiovascular health. *Nutrición Hospitalaria,* 27(1): 31-45.

Sankhala, A., Sankhala, A.K., Bhatnagar, B., Singh, A. (2005). Nutrient composition of less familiar leaves consumed by the tribals of Udaipur region. *Journal of Food Science and Technology*, 42(5): 446-48.

Verás, A.O.M., Béttega, R., Freire1, F.B., M. A. S. Barrozo, M.A.S., Freire, J.T. (2012). Drying kinetics, structural characteristics and vitamin C retention of pepper (*Capsicum baccatum*) during convective and freeze drying. *Brazilian Journal of Chemical Engineering*. 29(4): 741-750.

Zduńczyk, Z., Flis, M., Zieliński, H., Wróblewska, M., Antoszkiewicz, Z., Juśkiewicz, J. (2006). *In vitro* antioxidant activities of barley, husked oat, naked oat, triticale, and buckwheat wastes and their influence on the growth and biomarkers of antioxidant status in rats. *Journal of Agricultural and Food Chemistry*, 54(12): 4168-4175,

In: Dietary Fiber
Editors: D. Betancur-Ancona, L. Chel-Guerrero et al.
ISBN: 978-1-62808-931-8

Chapter 10

Fibrous Fraction of Hard-to-Cook Bean *Phaseolus vulgaris* as a Potential Additive in the Food Industry

Mukthar Sandoval-Peraza, M. R. Segura-Campos, Luis Chel-Guerrero and David Betancur-Ancona [*]
Facultad de Ingeniería Química. Campus de Ciencias Exactas e Ingenierías, Universidad Autónoma de Yucatán, Mérida, Yucatán, México

Abstract

The common bean (*Phaseolus vulgaris* L.) is the most widely consumed legume in the world, and in Latin America is a basic dietary component. However, poor handling and storage after harvest induces the hardening process in the seed. The objective of this study was to evaluate the physicochemical properties of a fiber-rich fraction (FRF) obtained by wet fractionation of hardened *Phaseolus vulgaris* seeds. The results show the quantity of total dietary fiber (TDF), insoluble dietary fiber (IDF), and soluble dietary fiber (SDF) in the FRF of hardened beans were 43.12, 35.21, and 7.91 g/100g, respectively. The water holding capacity (WHC), water adsorption capacity (WA_dC) and water absorption capacity (WA_bC) were 7.3, 0.29, and 3.45 g/g respectively. The oil-holding capacity (OHC), emulsifying activity (AE), and emulsion stability (ES) values were 1.53, 7.95, and 58.04 g/100g respectively. The fiber rich fraction extracted from hardened *Phaseolus vulgaris* L. possess interesting properties suggesting that it is possible for use in the development of functional food ingredients for reduction of calories or dietary fiber enrichment.

Keywords: Hard-to-cook, dietary fiber, soluble fiber, insoluble fiber, functional properties, *Phaseolus vulgaris*.

[*] Facultad de Ingeniería Química. Campus de Ciencias Exactas e Ingenierías. Universidad Autónoma de Yucatán. Periférico norte km 33.5, Tablaje catastral 13615 Col Chuburná de Hidalgo Inn, C.P. 97203, Mérida, Yucatán. México. E-mail: bancona@uady.mx.

Introduction

Seeds legumes are major sources of dietary proteins in the developing countries, as animal proteins are expensive. In addition to their protein contributions, legumes are also rich in other nutrients such as starch, dietary fiber, protective phytochemicals, oil, vitamins and mineral elements (Shimelis et al., 2006).

Dry beans of *Phaseolus vulgaris* are important food sources, especially in developing countries where they are a major source of dietary protein (Figure 1). For example, in Mexico the estimated annual per capita intake of beans is 22 kg (Gonzalez de Mejia et al., 2005). *Phaseolus* beans are a good source of proteins, vitamins, and certain minerals (Ca, Fe, Cu, Zn, P, K, and Mg). They have beneficial effects on human health, being an excellent source of complex carbohydrates and polyunsaturated fatty acids. However, in tropical countries, storage of common beans under adverse conditions of high temperatura and high humidity renders them susceptible to a hardening phenomenon, also known as the hard to- cook (HTC) defect. Beans with this defect are characterized by extended cooking times, are less acceptable to the consumer, and are of lower nutritive value. In addition, in the raw state, common beans contain antinutritional and toxic substances such as polyphenols, phytates, enzymatic inhibitors, and lectins which limit their acceptability and should be removed or eliminated for effective utilization (Martin-Cabrejas et al., 1997).

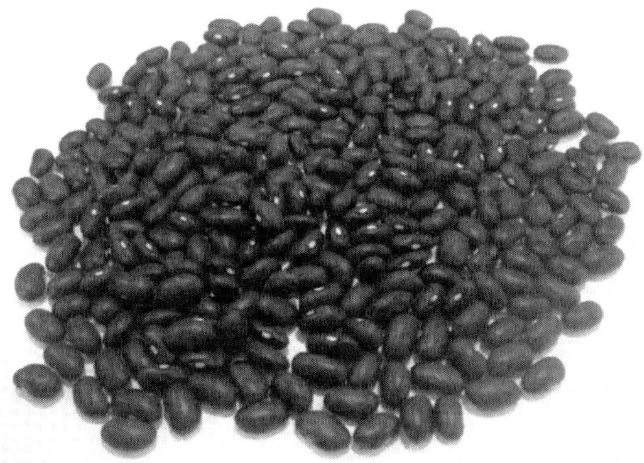

Figure 1. *Phaseolus vulgaris* seeds

Hardness of cooked seeds has been considered a fundamental textural quality of beans and other legumes. According to Hohlberg and Stanley (1987) hardness defects have been classified as hardshell, when the seeds do not absorb sufficient water during cooking and therefore do not soften when cooked, and as hard to-cook, when the seeds absorb enough water but fail to soften upon cooking. Many researchers have reported that extended storage under high temperature and high relative humidity conditions will promote hard-to-cook beans (Hohlberg and Stanley, 1987). All species are affected in this way, but especially common beans, cowpeas and chickpeas (Leterme, 2004).

Several hypotheses have been proposed to explain the cause of bean hardening: lipid oxidation and/or polymerization, formation of insoluble pectates, lignification of middle lamella, and multiple mechanisms. However, most researchers do agree that the defect develops mainly in the cotyledons (Maurer et al., 2004). It is thought that hardening of bean seeds is due to structural changes in the cotyledons, but the chemical reactions responsible are not completely understood. The hard-to-cook defect has been shown to be the result of physical and chemical changes that occur at the intercelular level during storage, resulting in an increase in stability of the middle lamella upon cooking. The most widely accepted explanation relates to the insolubilization of the pectic substances due to the enzyme phytase (Hohlberg and Stanley, 1987). At this respect, Hentges et al. (1991) suggest that the mechanism(s) responsible for the development of the hard-to-cook defect theory involves associations among phytic acid, minerals, and pectin. Phytic acid, located in the protein bodies of the cotyledons, chelates divalent cations. In high temperature, high relative humidity conditions, there would be increased metabolic activity, phytase activation, and membrane degradation. Phytase hydrolyzes phytin to release bound calcium and magnesium. Mattson (1946) related long cooking times of yellow peas to low phytate. Since membranes are degraded, these cations could diffuse to the pectic substances in the middle lamella forming insoluble pectic salts. A decrease in pectin solubility would increase cooking time. Jones and Boulter (1983) reported decreased pectin solubility and pectin esterification in hard-to-cook black beans. A cause and effect relationship, however, has not been clearly established. Other factors including carbohydrate solubility and protein solubility have possible roles in the development of the hard-to-cook defect. Cooking time has been negatively correlated with soluble sugar and positively correlated with protein content of dry legumes. Other enzymatic reactions have been suggested to contribute to hardening. These include removal of methyl groups from pectins by pectinesterases, hydrolysis of storage proteins by proteases, oxidation of polyphenols assisted by peroxidases or polyphenolases, and, less likely, oxidation of lipids by lipoxygenases (Hohlberg and Stanley, 1987).

Garcia et al. (1998) registered the scanning electron micrographs of cell wall isolates (Figure 2). They finded that samples prepared from HTC beans shows a thickening of the walls at the cell junction. Similar results were observed by Hincks and Stanley (1987), while searching for evidence of lignification in beans, and by Bhatty (1990) in poor-cooking lentils. At this respect, Varriano-Marston and Jackson (1981) had suggested the occurrence of a possible lignification of the middle lamella as an explanation for the HTC of beans. However, Garcia et al (1998) in isolated cell walls of dehulled normal and hard beans failed to confirm the presence of lignin (the phloroglucinol- HCl test was negative).

Despite the deterioration reactions that may occur in the seed, portions such as the fiber can still be used. Chim-Rodriguez et al. (2010) reported the use of fibrous residues of *Canavalia ensiformis* L. and *Phaseolus lunatus* L. in the production of cookies. The sensorial evaluation showed the acceptance of the cookies with fiber added compared to conventional wheat cookies. Fibrous fractions are used because of their functional properties such as retention, absorption and adsorption of water, oil-holding capacity, viscosity, antioxidant capacity, organic molecule absorption capacity, etc. Therefore the food industry uses this fiber in many products such as pastas, soups, beverages, meat, and bread because of its functional properties (Elleuch et al., 2011). Besides the functional properties of the fiber, its consumption also has a beneficial effect for the consumer. Recent studies indicate that dietary fiber may be protective against cardiovascular diseases, diabetes, obesity, colon cancer, and diverticular diseases among others (Kutoš et al., 2003). It has also been reported that the amount of indigestible carbohydrates that reach the colon can be degraded by the action of fermentation by intestinal bacteria. The metabolites produced by this degradation repair the colonic mucosa, reduce cholesterol levels in the blood, eliminate carcinogenic agents, and have vasodilator effects (Garcia and Infante, 2007).

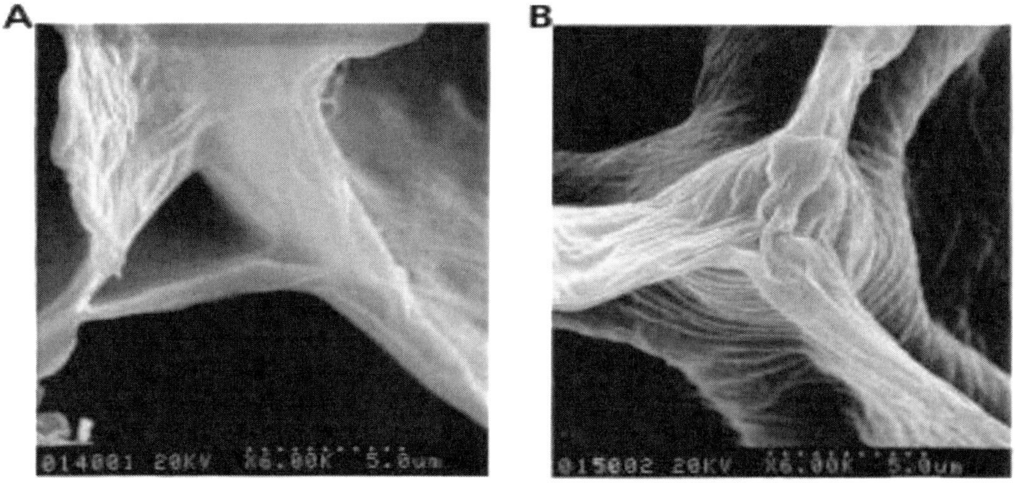

García et al., 1998.

Figura 2. Scanning electron micrographs of isolated walls of (A) control and (B) HTC bean cotyledons.

For the above mentioned, the objective of this study was to evaluate the physicochemical properties of a fiber-rich fraction extracted from hardened *Phaseolus vulgaris* L seeds as potential additive in functional foods.

Materials and Methods

Seeds and Chemicals

Twenty-five kilogrammes of common black beans (*P. vulgaris* L.), var. Jamapa, were used. Two lots (1 kg) were taken to measure cooking time and hardness following Mexican official methods (NMX-FF-038-SCFI-2002.). The use of a fibrous residue extracted from fresh beans was implemented as a control. All chemicals were reagent grade or better and acquired from Sigma Chemical Co. (St. Louis, MO, USA).

Degree of Hardness

Degree of hardness for freshly harvested and HTC beans were determined using a 300 g sample for each type. The respective samples were soaked in water for 12 h, this soak water discarded, fresh water added and the beans put to boil. Cooking was stopped at 55 min, according to the method dictated in applicable Mexican regulations (NMX-FF-038-SCFI-2002). Hardness was measured per bean type using 30 cooked beans (10 g) in an Instron 4411 Universal Testing Machine (10 mm/min compression speed; 8-mm diameter probe; 5 kg load cell), according to the method applicable in Mexican regulations (NMX-FF-038-SCFI-2002).

Flour Preparation

Selected seeds were ground in a disk mill (model 4-E Quaker, Mill Straub Co., Philadelphia, PA, USA) and then sifted through 4.76 and 2.38 mm screens in order to remove the smallest particles before the air classification. Hulls were removed with a fluidizing air bed and the flour resulted was milled in a Cyclotec mill (Tecator, Höganas, Sweden) until passing through a 0.841 mm screen.

Fibrous Residue

The fibrous residues of freshly and HTC beans were processed using the wet-fractionation method reported by Betancur-Ancona et al. (2001). Briefly, 1 kg of 0.841 mm screen grade flour was suspended in distilled water at a 1:6 (w/v) ratio. The pH was adjusted to 11 with 1 N NaOH and the dispersion stirred for 1 h at 400 rpm with a mechanical agitator (Caframo Rz-1). Wet milling was then done in a Kitchen-Aid mill, separating the fiber solids from the starch and protein mix with 0.173 and 0.104 mm screen. The fibrous residue was washed 5 times, using a 1:3 (w/v) solids to distilled water ratio. The resulting fiber fraction was dried at 60 °C in an air convection oven (Imperial V), and then weighed and milled in a Ciclotec mill, until it passed through a 0.841 mm screen.

Proximate Composition

The nitrogen (method 954.01), fat (method 920.39), ash (method 923.03), crude fiber (method 962.09), and moisture (method 925.09) contents of the fibrous residues were determined according to official AOAC procedures (1997). Nitrogen content (N_2) was determined with a Kjeltec Digestion System (Tecator, Sweden), using cupric sulfate and potassium sulfate as catalysts. Protein content was calculated as nitrogen x 6.25. Fat content was obtained from a 1 h hexane extraction. Ash content was calculated from the weight of the sample after burning at 550 °C for 2 h. Moisture content was measured, based on sample weight-loss after oven-drying at 110 °C for 2 h. Carbohydrate content was estimated as nitrogen-free extract (NFE).

Total (TDF), Soluble (SDF) and Insoluble (IDF) Dietary Fiber

Total Dietary Fiber

The dietary fiber fractions were determined using the Prosky et al. (1988) method. Briefly, 1 g (d.b.) fiber samples were placed in four Erlenmeyer flasks (W_1) and weighed. To each of these samples, 50 mL of phosphate buffer (0.08 M, pH 6) were added, and the pH adjusted to 6 with 0.325 HCl N or 0.275 N NaOH. These were then placed in a water bath at 100 °C for 10 min. Then, 0.1 mL α-amylase (Sigma A-3306) was added to each and they were left to incubate at the same temperature for 15 min under constant agitation. The flasks were then cooled rapidly and the samples adjusted to pH 7.5. After this, they were placed in a water bath at 60 °C for 10 min, 0.1 mL protease solution was added to each (Sigma P-3910,

50 mg in 1 mL phosphates buffer), and they were left to incubate at the same temperature for 30 min. The flasks were cooled and the samples adjusted to pH 4, and then returned to the water bath at 60 °C until they reached this temperature. After adding 0.3 mL amyloglucosidase (Sigma A-9913) to each, the samples were left to incubate for 30 min under constant agitation. Then, 95% ethanol at the same temperature was added at a 1:4 sample/ethanol ratio, and the mixture left in the water bath for 1 h. The samples were filtered at a constant weight into crucibles for fiber into which a 1 g cap of Celite had been previously placed. The flasks were rinsed three times with 20 mL of 78% ethanol, twice with 10 mL 95% ethanol, and twice with 10 mL acetone. The crucibles were then placed in a stove at 130 °C for 1.5 h, and weighed (W_2). Two of the crucibles were placed in a furnace at 550 °C for 4 h (W_3), and crude protein was determined using the contents of the remaining two (W_4). Calculations were done using the equation 1:

$$\%\text{TDF} = (W_2 - W_3 - W_4 - W_5)\ X\ 100/\ W_1 \qquad (1)$$

where W_5 is the reagent weight (blank).

Insoluble (IDF) and soluble dietary fiber (SDF)

The same Prosky et al. (1988) method was used to quantify IDF, the only difference being that alcohol was not added to precipitate IDF. Calculation of IDF percentage in the samples was the same as for TDF. The SDF was calculated by subtracting the IDF value from the TDF value.

Functional Properties

Water-holding (WHC) and Oil-Holding Capacity (OHC)

Both capacities were determined following Chau et al. (1997). Briefly, 1 g (d.b.) of sample was weighed and then stirred into 10 mL of distilled water or corn oil (Mazola, CPI International) for one minute. These fibrous suspensions were then centrifuged at 2200g for 30 min and the supernatant volume measured. Water holding capacity was expressed as g of water held per g of sample, and oil-holding capacity was expressed as g of oil held per g of fiber. Corn oil density was 0.92 g/mL.

Water Absorption Capacity (WA_bC)

This property was determined according to AACC method 88-04 (AACC, 1984). Approximate water absorption capacity was first determined by weighing out 2 g (d.b.) of sample, adding water until saturation (approx. 40 mL) and centrifuging at 2000g for 10 min in a Beckman GS-15R centrifuge. Excess water was discarded and the residue weighed. Approximate water absorption capacity was calculated by dividing the increase in sample weight (g) by the quantity of water needed to complete original sample weight (2 g d.b.) to 15 g. Water absorption capacity (WA_bC) was then determined by placing samples in four tubes, adding different quantities of water to bracket the measurement (1.5 and 0.5 mL water above original weight, and 1.5 and 0.5 mL water below; one in each tube), agitating vigorously in a vortex for 2 min, and centrifuging at 2000 g for 10 min in a Beckman GS-15R centrifuge. The supernatant was discarded and the residue weighed. Average water absorbed was calculated and the WA_bC calculated, expressed as g water absorbed per g of sample.

Water Adsorption capacity (WA_dC)

This property was determined according to Chen et al. (1984). Briefly, 1 g (d.b.) of sample was placed in an equilibrium micro-environment at 98% relative humidity, generated by placing 20 mL of saturated potassium sulfate saline solution in tightly sealed glass flasks and placing these in desiccators at 25 °C. The sample was left in the micro-environment until reaching constant weight (72 h). Water adsorption capacity was expressed as g of water per g of sample.

Emulsifying Activity (AE) and Emulsion Stability (ES)

These properties were evaluated following Chau et al. (1997). Briefly, 100 mL of 2% (w/v) fibrous suspension were homogenized using a Caframo RZ-1 homogenizer at 2000 rpm for 2 min. Then, 100 mL of corn oil (Mazola, CPI International) were added to each sample and homogenized for 1 min. The emulsions were then centrifuged in 15 mL, graduated centrifuge tubes at 1200g for 5 min, and the emulsion volume measured. Emulsifying activity was expressed as percentage of the emulsified layer volume of the entire layer in the centrifuge tube. To determine emulsion stability, the prepared emulsions were heated at 80 °C for 30 min, cooled at room temperature and centrifuged at 1200g for 5 min. Emulsion stability was expressed as percentage of the remaining emulsified layer volume of the original emulsion volume.

Statistical Analysis

All determinations were done in triplicate. Statistical analysis was done to determinate the data's central tendency and standard deviation. The differences between fiber-rich fraction from fresh and hardened beans was established according to Montgomery (2003) using the statistic t-student using the Statgraphics plus 5.1 computer software.

Results and Discussion

Degree of Hardness

Cooking time and hardness was compared between fresh and hard beans. The fresh bean had values of 50 minutes of cooking and 0.38 kgf of texture. The hard bean had 70 minutes of cooking and 0.76 kfg of texture these values exceeded acceptable values and are indicative of the development of the HTC phenomenon (NMX-FF-038-SCFI-2002; ≤ 55 minutes of cook and ≤0.5 kfg of texture) (NMX-FF-038-SCFI, 2002). The increase in cooking time of hardened beans may be caused because by the difficulty of the cotyledons to soften. Due to the insolubilization of pectin and cell wall lignification, water takes longer to penetrate into the seed interior (Liu et al., 1992).

Proximate Composition

The proximate composition analysis between FRF from fresh and hard beans is shown in Table 1.

Table 1. Proximate composition (g/100g d.b.) from the FRF of *P. vulgaris* from fresh and hard beans

Component	FRF *P. vulgaris* fresh	FRF *P. vulgaris* hard
Moisture	(10.43 ^{a} ± 0.01)	(6.34 ^{b} ± 0.08)
Protein	12.25 ^{a} ± 0.17	15.93 ^{b} ± 0.07
Fat	1.92 ^{a} ± 0.08	1.74 ^{a} ± 0.22
Crude fiber	5.68 ^{a} ± 0.05	4.62 ^{b} ± 0.09
Ash	1.66 ^{a} ± 0.02	2.55 ^{a} ± 0.42
Nitrogen-free extract (NFE)	78.37^{a} ± 0.01	75.25^{b} ± 0.58

$^{a-b}$ Different lowercase in the same row indicate statistical difference (P< 0.05).

The process that they went through may cause the high value of protein shown in both cases: the seeds were peeled leaving only the cotyledon, which contains the highest amount of protein. The FRF from hard bean has the highest value of protein (15.93%) in comparison with the FRF from fresh bean (12.15%). This can be explained because in the hardening process some proteases can hydrolyze storage proteins. This hydrolysis produces reactive peptides that can react with FRF; this link may be responsible for the insolubilization of proteins from the FRF. The hardness process may be the responsible the proteins remain on high value despite the fact that we made a solubilization in alkaline pH.

Total (TDF), Soluble (SDF) and Insoluble (IDF) Dietary Fiber

Chemical composition of FRF from fresh and hard beans is presented in Table 2. The FRF from hard bean had the higher percentage of total dietary fiber. In both cases of FRF, the highest portion of fiber was in the insoluble fraction. However, FRF from hard bean showed the highest amount of soluble dietary fiber.

Table 2. TDF, IDF, and SDF (g/100g d.b.) to the FRF of *P. vulgaris* from fresh and hard beans

Component	FRF *P. vulgaris* fresh	FRF *P. vulgaris* Hard
TDF	40.52 [a] ± 0.66	43.12 [b] ± 0.46
IDF	37.91 [a] ± 0.6	35.21 [b] ± 0.46
SDF	2.6 [a] ± 0.56	7.91 [a] ± 0.28

[a-b] Different lowercase in the same row indicate statistical difference ($P< 0.05$).

Betancur-Ancona et al. (2004) reported the values of TDF, IDF and SDF in FRF from *Phaseolus lunatus,* which were 29.4, 28.6, and 0.77% respectively, *i.e.*, the amount of fiber present in *Phaseolus vulgaris* was higher. These values indicated that the FRF from hard bean is a good source of soluble dietary fiber. This portion aids in the decrease of cholesterol levels in blood, control of glucose in the bloodstream in the case of diabetics, and this fraction can be an ingredient in diet food products against obesity. The insoluble residue is linked to the ability to decrease the incidence of colon/rectal cancer and diverticulitis (Elleuch et al., 2011).

Functional Properties

Water-Holding (WHC) and Oil-Holding Capacity (OHC)

The highest water-holding capacity (WHC) was shown by the FRF from hard bean (7.3g/g) in comparison with the FRF from fresh bean (5.01g/g) (Figure 3). This may be because the FRF from hard bean has a higher value of SDF (7.91%), which is the portion responsible in great part for the WHC. Steel et al. (1995) reported the values of WHC obtained in extruded flours from *Phaseolus vulgaris* fresh, hardness and mixed flours of hardness bean and rice reporting 4.82, 4.78 y 7.12 g/g respectively. Zambrano et al. (2001) indicated that the WHC obtained in maize hulls (2.32 g/g), wheat hulls (2.48 g/g), and soybean hulls (1.27 g/g), were lower than the FRF from hard bean in this study. This may be caused by too many factors like the chemical composition in the fiber, the source of which is extracted, the ratio of insoluble/soluble fiber present in the dietary fiber, as well as the particle size (Escudero and Gonzalez, 2006). The fiber with a high WHC can be an advantage, because physiologically the fiber can form viscous solutions in the small intestine decreasing the transit time of nutrients; it also increases the thickness of water that has to transfer the solutes to reach the intestinal membrane, which produces a decrease in the absorption of glucose, lipids and amino acids. Likewise, there will be a decrease in the absorption of bile acids, and so these acids will be synthesized from cholesterol thus decreasing the cholesterol levels in the blood (Escudero and Gonzalez, 2006). In the manufacturing of foods, the water-holding capacity is very important because this ability is related to the formulation of low calorie foods (Elleuch et al., 2011).

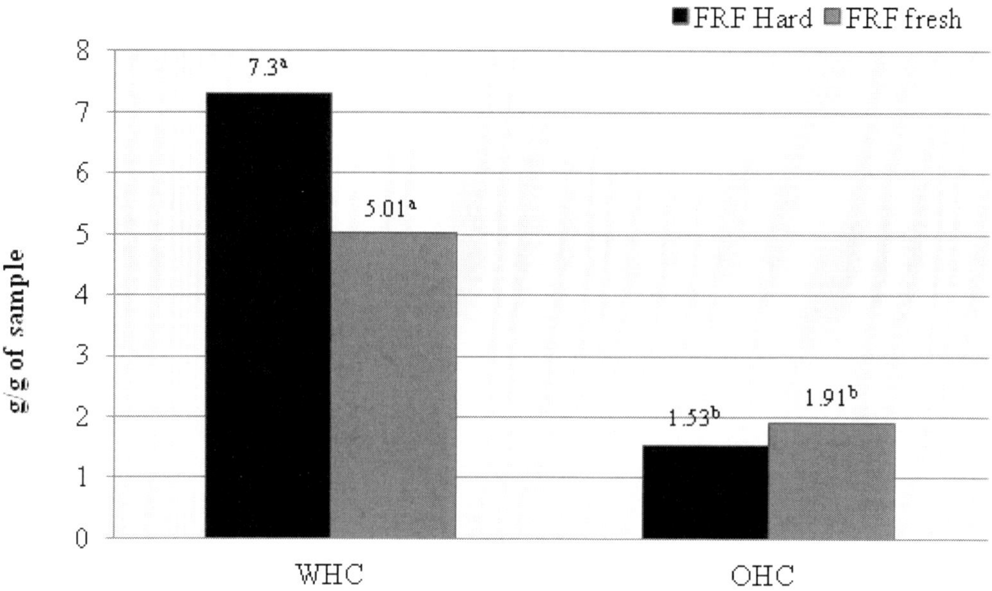

[a-b] Different lowercase in the column indicate statistical difference (P< 0.05).

Figure 3. Water holding capacity (WHC) and oil holding capacity (OHC) of FRF from hard and fresh bean (g /g of sample).

In the oil-holding capacity the FRF from fresh bean has the highest value (1.91 g/g) with respect to the FRF from hard bean, which had 1.53 g/g of retention (15.3 in percent). Betancur-Ancona et al. (2004) reported the oil-holding capacity in the fibrous fraction extracted from *Phaseolus lunatus* and *Canavalia ensiformis,* obtaining values of 18 and 23% respectively; these values were highest in comparison with the result of this study (15.3%). These authors suggested that oil-holding capacity is caused by the amount of lignin and SDF present in the food. Vázquez-Ovando et al. (2009) reported 2.02 g/g for oil-holding capacity in the fibrous fraction extracted from *Salvia hispanica, i.e.,* a higher value than the result of this study. Sangronis et al. (2004) obtained values of 2.2 and 2.4 g/g of oil-holding capacity in flours from fresh and germinated common black *Phaseolus vulgaris*, respectively. López et al. (1997) mentioned that the ability of the fiber to interact with oiling compounds depends in part on the surface characteristics, particles thickness of the compound, and the amount of lignin present in the fiber. Taking into consideration the enzymatic and molecular reactions occurring in the hardening process, it is possible that these reactions may produce chemical and physical changes in the fiber affecting the values of oil compounds retention.

Water Absorption Capacity (Wa_bC) and Water Adsorption Capacity (Wa_dC)

In the water absorption capacity (Figure 4), the FRF from hard bean has a slightly higher value (3.45g/g) but was statistically different (P<0.05) with respect to the FRF from fresh bean (3.3g/g). Zambrano et al. (2001) reported the WA_bC of maize hulls (3.17 g/g), wheat hulls (2.91 g/g), and soybean fiber (1.42 g/g), showing that the WA_bC of the FRF from hard bean is mostly higher in comparison with all materials mentioned. Gaamangwe et al. (2010) reported the WA_bC in dehulled flours from *T. esculentum* (1.5 g/g), and observed that the FRF from hard bean showed a better WA_bC. Vázquez-Ovando et al. (2009) reported 11.73 g/g of WA_bC in fibrous residues of *Salvia hispanica,* which is higher compared to this study. This could be caused by the chemical composition of the fiber, since it can form a lattice trapping the water of the medium, or can associate with their structural water matrix (Escudero and Gonzalez 2006). In the water adsorption capacity the FRF from hard bean has the highest value (0.29g/g) in comparison with the FRF from fresh bean (0.23g/g). Vázquez-Ovando et al. (2009) reported the values for WA_dC obtained in fibrous residue extracted from *Salvia hispanica* as 0.3 g/g, which is similar to the FRF from hard bean (0.29 g/g) of this study. Zambrano et al. (2001) also reported the WA_dC in maize hulls, wheat hulls, and soybean fiber, obtaining 0.41, 0.3 and 0.38 g/g respectively; the value of WA_dC in wheat hulls is very similar to the WA_dC of the FRF from hard bean but lower than the other materials. The determination of this parameter is important, considering its relationship to stability and deteriorative changes in the source of fiber during storage, where the water can produce molecular changes because it may act as a plasticizer modifying the physiologic function of the dietetic fiber (Zambrano et al., 2001). Physiologically, the WA_dC has a very important role, as it has been demonstrated that compounds present in the fiber have the capacity to absorb organic molecules like acids and biliary salts. López et al. (1997) mentioned that the adsorption process in the fibers limits the absorption of bile acid in the intestine forcing the organism to produce the synthesis of new bile acids from cholesterol, which results in reduced levels of this compound in the blood.

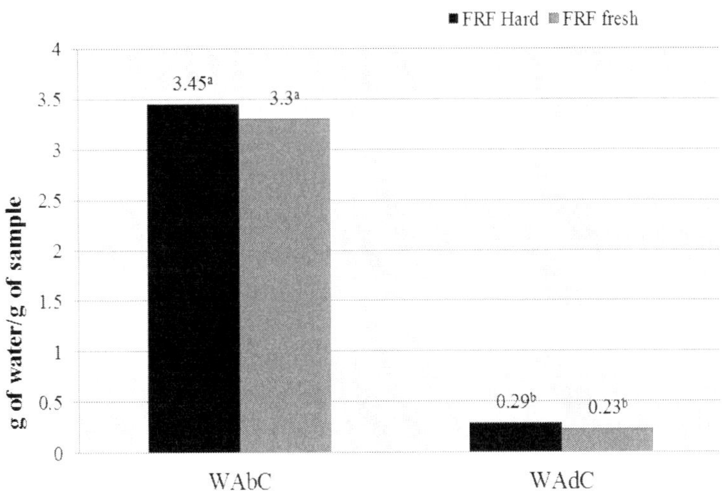

[a-b] Different lowercase in the column indicate statistical difference (P< 0.05).

Figure 4. Water absorption capacity (WA_bC) adsorption capacity (WA_dC) of FRF from hard and fresh beans (g of water/g of sample).

Emulsifying Activity (AE) and Emulsion Stability (ES)

Emulsifying capacity is the ability of a molecule to act, as an agent that facilitate the solubilization or dispersion of two immiscible liquids, and emulsion stability is the ability to maintain an emulsion and it resistance to rupture. Therefore, it was noted that the FRF from hard bean showed the highest AE and ES with respect to the FRF from fresh bean (Figure 5). This behavior is directly related to fiber type and the percentage of the soluble and insoluble fiber fractions. In this case, the FRF from hard bean was a high percentage of IDF (35.21%) and SDF (7.91%) in comparison to the FRF from fresh bean (37.91% of IDF and 2.6% of SDF), thus indicating that the compounds of the soluble fraction present in the FRF from hard bean may be responsible for emulsion stability. Betancur-Ancona et al. (2004) reported the AE and ES of the fibrous residue from *P. lunatus* obtaining 49.3% of AE and 28.25% of ES, *i.e.*, the fibrous residue of *P. lunatus* had the highest AE in comparison with the FRF from hard bean; however, the hardened FRF showed a better ES with respect to the *P. lunatus* fibrous residue.

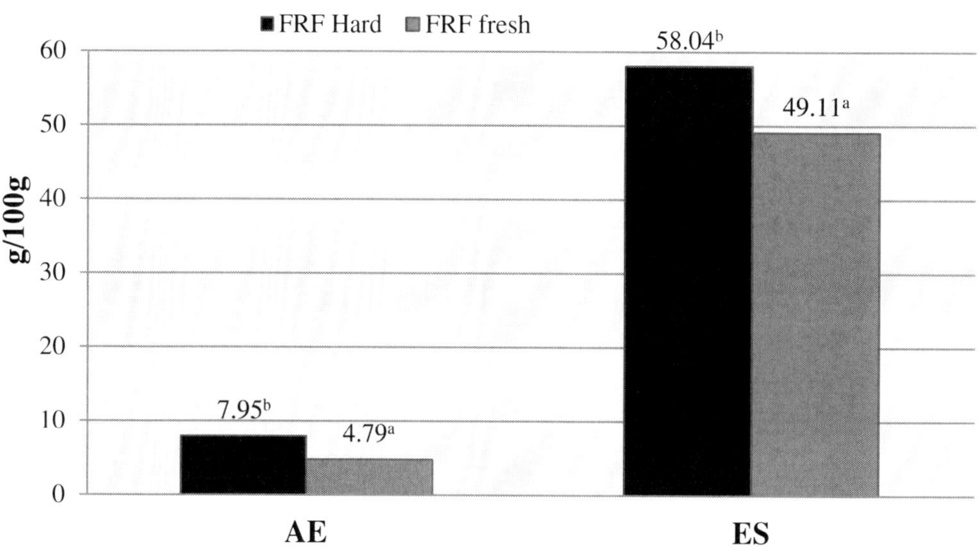

a-b Different lowercase in the column indicate statistical difference ($P < 0.05$).

Figure 5. Emulsifying activity (AE) and emulsion stability (ES) (g/100g d.b.) to the FRF from *Phaseolus vulgaris* fresh and hard.

Most fractions (cellulose, lignin, hemicellulose, pectins, gums and mucilages) of dietary fiber are the major constituents of plant cell walls. Although some authors recommend dropping the terms "soluble" and "insoluble" fiber, the physiological effects of this indigestible component of foods is being increasingly recognized (Punna et al., 2003). According to Romero-López et al. (2012) the development of new products with substantial dietary fiber contents is a strategic area for the food industry. Consumers are demanding foods that show two main properties: the first one refers to the traditional nutritional aspects of the food, whereas, as a second feature, additional health benefits are expected from its regular ingestion. Foods complying with these requisites are often called functional or nutraceutical foods. Huang et al. (2011) suggest that in addition to the physicochemical properties given by fiber-rich food, studies in experimental animals and humans have suggested that fiber component can provide physiological effect such as reducing blood sugar content and decreasing serum lipid concentration. For the above mentioned and in view of the potential benefits of the fibrous fraction from hard bean (*Phaseolus vulgaris*) a wide range of fiber-rich products could be developed as functional food ingredients.

Conclusion

This study revealed that the fibrous residue from hard bean (*Phaseolus vulgaris*) have a 43.12% of total dietary fiber. It was discovered that 35.21% consisted of the insoluble fraction and 7.91% for the soluble fraction. It was observed that this residue has elevated values in retention, absorption and adsorption of water, but relatively low levels in the retention of oil, emulsifying capacity and emulsion stability. The results of our study confirmed that fibrous residue from hard bean has excellent potential in food applications as a functional ingredient, especially in the development of reduced calorie food and dietary fiber enriched food products.

References

AACC. (1984). Official methods of analysis, 12th ed. *American Association of Cereal Chemists*, St. Paul, MN, USA.

AOAC. (1997). Official Methods of analysis. *Association of official analytical chemists*, 15th ed., William Horwitz Editor: Washington, D.C., USA.

Bhatty, R. S. (1990). Cooking quality of lentils. The role of structure and composition of cell walls. *Journal of Agricultural and food Chemistry, 38*, 376-383.

Betancur-Ancona, D., Camelo-Matos, R., Chel-Guerrero, L. and Dávila-Ortíz, G. (2001). Physicochemical and functional characterization of Baby Lima bean (*Phaseolus lunatus*) starch. *Starch/Stärke, 53(5),* 219–226.

Betancur-Ancona, D., Peraza-Mercado, G., Moguel-Ordoñez, Y. and Fuertes-Blanco, S. (2004). Physicochemical characterization of lima bean (*Phaseolus lunatus*) and Jack bean (*Canavalia ensiformis*) fibrous residues. *Food Chemistry, 84*, 287-295.

Chau, C.F., Cheung, K. and Wong, Y.S. (1997). Functional properties of protein concentrates from three Chinese indigenous legume seeds. *Journal of Agricultural and Food Chemistry, 45(7),* 2500–2503.

Chen, J., Piva, M. and Labuza, T.P. (1984). Evaluation of water binding capacity (WBC) of food fiber sources. *Journal of Food Science, 49(1)*, 59–63.

Chim Rodriguez, A., Chel Guerrero, L., Betancur-Ancona, D. (2010). Incorporacion de almidones primarios y secundarios de *Canavalia ensiformis* y *Phaseolus lunatus* en galletas. In: Utilización de recursos naturales tropicales para el desarrollo de alimentos. Editores: David A. Betancur Ancona, Luis A Chel Guerrero, Arturo F. Castellanos Ruelas. PRIORI-UADY. ISBN:978-607-7573-77-7. Mérida, Yucatán, México.

Elleuch, M., Bedigian, D., Roiseux, O., Besbes, S., Blecker, C. and Attia, H. (2011). Dietary fiber and fiber-rich by-products of food processing: characterization, technological functionality and commercial applications: A review. *Food Chemistry*, *124*, 411-421.

Escudero, A.E. and González, S.P. (2006). La fibra dietética. *Nutrición Hospitalaria, 21(2)*, 61-72.

García, O. and Infante, R.B. (2007). La fibra alimentaria y sus aspectos nutricionales. Una visión de los alimentos Venezolanos. *INFORMED, 9(6)*, 285-294.

García, E., Filisetti, T.M.C.C., Udaeta, J.E.M., Lajolo, F.M. (1998). Hard-to-cook beans (*Phaseolus vulgaris*): Involvement of phenolic compounds and pectates. *Journal of Agricultural and Food Chemistry, 46*, 2110-2116.

Gonzalez de Mejía, E., Valadez-Vega, M.C., Reynoso-Camacho, R., Loarca-Pina, G. (2005). Tannins, trypsin inhibitors and lectin cytotoxicity in tepary (*Phaseolus acutifolius*) and common (*Phaseolus vulgaris*) beans. *Plant Foods for Human Nutrition, 60*, 137-145.

Gaamangwe, N., Kwaku, G. and Minnaar, A. (2010). Physicochemical, nutricional and functional properties of marama bean flour. *Food Chemistry, 121*, 400-405.

Hentges, D.L., Weaver, C.M., Nielsen, SS. (1991). Changes of selected physical and chemical components in teh development of the hard-to-cook bean defect. *Journal of Food Science, 56(2)*, 436-442.

Hincks, M. J., Stanley, D. W. (1987). Lignification: evidence for a role in hard-to-cook beans. *Journal of Food Biochemistry, 11*, 41-58.

Hohlberg, A.I. and Stanley, W. (1987). Hard-to-cook defect in black beans. protein and starch consideartions. *Journal of Agricultural and Food Chemistry, 35*, 571-576.

Huang, Y.L., Chow, C.J., Fang, Y.J. (2011). Preparation and physicochemical properties of fiber-rich fraction from pineapple peels as a potential ingredient. *Journal of Food and Drug Analysis, 19 (3)*, 318-323.

Jones, P.M.B. and Boulter, D. (1983). The cause of reduced cooking rate in Phaseolus vulgaris following adverse storage conditions. *Journal of Food Science, 48*, 623.

Kutoš, T., Golob, T., Kač, M. and Plenstenjak, A. (2003). Dietary fiber content of dry and processed bean. *Food Chemistry, 80*, 231-235.

Leterme, P. (2004). Hard-to-cook defect in grain legumes: scientists try to explain. *Grain Legumes, 39*, 8-9.

Liu, K., McWatters, K.H. and Dixon, P.R. (1992). Protein insolubilization and thermal destabilization during storage as related to hard-to-cook defect in cowpeas. *Journal of Agricultural and Food Chemistry, 40*, 2483-2487.

López, G., Ros, G., Rincón, F., Periago, M., Martínez, C. and Ortuño, J. (1997). Propiedades funcionales de la fibra dietética. Mecanismos de acción en el tracto gastrointestinal. *Archivos Latinoamericanos de Nutricion, 47(3)*, 203-207.

Martin-Cabrejas, M.A., Esteban, R.M., Perez, P., Maina, G., Waldron, K.W. (1997). Changes in physicochemical properties of dry beans (*Phaseolus vulgaris*) during long-term storage. *Journal of Agricultural and Food Chemistry, 45*, 3223-3227.

Mattson. S. (1946). The cookabilitv of vellow neas. A colloid-chemical and biochemical study. Acta A griculture Suecaha II. 2, 185.

Maurer, G.A., Ozen, B.F., Mauer, L.J., Nielsen, S.S. (2004). *Journal of agricultural and food chemistry, 52*, 1470-1477.

Montgomery, D. (2003). *Diseño y Análisis de experimentos*. Ed. Iberoamericana: México D.F., México.

NMX-FF-038-SCFI-2002. Productos alimenticios no industrializados para consumo humano, fabáceas, frijol (*Phaseolus vulgaris*) especificaciones y métodos de prueba. Available online:http://www.sagarpa.gob.mx/agronegocios/Lists/Instrumentos%20Tcnicos%20Normalizacin%20y%20Marcas%20Colecti/Attachments/91/NMX_FRIJOL.pdf.

Punna, R., Paruchuri, U.R. (2003). Total, insoluble and soluble fiber contents in Indian fruits. *Journal of Food Compition and Analysis, 16*, 677–685.

Prosky, L., Asp, N.G., Schweizer, T.F., DeVries, J.W. and Furda, I. (1988). Determination of insoluble, soluble and total dietary fiber in foods and food products: interlaboratory study. *Journal of the Association of Official Analytical Chemists, 71(5)*, 1017–1023.

Romero-López, M., Osorio-Diaz, P., Bello-Perez, L.A., Tovar, J., Bernardino-Nicanor, A. (2011). Fiber concentrate from orange (*Citrus sinensis* L.) bagasse: Characterization and application as bakery product ingredient. *International Journal of Molecular Sciences, 12*, 2174-2186.

Sangronis, E., Machado, C. and Cava, R. (2004). Propiedades funcionales de las harinas de leguminosas (*Phaseolus vulgaris y Cajan cajan*) germinadas. *INTERCIENCIA, 29(2)*, 80-85.

Steel, C.J., Sgarbieri, V.C. and Jackix, M.H. (1995). Use of extrusion technology to overcome undesirable properties of hard-to-cook dry beans (*Phaseolus vulgaris L.*). *Journal of Agricultural and Food Chemistry, 43*, 2487-2492.

Shimelis, E., Meaza, M. and Rakshit, S. (2006). Physico-chemical Properties, Pasting Behavior and Functional Characteristics of Flours and Starches from Improved Bean (*Phaseolus vulgaris* L.) Varieties Grown in East Africa. Agricultural Engineering International: the CIGR Ejournal. Manuscript FP 05 015. Vol. VIII. February.

Varriano-Marston, E., Jackson, G. M. (1981). Hard-to-cook phenom- enon in beans: structural changes during storage and imbibition. *Journal of Food Science, 46*, 1379-1385.

Vázquez-Ovando, A., Rosado-Rubio, G., Chel-Guerrero, L. and Betancur-Ancona, D. (2009). Physicochemical properties of a fibrous fraction from chia (*Salvia hispanica L.*). *Food Science and Technology, 42*, 168-173.

Zambrano, Z.M., Meléndez, P.R. and Gallardo, N.Y. (2001). Propiedades funcionales y metodología para su evaluación en fibra dietética. In *Fibra dietética en Iberoamérica: Tecnología y Salud.* Lajolo, F.M.; Saura-Calixto, F.; Witting de Penna, E. and Wenzel de Menezes, E., Eds.; Livraría: São Paulo, Brasil, 2001; Chapter 14, pp. 195–209.

In: Dietary Fiber
Editors: D. Betancur-Ancona, L. Chel-Guerrero et al.
ISBN: 978-1-62808-931-8

Chapter 11

Dietary Fiber: From Concept to Realization

Angela Zuleta[*]
Department of Food Science, Faculty of Pharmacy and Biochemistry, University of Buenos Aires, Buenos Aires, Argentina

Abstract

The concept of dietary fiber appeared in 1953 in order to describe the components of the cell walls of edible plants. Since then, and particularly in recent years, the definition of dietary fiber has changed in order to include a growing number of substances and to recognize its physiological effects. Establishing a definition for dietary fiber has historically been a balance between nutritional knowledge and analytical method capabilities. Due to the complexity of the issue caused by the diversity of the structures, physical, chemical and physiological properties of these compounds, it has been very difficult to arrive at a definition and an analytical method to identify this fraction. In 2008 the Codex Committee on Nutrition and Foods for Special Dietary Uses (CCNFSDU) agreed on a definition of dietary fiber: "*Dietary fiber means carbohydrate polymers with ten or more monomeric units, which are not hydrolyzed by endogenous enzymes in the small intestine of the human.*" Basically, the term fiber refers to carbohydrates that cannot be digested. Fiber is present in all edible plants, including fruits, vegetables, grains, and legumes. However, not all fiber is the same, and there are a number of ways to categorize it. The physicochemical and biological properties of these compounds, as they relate to dietary fiber, are associated with physiological actions in the small and large intestine, having important implications in human health. Despite the healthful influence, dietary fiber can be helpful in reducing the risk of chronic diseases; the intake remains low in many populations worldwide. However, increasing fiber consumption in the diet has been a difficult challenge. This is mainly because fiber sources usually used in foods have not made high-fiber foods with high quality taste properties. In order to make a hypothesis and definition into labeling regulations that will benefit the consumer of high-fiber foods, appropriate analytical methodology was needed. Both the definition

[*] Email: azuleta@ffyb.uba.ar.

and the analytical method are necessary elements from the legal point of view, in terms of nutritional labeling of foods and, from the health point of view so as to have actual data for the design of diets in epidemiological research studies. It is the purpose of this chapter to give an overview of important oligosaccharides and polysaccharides that function as dietary fibers, to discuss their occurrence and structures and their various physiological effects and health implications, and to define and analyze these methods in order to further describe the role high fiber ingredients play in food development.

Introduction

Until recently, the interest of the nutritional recommendations focused on lipids and proteins, making the treatment of carbohydrates (CHO) rather secondary. Currently, macronutrient nutritional goals are directed not only to reduce the risk of malnutrition, but also the risks of developing chronic non-communicable diseases (NCDs) related to food. For example, a moderate consumption of fat is suggested to be a daily maximum of 30% of calories; proteins remain constant, and consequently the increase of calories is derived from CHO.

The CHO constitutes the largest proportion of macronutrients in the diet of the world's population in developed countries reaching 50% to 70% of the daily calories in developing countries. This includes a wide variety of compounds present in foods, with different molecular weights, different degrees of polymerization and various structures. Integrate simple sugars, such as monosaccharides, disaccharides, and polyols, oligosaccharides with a polymerization degree between 3 and 9, as maltodextrins, raffinose, stachyose and verbascose, present in the beans, and polysaccharides with a degree of polymerization higher than 9, and starch, cellulose, hemicellulose and pectin.

The meeting FAO / WHO in human nutrition CHO agreed that CHO intake should be at least 55% of total calories, and caloric intake should be mainly complex CHO with a low glycemic index (GI) (FAO/OMS, 1998). This recommendation emphasizes the consumption of foods that meet this condition and distance of the conceptual framework that regarded all complex CHO as having similar physiological properties.

The importance of high-CHO foods in the diets of populations tends to increase due to current recommendations, which are based on the need to lower the risk factors of NCDs such as cardiovascular disease, cancer and obesity (Araya and Lutz, 2003).It is shown that higher fat intake increases energy consumption because of the difficulty of humans to regulate energy intake (Flatt, 1996). It is clear that the decrease in fat consumption inevitably leads to increased consumption of CHO, as the concentration of dietary protein remains constant. Consequently, food that is high in starch is of particular importance, as it helps to meet nutritional goals. This is accompanied by other specific recommendations, such as reducing the consumption of simple sugars and increasing dietary fiber (Stubbs et al., 2001). This implies the need for better understanding of this component of the diet, and has been central in many research papers (Zuleta and Araya, 2009).

Dietary Fiber (DF)

The first reference to the properties of the fiber, which is attributed to Aretaeus of Cappadocia (second century BC), relates the properties of wheat mixed with milk and wine on the stomach. Hippocrates and Galen in turn related cereal grains with intestinal physiology (constipation), while Cleave, commander of the British navy surgeon, observed that Aborigines who ate diets high in raw vegetables with low consumption of meat proved the existence of a relationship between the consumption of vegetables (fiber) and metabolic or degenerative diseases (Dreher, 2001).

However, the first reference to the definition of DF appears in 1953 when Hipsley defines it as "not available CHO in foods from plants, which have no nutritional value". In 1975, Trowell postulates the "dietary fiber hypothesis", which states that diets rich in foods containing material of the plant cell wall in a relatively natural state, have a protective action against a number of diseases that are prevalent in Western society (Dreher 2001).

One must consider that the main source of DF constitutes the cell walls of plants (Theander and Westerlund, 1986). Its composition is highly variable in different plants and even within the same plant, depending on the degree of maturation and tissue.

As mentioned above, the components of the DF by definition are resistant to hydrolysis and absorption in the small intestine. They pass through the upper gastrointestinal tract, entering the colon virtually unchanged.

Two fractions traditionally recognized DF as "soluble fiber" (SF) and "insoluble fiber" (IF); to differentiate between the soluble components, which will form gels or viscous solutions (e.g., pectins) that are insoluble and will produce a bulk effect (e.g., cellulose). However, this difference does not always predict the physiological effects. For this last FAO / WHO the distinction between soluble and insoluble fiber is to be replaced by fermentable and non-fermentable. The non-fermentable fiber types, such as lignified outer layers of cereal grains, generally have a fecal bulking effect by its ability to bind water in the distal colon. Fermentable fiber also contributes to the formation of package through increased microbial mass (EFSA, 2010).

The DF components are fermentable substrates of anaerobic fermentation by colonic microflora and produce AGCC. The main fiber types involved in resistant starch (AR) are maltodrextinas resistant, inulin, polydextrose and hemicellulose. The degree of fermentation depends on both the substrate (molecular structure and physical form) and host factors (bacterial flora and transit time).

Fully digestible starch has always been considered, but it has been found that, for various reasons (biological origin by technological processes and/or food preparation) some of the starch remaining in the residue is not digestible by enzymes in the thin intestine, i.e. it passes into the colon along with the polysaccharide to form the fiber. Therefore, the concept changed this nutrient that is believed fully digestible, a fact confirmed in vivo when tested in patients ileostomised (Englyst et al., 1992).

The digestion rate of the starch is affected by the inherent and acquired through food. The physical matrix is highlighted, which influences the accessibility of digestive enzymes. This rigid matrix is relevant in the amylose content, which in the majority of starches reaches about 25%.

Another factor is the ratio of amylose and amylopectin starch: the amylose molecule is mainly linear, which is stiffer and less sensitive to the action of amylase, whereas amylopectin is a branched structure that facilitates the enzymatic action (Grandfelt and Bjork, 1991). The higher the amylose content, with greater the difficulty in gelatinized starch is, which is more susceptible to retrogradation (Colonna and Mercier, 1985).

Corn starches, commonly referred to as high amylose starches, which are obtained by genetic techniques, have amounts up to 70-75%. Amylopectin, meanwhile, is about 75% of most common starches. Some starches are composed exclusively of amylopectin, and are known as wax or waxy starches (Bello-Pérez et al., 2006).

Starches are found in foods that need to be processed, except for most fruits. When cooked in water the semicrystalline structure of the starch granules is altered, causing gelatinization, which is a process with an irreversible loss of the crystalline region, making it more sensitive to enzymatic action. The granules do not dissolve during processing, remaining a dispersion. Moreover, during extrusion it forms covalent molecular bonds between starch and lipids or proteins, producing a decrease in the rate of digestion, but predominantly gelatinization.

Forms of consumption that maintain their integrity, such as whole grain (corn and beans), slow the rate of digestion. The refined foods, such as polished rice, wheat flour or legumes in flour form, allow a rapid rate of digestion (Elliasson and others 1996). The ground particle size of the consumed food is important; the finer material is mostly digested by digestive enzymes (Holt et al., 1992, 1995).

When cooling a food already cooked retrogradation occurs, a process in which the gelatinized starch takes a new semi-crystalline structure by intramolecular bond formation. A higher amount of amylose facilitates this reversal, slowing the rate of digestion. (Topping et al., 2003).

As mentioned above, studios performed both in vitro and in vivo for classifying starches according to their availability. Englyst et al., (1992) proposes a nutritional classification of starch based on the glycemic response that is obtained after hydrolysis:

- Quickly digested (20 min), abundant in freshly cooked food
- Slowly digestible (120 min), abundant in ground raw cereals
- Resistant starch (AR). In turn, this is classified into three types:
- -Type 1 or AR1: starch physically trapped within structures such as plant cell walls, making it inaccessible to the intestinal enzymes. It comes in the partially milled cereal grains and legumes.
- Type 2 or AR2: starch crystallized enzymes cannot be attacked unless previously gelatinized. It comes in raw potatoes, green bananas and cornmeal.
- Type 3, retrograded or AR3: starch changes its conformation to physical phenomena such as heat and cold, resulting in resistance to intestinal enzymatic degradation. It is usually present in starchy foods after cooking and subsequent cooling, such as bread, cereal flakes and potatoes cooked and cooled (Englystet al., 1992). AR3 content increases when foods are subjected to an increasing number of cycles of heating and cooling (Topping et al., 2003).
- Some authors added to this Type 4 list (Brown, 2004) of chemically modified starch (by the action of acids, dextrinization enzymatic acetylation, hydroxyethylation, etc.).

These starches reach the large intestine intact, so they are considered part of the DF. While the AR is part of the insoluble fiber, its effects are similar to those of the soluble fiber.

As described, not only the botanical origin of the starch hydrolysis rate is affected, but the processes that have been subjected as well. The rapid digestion rate of starch is gelatinized, including foods subjected to firing in liquid or that have been autoclaved. The slowly digestible starches are those that, by the structure of the food matrix hamper access to the hydrolytic enzymes found in seeds and grains, in highly dense foods like pasta, and raw foods, as mentioned above. The retrograded starch that is formed on cooling the gelatinized starch may be part of this fraction refractory to enzymatic action.

Technological processes used in the production of products that do not require cooking for consumption and dissolve quickly in water, accelerate the digestion of starches. Spaghetti production is a process that induces a slow digestion, due to the encapsulated structure and bonding of starch to gluten, factors that decrease the gelatinization (Grandfelt and Bjork, 1991).

In rice, the rate of digestion depends on the concentrations of amylose and technological and culinary processes that apply. For example, rice and parboiled rice graining, which is fried in oil prior to cooking in water, slow digestion (Araya et al., 1998).

Raw cereal starch is digested very slowly, so its gelatinization in cooking water allows greater access to the intestinal amylases. Raw potato starch, which is indigestible by its crystallographic structure, is completely digested by the same process. Altering the structure of the food by spraying or other cooking processes and also chewing, increases digestion, allowing access to the digestive enzymes. A process which delays the digestion of starch is spaghetti, in which there is a protein network that encompasses the granules absorbing water, preventing and delaying the hydrolysis. Moreover, cooking with small amounts of liquid, such as cookies, hinders complete gelatinization of the granules, slowing hydrolysis (Colonna et al., 1992).

Ungelatinized starches from corn hybrids with high amylose content of approximately 60 to 70%, are resistant to amylolysis (i.e., AR2) and are commercially used as an ingredient in various processed foods.

The products obtained from these starches by physical treatments and enzymatic ingredients retain a high content in foods where AR sterilization, baking, etc. are used (Sajilata et al., 2006). Some authors have produced chemically modified starches such as phosphate di-or polyfunctional (i.e., AR4), which may become resistant to the level of phosphorus that is incorporated. While these modified starches can be used as thickening additives in amounts generally 0.5% to 2%, there are no clinical data to support its use as an ingredient in common starch replacement (Brown, 2004).

The progress of studies on the properties and new sources of DF has been aided by the advance in the development of new analytical methodologies that allow the discovery of new indigestible compounds. Resistant dextrins are new products related to the AR, which is obtained by treating starch with acid and heat, followed by an enzymatic process.

Polydextrose is another product that, not being hydrolyzed in the small intestine, can be part of the fiber. It is obtained by thermal polymerization of glucose with citric acid as a catalyst and sorbitol as a plasticizer. It is used as a bulking agent and humectant in formulations to eliminate or replace fat and sugar. Indigestible oligosaccharides, are compounds of low molecular weight, from 3 to 9 units, which have joints resistant to the hydrolysis of human digestive enzymes, so they are considered part of the DF from the physiological standpoint, but are not quantified by conventional methods of analysis, and are not included in the definition.

The components that fall within this fraction are (AACC, 2001):

- Galactooligosaccharides or transgalacto-oligosaccharides (TOS) synthetic: obtained from lactose by transglucosylation by β-galactosidase.
- Galacto-oligosaccharides (GOS) from soybeans and other legumes: comprise the raffinose (DP3), stachyose (DP4) and verbascose (DP5). Serum obtained in the process of isolating soy proteinare α-galacto-oligosaccharides, but as human intestine lacks α-galactosidase, hydrolysis resistance and reach the colon.
- Fructans: are widely distributed in nature in plants, algae, bacteria and fungi. However, its knowledge has been limited due to the difficulty of analytical determination. In plants CHO is stored as backup in different organs such as leaves, roots, tubers, rhizomes and fruits. As fructans are located, other physiological functions in addition to the reservationpredominantly against starch, which meets this goal in most species. It has been suggested that fructans contribute to the stability of proteins and membranes during the drying process, replacing the hydration layer. This feature may be related to the structural flexibility possessed by the fructans, which makes it unique among all the polysaccharides (Pontis and Del Campillo, 1985).
- Inulin and fructo-oligosaccharides (FOS) are the most studied fructans from a nutritional standpoint and technology. Both differ in the degree of polymerization of the polymer blends they contain, which is between 2 and 60 for inulin and between 2 and 10 for FOS. They are formed by a sucrose molecule to which they are attached by successive fructose molecules linked β 2-1, resistant to enzyme hydrolysis in the human digestive tract, reaching the colon intact. Thus, fructans are considered part of the DF (Prosky, 1999; AACC, 2001).

In the colon, these compounds are completely fermented by bacteria, giving rise to short chain AG (acetate, propionate, butyrate, lactate) and bacterial biomass gases (CO2, H2, methane). Even high doses were not detected in significant amounts as fructans in stool (Cherbut, 2002). As a result of this fermentation there is an increase in bacterial mass, which results in an increase of stool weight and size, promoting bowel motility. The volume index (increase in stool weight expressed as g / g indigestible ingested CHO) is 1.2 to 2.1, a value similar to that produced with other fibers such as pectins and easily fermented gums, mainly due to an increase in microbial biomass.

Increased stool frequency, particularly in slightly constipated individuals, with decreased fecal pH, which is linked to the suppression of the production of putrefactive substances in the colon (Nyman, 2002). By their ability to ferment, inulin and FOS can modulate various aspects of intestinal epithelial integrity, reducing the risk of gastrointestinal diseases (Cherbut, 2002).

As a result of this fermentation there is an increase in bacterial mass, which results in an increase of stool weight and size, promoting bowel motility. The volume index (increase in stool weight expressed as g / g indigestible ingested CHO) is 1.2 to 2.1, this value is similar to that produced with other fibers such as pectins and easily fermented gums, mainly due to the increase in microbial biomass.

Increased stool frequency, particularly in slightly constipated individuals with decreased fecal pH, is linked to the suppression of the production of putrefactive substances in the colon (Nyman, 2002). By their ability to ferment, inulin and FOS can modulate various aspects of intestinal epithelial integrity, reducing the risk of gastrointestinal diseases (Cherbut, 2002).

Definitions

Initially the term "dietary fiber" (DF) defined as a "food portion derived from the cell wall of plants poorly digested by humans" 13. The recognition that the polysaccharides are added to foods, especially hydrocolloids, could have similar effects to those from cell walls led to the redefinition of DF to include "the polysaccharides and lignin that are not digested in the human gut intestine. (EFSA, 2010; American Dietetic Association, 2008) Given the importance of the digestibility in the small intestine of the HC for its nutritional effects, it is considered that DF should include all non-digestible carbohydrates plus lignin.

These includes:

- Non-starch polysaccharides (PSNA): cellulose, hemicellulose, pectin, hydrocolloids (gums, mucilages, ß-glucans),
- Oligosaccharides resistant to three or more monomeric units: FOS, GOS,
- Lignin resistant starch.

Some of these compounds are substrates for the anaerobic fermentation by colonic microflora. As a result of scientific debate organized by the AACC (American Association of Cereal Chemists), in 2001 we established a definition: "Dietary fiber is the edible part of plants or CHO analogues that are resistant to digestion and absorption in the human intestine, with complete or partial fermentation in the large intestine. The DF includes polysaccharides, oligosaccharides, lignin and associated substances. DF promotes the beneficial physiological effects including laxation, and/or decrease of cholesterol and/or glucose. "As can be seen, this definition content extends DF and CHO in those analogs, i.e., those that are produced in food processing, or by chemical, physical or enzymatic processes. In addition the explicit physiological benefits provided are to be considered as fiber.

Codex Alimentarius (2009)

The term "fiber" means carbohydrate polymers with nine or more monomeric units, which are neither digested nor absorbed in the human small intestine and belong to the following categories:

- Carbohydrate polymers naturally occurring in food as consumed,

- Edible carbohydrates polymers have been obtained from raw food material by physical, enzymatic or chemicals and have a beneficial physiological effect demonstrated by generally accepted scientific evidence,
- Edible synthetic carbohydrate polymers have a beneficial physiological effect demonstrated by generally accepted scientific evidence.

European Union (EU) Directive 2008/100/Ec

For the purposes of this Directive, the term "fiber" means carbohydrate polymers with three or more monomeric units, which are neither digested nor absorbed in the human small intestine and belong to the following categories:

- Carbohydrate polymers naturally occurring in food as consumed,
- Edible carbohydrate polymers have been obtained from food raw material by physical, enzymatic or chemical processes and have a beneficial physiological effect demonstrated by generally accepted scientific evidence,
- Edible synthetic carbohydrate polymers having a beneficial physiological effect demonstrated by generally accepted scientific evidence.

In order to take into account new scientific and technological knowledge it is necessary to amend the list of energy conversion factors. In the report of an FAO technical workshop entitled Food energy, methods of analysis and conversion factors ("Food energy, methods of analysis and conversion factors"), indicated that 70% considered fermentable dietary fiber in traditional foods. It is therefore desirable that the average energy value for dietary fiber is 8kJ/g (2kcal/g).

To calculate the Calories we will consider the following factors: Fiber: 2kcal/g.

However, this decision is very controversial because, although the FAO document indicates that value, this is for a mixed diet. The same document states that this depends on the degree of fermentation, in the case of a non-fermentable fiber the value should be considered 0 Kcal/g.18.

If there is not a method for measuring the fermentability of the fiber, it is advised to keep the value of 0 kcal/g, and only increase it if you know the degree of fermentation, so the Argentine Food Code stipulates a value of 0 kcal, as reported in the following paragraph.

Argentine Food Code

Section 1385: Fiber means any edible material that is not hydrolyzed by the endogenous enzymes of the human digestive tract.

To calculate the Calories we will consider the following factors:

- Fiber: 0 Kcal/g.

Article 1386: modified food means the fiber added to those products must be covered by this Code and in the future incorporate the National Health Authority. Must contain a minimum of dietary fiber:

3g/100g solids and 1g/100 ml liquid (Argentine Food Code, 2013).

The definitions represent the latest decisions taken on the subject, so there is remarkable controversy generated by the difference of monomers nine to CODEX and three EU as a lower limit for the Indigestibility of the compounds.We suggest leaving it to the consideration of each country, excluding all the resistant oligosaccharides with between 3 and 10 monomers, among which are most prebiotic compounds such as fructans, GOS or GOS trans.

Committees ILSI ILSI Europe and North America held a Forum at the Ninth Symposium on Fiber Vahouny 2010 to discuss the way in which these issues can be resolved to reach a scientific consensus on the subject. According to the conclusions of this session most experts agreed on maintaining a global consensus on the inclusion of non-digestible HC with> GP3 as FD since no methodological reasons or physiological effects make a difference between the HC with GP 3-9 and> 10 (Howlett et al. 2010).

Physiological Effects of Dietary Fiber

a) At Intestinal Level

Positive effects caused by the ingestion of DF include increasing stool volume, reducing the transit time and the number of bowel movements per day. The analysis of numerous studies on fecal weight gain showed that the effect is variable, according to their source, and established the decreasing order of activity as follows: wheat bran> Fruits and Vegetables> cellulose isolated > pectin. Wheat bran is more effective due to its larger particle size. By keeping the water-retaining structure thus it produced softer stools and accelerates intestinal transit (Gibson et al., 1990). Furthermore, increasing fecal volume and, consequently, the diameter of the colon without increasing the intrinsic tension wall, reduces the pressure required for the propulsion of stool, preventing the formation of diverticula. This property of the DF drew attention to its use in the treatment of irritable bowel syndrome, constipation and diverticulosis, a disease that has a special place in the annals of the fiber, as it was the first disease in which this therapeutic effect was observed.

The majority of polysaccharides comprising the DF, with a small proportion of the starch, passes through the small intestine without being degraded in the colon but can be metabolized by the bacteria and exert various physiological effects which depend on the interaction with bacteria. The human gut microflora containing 10^{10}-10^{11} cells / g of feces, mainly anaerobic and saccharolytic and its composition depends on the individual characteristics of the intestine. Most fermentable fibers can produce increasing fecal weight, to some degree, due to an increase in daily bacterial mass excretion. Soluble fibers are the most fermentable and it was observed that the DF of carrots, peas (peas) and cabbage is digested in 80 to 93%, while the wheat bran fermented between 30 and 50% and barely reaches cellulose 6% (Nordgaardet al., 1995).

Other beneficial effects especially related to the fermentation of DF include:

- Encourage the resistance to colonization by pathogenic bacteria and viruses, by competition with normal flora abundant with the prevailing lactic acid bacteria (Goñi 2005).
- Exert a protective effect on the colon, especially through a dilution effect of the luminal contents, reduces the risk associated with the presence of carcinogens. Also generates fatty acids (FA) protectors, such as butyric acid, by fermentation and acidified decreases in the colonic contents generation of potential tumor promoting agents (American Gastroenterological Association, 2000). A more acidic intestinal content reduces the action of putrefactive bacteria, producing potentially toxic ammonia and nitrosamines. In addition, butyrate is a substrate for the colonocytes, which uses it for its growth and reproduction, helps rebuild the mucosa and protects it. Acetate and propionate are short chain FA through the intestinal wall, heading via blood to the liver and peripheral tissues (Goñi et al., 1996). Lowering the pH of the intestinal content and the concentration of secondary bile acids (deoxycholic, lithocholic) is associated with a decreased risk of colorectal cancer (Kritchevsky, 1995).

b) On the Glycemia and Insulinemia

It was observed that food containing significant amounts of soluble DF such as oats, barley, rye, soybeans, beans and lentils reduces postprandial hyperglycemia and insulin. Due to this property, this food can help improve diabetic control. This effect is explained because the bulk of soluble fibers slow the gastric emptying time. Food with high DF levels has a slow rate of digestion, in particular by the action of water-soluble components comprising the soluble fiber (Bjorck et al., 1994). In addition, the viscosity hinders the diffusion of nutrients to the intestinal epithelium to resist the effects of intestinal contractions of mixing and propulsion of the luminal contents, absorption delaying (Jenkins, 1978, Meier and Gassull, 2004). Another feature that complicates the picture of the cause-effect of DF on glycemia is the role of starch. All foods containing starches exhibit a speed ratio of fast and slow digestion, but not all contain AR. Moreover, some have free glucose which, when added to the rapidly digestible starch, constitutes the indicator called "rapidly available glucose" (Englyst et al., 1999). Therefore, food speaks fast or slow digestion when characterized by the highest proportion of starches in that category. If the distribution is homogeneous, they are classified as intermediate speed.

Quickly absorbed foods such as low molecular weight dextrins, maltose, sucrose, mashed potatoes and white bread, which show a rapid digestion of its starch, produces high glycemic and insulinemic responses (Englyst et al., 1999; Roberts, 2000; Araya et al., 2002). Thereafter there is a rapid decrease in both blood parameters values leading to levels lower than baseline (Ludwig, 2000).

c) Fiber and Cancer

Regarding the relationship between fiber and cancer the evidence is conflicting, although some studies showed an indirect relationship between fiber intake and the risk of certain cancers such as breast cancer. In a meta-analysis of 10 cohort studies of fiber and cancer, there was an 11% decrease in cancer risk between the highest and lowest quartiles of fiber intake (Dong et al., 2011). As to the relationship between fiber intake and risk of colorectal cancer (CRC), the results are still contradictory studies. Since the 1970s there have been many epidemiological studies. Burkitt raised the hypothesis that DF decreased the CRC risk, based on the observation of rural African populations having a high fiber intake and a lower risk of cancer. General studies with a case-control design show a protective association; while in the cohort studies the results are different (Aune et al., 2011). A cohort study conducted in the Nurses' Health Study (NHS) and the Health Professionals' Follow-up Study (HPFS), which included 76,947 women and 47,279 men, has not found a statistically significant relationship between the two variables (Michels et al., 2005).

In a systematic review that included 13 cohort studies, in which 725,000 people participated, showed that fiber intake was inversely associated with the risk of developing CRC in an analysis adjusted for age, but this effect disappeared after adjusting for other dietary risk factors (folate intake, red meat, milk, alcohol, etc.) (Park et al., 2005).

The protective effect of DF and grain consumption in CRC risk is biologically explicable. Whole foods are important sources of DF and may decrease the risk of CRC by increasing stool bulk, diluting fecal carcinogens, and decreased transit time, which reduces the contact between carcinogens and the colorectal mucosa. Moreover, the DF bacterial fermentation results in the production of SCFA, which may have protective effects against CRC (Auneet al., 2011).

Other components of whole grains may also protect against CRC including antioxidants, vitamins, minerals, phytate, phenolic acids, lignans and phytoestrogens. Whole grains have high folic acid and magnesium levels, which have been independently associated with a reduced risk of CRC (Aune et al., 2011). This effect has been studied in anticarcinogenic colonic level with butyrate, one of the AGCC, which is capable of modulating gene expression and having a regulatory impact on apoptosis, together with propionate protection against the development of cancer in general and in particular CCR. Butyrate is used primarily in the colonic energy source. Ethyl propionate is in greater concentrations to reach the circulation, and is captured 60% by the liver. Thus the antineoplastic effect of the colon transcends propionate, reaching other organs (Hosseini et al., 2011).

d) Fiber and Body Weight Regulation

DF as reducing body weight: The effect of fiber on the utilization of dietary energy, which is related to the promotion of the expression of appetite and satiety, determines the amount of energy consumed. These physiological processes result from the interaction of different types of factors: genetic, cultural and biological. Appetite and satiety mediated by CHO are related to energy regulation and proper body weight. CHO may influence the food intake through the flavor, mastication time, stomach distention, digestibility, absorption rate, hormonal changes and metabolic signals indicating the use of different tissues (Rolls et al., 1997).

There are several observational and interventional studies that show an inverse relationship between consumption of DF, and weight and body fat, considering the usefulness of DF in the prevention and treatment of obesity (Papathanasopoulos and Camilleri, 2010).

Different mechanisms have been proposed:

- DF-rich diets tend to be lower in energy density, without altering the volume, displaces other nutrients and calories available.
- requires more chewing time, limiting intake to promote secretion of saliva and gastric juices resulting in gastric distention and satiety.
- slows gastric emptying generating satiety, and slows the rate of absorption of lipids and glucose, insulin secretion less secondary.

Fermentable fibers, through the formation of peptides modulate propionate such as ghrelin, glucagon-similar peptide (GLP-1) and peptide YY (PYY), lowering the first and increasing the latter. GLP-1 stimulates insulin secretion, whereas PYY delays gastric emptying. In contrast, ghrelin stimulates appetite (Hosseini et al., 2011).

e) Effect on the Bioavailability of Nutrients

Foods high in phytate-containing DF, oxalates or tannins, such as wheat bran, reduce the bioavailability of nutrients, especially calcium, iron and zinc. This effect would be irrelevant in the case of adults eating nutritionally adequate diets. However, it may constitute a risk in the case of children, especially related to iron and even total caloric intake (Lairon et al., 2003).

f) Prebiotic Effect

The colon is a complex ecosystem, consisting of a delicate balance of beneficial bacteria and other pathogenic effect strains capable of generating toxins and carcinogens. Among the beneficial bacteria are bifidobacteria and lactobacilli. When these bacteria preferential substrates, fructans contribute to the health of the host, through the intestinal pH decrease little tolerated by bacteroides, which are not a conducive environment for proliferation. The health benefits attributed to bifidobacteria include inhibition of growth of harmful bacteria, stimulation of immune system components, better absorption of certain ions, such as calcium, and the synthesis of vitamins B (Niness, 1999). The bifidogenic effect, which causes positive changes in the composition of the microflora has been shown in vivo in humans eating doses between 5 and 20g/day, generally over a period of 15 days (Gibson and Roberfroid, 1995).

Inulin and FOS have been termed prebiotics (Gibson and Roberfroid, 1995), i.e., "non-digestible ingredients of foods that selectively stimulate the growth and/or activity of intestinal bacteria that promote health." They are often used in combination with probiotics or live bacteria that are added to the diet to promote health. The pre and probiotic combinations have synergistic effects and are called symbiotic.

Indigestibility of fructans in the upper gastrointestinal tract is the basis of their reduced caloric value compared to their monosaccharide components. As mentioned above, in the colon flora AG becomes a short chain by the action of bacteria, which contributes to metabolize energy of the host. The energy value estimated for both insulin and FOS is 1.5 kcal of useful energy (Roberfroid, 1999).

Due to their resistance to hydrolysis, fructose and glucose molecules that make up the FOS appears in portal blood when they are ingested orally and have been found to be suitable for consumption by diabetics (Roberfroid, 2000). Inulin has a long history of use by diabetics and in fact, high dose benefits are reported (40-100g/day) (Niness 1999). The studies draw attention to a significant reduction of glycemia in insulin-dependent diabetics; a 2 weeks treatment with 8 g of FOS (sucrose) also decreased total cholesterol and LDL (Yamashita et al., 1984).

The potential effect of FOS on glucose and lipid levels based on the hypothetical effect of colon AG produced during fermentation can influence the metabolism of lipids and CHO (Alleset al., 1999). The effects of fructans on glycemia and insulin are not yet fully elucidated, and the available data are contradictory, indicating that these effects may depend on physiological conditions (fasting state compared with post prandial) or diseases (e.g. diabetes).

Studies on the effect of the consumption of fructans on lipid metabolism point to a decrease in blood triglycerides (Brighenti, 2007), while the effect on the reduction of cholesterol is more evident in hypercholesterolemic subjects. Oral administration of 7g/day of inulin in individuals with obesity and dyslipidemia decreased concentrations of total cholesterol, LDL, VLDL and triglycerides (Balcazar et al., 2003). This is due to the decrease of de novo lipogenesis in the liver, whereas decreasing colonic pH causes deconjugation and removal of bile acids and cholesterol utilization for the synthesis of new bile acids. It is also noted that the presence of propionate could interfere with the formation of cholesterol in the liver (Jackson et al., 1999). To interpret the results of human studies it is necessary to consider a number of factors, such as the duration of treatment, CHO intake compared with lipid and serum lipid composition at the beginning of treatment.

The effect of fructans on mineral absorption has been studied (Ohta et al., 1998). Lowering the pH of the colon by fermentation, the production of short chain FA and the increase in calbindin protein concentration in the colon have been hypothesized to explain this effect. Increasing the bioavailability of calcium in rats has shown that feeding FOS calcium concentration increases and improves bone structure. It has also been demonstrated in rats that inulin growth increases mineral content and bone density (Roberfroid, 2002). The administration of a diet containing 16.8 g of FOS or inulin 40 g, increases calcium absorption by 12% and 11%, respectively (Coudray et al., 1997, Van den Heuvel et al., 1999). A mixture of inulin and FOS (8 g) increased calcium absorption in girls near menarche and in women with more than six years of menopause, with adequate or high calcium intake without a compensatory increase in urinary excretion calcium, suggesting that these ingredients may affect the absorption of calcium in the prolonged postmenopausal phase (Tahiri et al., 2003). Different results were obtained using FOS with degree of polymerization GP4, inulin GP25, or a mixture of both (50% each), and branched-chain inulin at a level of 10% in adult rats on experimental diets for 28 days (Coudray et al., 2003). All compounds studied increased intestinal absorption and balance of calcium, but it was only significant for the mixture of FOS and inulin HP. This effect is explained by the fermentation produced throughout the colon, the lower degree of polymerization of the first fermentation, whereas inulin of polymerization was more fermented in the distal colon. The results provide promising evidence that inulin and FOS increase the absorption of calcium, magnesium and iron in humans (Coudray et al., 1997, 2003).

The increase of Bifidobacteria caused by consumption of inulin and FOS fermentation is responsible for more benefits than that produced by proteolytic bacterioas, which cause genotoxins detoxification in the intestine, production of AG intestinal pH decreases, thus creating a bactericidal to the enteric environment such as E coli and Clostridium perfringens. Developing a favorable microenvironment may also involve modulation of bacterial enzymes. Butyric acid has a protective effect on the colonic mucosa, increasing the proliferation of normal cells and causing increased secretion of mucin, a barrier that can protect epithelial cells from attack by reactive compounds (Pool-Zobel et al., 2002).

Whole Grains

The FDA defines whole grains as the intact grain, ground or rolled, the main components, endosperm, germ and bran, are present in the same proportions as in the intact grain.

Among the commonly used whole grains are wheat, oats, barley, brown rice, corn, rye, millet, sorghum, triticale, amaranth, buckwheat and quinoa (Jonnalagadda et al., 2011).

Evidence of the benefits of eating whole grains:

- Consuming 3 or more servings of whole grains per day is associated with lower BMI, lower abdominal adiposity and a trend toward less weight gain over time. However, evidence is inconsistent regarding weight loss.
- Reduced risk of heart disease and death secondary to it, lower risk of hypertension, and reduced progression of atherosclerotic lesions.
- It has been shown to reduce plasma lipid levels, including the low-density lipoprotein (LDL Low-density lipoprotein), the results of the studies are variables.
- Improved insulin sensitivity with lower fasting insulin levels and the area under the insulin curve 2 hours post ingestion, and less risk of DBT 2.
- Reduced risk of colorectal cancer and improvement of gastrointestinal immune response.

These effects have been attributed to the presence of vitamins, minerals, DF, lignin, beta-glucans, insulin, phytosterols, and numerous phytochemicals, many of which are present in the germ and bran of the grain, and processing typically loses some of them (Jonnalagadda et al., 2011). According to FDA regulations, a product must contain at least 51% whole grains in order to receive that designation. (U.S. Food and Drugs Administration).

Consumer Recommendations

Various institutions dealing with public health in countries like the United States, Canada, England, Sweden, Norway and Denmark recommend, for adults, an increase in food fiber intake through contributors such as vegetables/legumes, fruits and whole grains, or ingesting more supplements. Current recommendations of dietary fiber (DF) for adults are in the range of 25 to 30 g/day, or 10 and 13 g/1000 kcal, with a ratio of DF insoluble/DF soluble than 3/1 (FAO, 2003).

There is still no consensus on the caloric value of the fiber. It is now considered not to provide energy, but it raises some fermentable fibers contributing between 1 and 2 kcal/g, from the short chain FA produced by the fermentation. When creating a balanced diet with adequate fiber proportion, it should be noted that not only cereals are rich in it. DF in fruit has a more balanced composition that grain and a higher proportion of soluble fiber, so it has a greater capacity to retain water. Also, as previously mentioned, grains contain phytic acid in varying amounts, and this can affect the bioavailability of certain minerals.

Labeling: Health Claims

In our country the inclusion of health claims (Health Claims) in the labeling of food is not yet permitted.

The EFSA has completed its study of the health claims of more than 2,758 substances that the food industry has used or wants to use to advertise their products. The result is devastating: almost 80% were not scientifically tested or were too general. The study began in 2008, and the results in relation to health claims and consumption of DF are:

- DF, in amounts greater than 25 g/day, reduces risk of heart disease, DBT 2 and weight control. True. Enough evidence.
- Beta-glucan rye and oats help control cholesterol. True. Enough evidence.
- Wheat fiber helps maintain weight or lose weight. False. The studies presented do not prove it.
- Beta-glucan rye and oats increase the feeling of satiety. False. The studies presented do not prove it.
- The FS helps control blood cholesterol. False. The studies presented do not prove it. (EFSA, 2013)

Analytical Methods

Dietary Fiber

The oldest method, whose origins date from the early nineteenth century, is based on a strong acid and alkali treatment, and expressed their results as Crude Fiber (AOAC 962.09). In the last decade other methods to obtain actual data were perfected, and the results differ from those obtained with the previous method by the expression of dietary fiber or dietary (DF), which corresponds to the English name dietary fiber,

1) Gravimetric methods:

   a) Crude Fiber: based on sequential treatment with acids and alkalis in standardized conditions. Unfortunately this method underestimated the real amount of the non-digestible fraction of plant cell walls as pectins, completely losing much of the cellulose, hemicellulose and lignin and all soluble fiber.

Crude fiber values have no relation to the true value of DF of food for humans. DF values are usually 3 to 5 times greater than the values of crude fiber, but a correction factor cannot be applied for the relationship between DF crude fibers, which vary depending on the chemical components. Crude fiber has little physiological significance in human nutrition, and the information should not be used to describe the fiber content of foods (AOAC 962.09).

   b) A neutral detergent method (Van Soest and Wine, 1967) represents the insoluble fraction of the fiber, since treatment with neutral detergent solutions lose soluble polysaccharides,
   c) Enzymatic gravimetric methods: simulating the human digestive process. This exceeded the previous technique, since it determines the total fiber, through modifications, and can differentiate the insoluble soluble fiber (Asp, 1987; Prosky et al., 1988)

2) Colorimetric and chromatographic methods: quantified monomeric constituent fiber. After enzymatic treatment to remove the starch, the residue is fractionated in the soluble and insoluble components, which are then subjected to selective acid hydrolysis to release sugars from non-cellulosic polysaccharides and cellulose. Sugars can be quantified by colorimetric methods or by chromatographic methods (Theander and Westerlund, 1986, Englyst and Cummings, 1988), which are more specific than in the previous case. Uronic acids, pectins components and some thickeners can be measured by colorimetric methods. The sum of the 7 or 8 monomers arise certain results that can be expressed as total fiber, soluble fiber, insoluble fiber, or in some tables, such as non-starch polysaccharides (NSP), non-cellulosic polysaccharides (NCP) and cellulose. Lignin is not included in these values.

Finally, it is worth noting that the method most credited for determining the fiber content of foods is the AOAC 991.43 (AOAC, 2000). However this method does not quantify the fiber as oligosaccharides, perhaps because of their relatively low molecular weight and high solubility in water and alcohol.

Resistant Starch (RS)

The RS includes the latest definitions proposed for fiber, which in many countries is determined by RS and DF Total AOAC 985.29 method. However, its determination is required separately for studies conducted on its functions. During the European program for the study of resistant starch Euresta developed several methods (Champ and Faisant, 1996).

Muir and O´Dea (1992) developed a method of chewing prior to treatment with pepsin, pancreatic amylase and amyloglucosidase.

Finally, Goñi et al., (1996) developed an enzymatic-colorimetric method with pepsin, pancreatic amylase and amyloglucosidase at 37°C, which was the basis of the AOAC method 2002.02.

The *in vivo* method is the most accurate, but presents many challenges for implementation, so it is used only in research because it involves intubation of individuals to collect duodenal contents and the subsequent extent of the same starch content resisted digestion and was not absorbed (Champ et al., 2003).

Fructan

This analysis has gained great interest because of the importance acquired from the point of view of health and, therefore, in the food industry to comply with legal requirements for nutritional labeling, which includes the statement of the energy value, protein, fat, and fiber CHO, fructans from which are part of the soluble fraction. Moreover, it is important to plant analysis to search for new sources of fructans. There is very little information about the content of these compounds in plants, since their identification, separation and quantification have traditionally been incomplete and tedious. The variety of structures, sources and factors that may affect this conformation, greatly hinders the finding of a suitable method. Numerous studies have been devised to measure fructans in plants and products. It is generally accepted that the best route is the hydrolysis of the polymers and the subsequent measurement of generated compounds, so that the results will be influenced by the effectiveness of the methodology and instrumentation with which they are separated and measured (Zuleta & Sambucetti, 2005).

The emergence of new sources of fiber, which are not determined by the official method, since by its low molecular weight are soluble in alcohol and non-digestible oligosaccharides, has led to the development of new methods that already have acceptance by the AOAC.

Conclusion

As described, there are a wide variety of compounds that share the indigestibility criterion so many efforts are made to ensure the definition of the fiber. Moreover, the difficulty is to use a single method for proximate analysis of this fraction, as well as various analytical or physiological criteria and naming, even adopting different researchers. Both the definition and the analytical method used are very necessary from a legal standpoint, in terms of nutritional labeling of food and, from the point of view of health, to have actual data for the design of diets and research. The study of DF has great interest from different points of view, analytical, health or technology, as reflected in the numerous studies on the subject. Heaton (1981) makes it clear why there is still no agreement on the definition of DF and there is still long way to go: "Fiber is not a substance but a concept. *Moreover a number of different concepts in the mind of the botanist, chemist, physiologist, dietitian or gastroenterologist".*

References

AACC (2001). Dietary Fiber Definition Committee of the American Association of Cereal Chemists. The definition of dietary fiber. *Cereal Foods World*, 46, 112-126.

Alles M.S. De Roos N.M., Bakx J.C., Van de Lisdonk E., Zock P.L. & Hautvas J.G. (1999). Consumption of fructooligosaccharides does not favorably affect blood glucose and serum lipid concentrations in patients with type 2 diabetes. *American Journal of Clinical Nutrition*, 69, 64-69.

American Dietetic Association (2008). Health implications of dietary fiber. *Journal of American Dietetic Association*, 108, 1716-1731.

American Gastroenterological Association. (2000). Impact of dietary fiber on colon cancer occurrence. *Gastroenterology*, 118, 1235-1257.

Araya H., Contreras P., Vera G., Alviña M. & Pak N. (2002). A comparison between an *in vitro* method to determine carbohydrate digestion rate and the glycemic response in young men. European *Journal of Clinical Nutrition*, 56, 735-739.

Araya H. & Lutz M. (2003). Alimentos funcionales y saludables. Revista Chilena de Nutrición, 30: 8-14.

Araya H., Vera G., Alviña M. & Pak N. (1998). Nuevas perspectivas acerca de la calidad nutricional de los hidratos de carbono complejos disponibles. *Revista Chilena de Nutrición*, 25, 35-44.

Asp N.G. (1987). Dietary Fiber, definition, chemistry and analytical determination. *Molecular Aspect of Medicine*, 9, 17-29.

Association of Agricultural Chemists (AOAC). (2000). Method 985.29, 944.29.Volume II. 17 h Ed Editor Dr William Hororwitz, Maryland USA.

Aune D., Chan D., Lau R., Vieria R. Greenwood D.C., Kampman E., & Norat T. (2011) Dietary Fiber, whole grains, and risk of colorectal cancer: systematic review and dose-response meta-analysis of prospective studies. *BMJ,* 343:d6617.

Balcázar B.R., Martínez E. & González M. (2003). Efecto de la administración oral de inulina sobre el perfil de lípidos y la sensibilidad a la insulina en individuos con obesidad y dislipidemia. *Revista Médica de Chile*, 131, 59-604.

Bjorck I. Grandfeldt Y., Liljeberg H. Tovar J. & Asp N-G. (1994). Food properties affecting the digestion and absorption of carbohydrates. *American Journal of Clinical Nutrition*, 59 (suppl), 699S-705S.

Brighenti F. (2007). Dietary fructans and serum triacylglycerols: A meta analysis of randomized controlled trials. *Journal of Nutrition*, 137, 2552S-2556S.

Brown I.L. (2004). Applications and uses of resistant starch. *Journal of AOAC International*, 87,727-732.

Champ M. & Faisant N. (1996). Resistant starch. En: Carbohydrates as organic raw materials. Edby F.W. Lichtenthaler, VCH Verlagsgesellschaft, Weinheim, Vol 3: 189-215.

Champ M., Langkilde A.M., Brouns F., Kettlitz B. & Be Bail Collet Y. (2003.) Advances in dietary fibre characterization. 1. Definition of dietary fibre, physiological relevance, health benefits and analytical aspects. *Nutrition Research Reviews*. 16: 71-82.

Cherbut C. (2002). Inulin and oligofructose in the dietary fibre concept. *British Journal of Nutrition*, 87 (Suppl 2), 159S-162S.

Codex Alimentarius, FAO-OMS(2009) Documento CL 2009/3-NFSDU.

Código Alimentario Argentino. Ley 18.284, Decreto 2126/71.www.anmat.gov.ar.

Colonna P. & Mercier C. (1985). Gelatinization and meeting of the maize and pea starches with normal and high-amylose genotypes. *Phytochemistry*. 24, 1667-1674.

Colonna P., Leloup V. &Buleon A. (1992). Limiting factors of starch hydrolysis. *American Journal of Clinical Nutrition*. 46: S17-S32.

Coudray C., Bellange J. & Castiglia-Delahaut C. (1997). Effect of soluble and partly soluble dietary fiber supplementation on absorption and balance of calcium, magnesium, iron and zinc in healthy young men. *European Journal of Clinical Nutrition*, 512: 375-380.

Coudray C., Tressol J.C., Gueux E. & Raysseguier Y. (2003). Effects of inulin-type fructans of different chain length and type of branching on intestinal absorption and balance of calcium and magnesium in rats. *European Journal of Nutrition*, 42: 91-98.

Dong Jia-Yi, Ka He, Peiyu Wang & Li-Qiang Qin. (2011). Dietary fiber intake and risk of breast cancer: a meta-analysis of prospective cohort studies. *American Journal of Clinical Nutrition,* 94, 900-905.

Dreher M. (2001) Dietary Fiber overview. In: Handbook of Dietary Fiber. Cho S.S. & Dreher M., (Eds). Cap 1. Marcel Drekker Inc., New York, pp. 1-17.

EFSA (2013). available in: http://www.efsa.europa.eu

EFSA (2010). Scientific Opinion on Dietary Reference Values for carbohydrates and dietary fibre. *EFSA Journal*; 8(3):1462.

Englyst H.N., Kingsman S.M. & Cummings J.H. (1992). Classification and measurement of nutritionally important starch fractions. European Journal of Clinical Nutrition, 46 (supp): 33S-350S.

Englyst K.N., Englyst H.N. Hudson G.J., Cole T.J. & Cummings J.H. (1999). Rapid available glucose in foods: an *in vitro* measurement that reflects the glycemic response. *American Journal of Clinical Nutrition*, 69: 448-454.

Englyst H.N. & Cummings J.H. (1988). Improved method for the measurement of dietary fiber as non starchpolysacharides in plant foods. *Journal of AOAC International*, 71, 808-814.

FAO/WHO. (1998). Carbohydrates in Human Nutrition: Report of a Joint FAO/WHO Expert Consultation, 14-18 April 1997, Rome. FAO Food and Nutrition Paper No. 66. Chap 4. The role of the glycemic index in food choice.

FAO/WHO. (2003) Expert Consultation: Carbohydrates in human nutrition.

Flatt SP. (1996). Glycogen levels and obesity. *International Journal of Obesity*, 20 (suppl 2): S1-S11.

Gibson G. R., Macfarlane S. & Cummings J. H (1990). The fermentability of polysacharides by mixed faecal bacterias in relation to their suitability as bulk-forming laxatives. Letters in Applied Microbiology.11, 251-254.

Gibson G.R. & Roberfroid M.B. (1995). Dietary modulation of the human colon microbiota. Introducing the concept of prebiotics. *Journal of Nutrition*, 125, 1401-1412.

Goñi I. (2005). Carbohidratos y salud intestinal. In: Carbohidratos en Alimentos Iberoamericanos. Ed Wenzel, Lajolo, Editora da Universidade de São Paulo, Cap12, pp. 287- 307.

Goni I., Garcia-Diz E. Manas E. & Saura-Calixto F. (1996). Analysis of resistant starch: a method for foods and food products. *Food Chemistry*, 56, 4, 445449.

Grandfelt Y. & Bjork I. (1991). Glycemic response to starch in pasta: a study of mechanisms of limited enzyme susceptibility. *Journal of Cereal Science*, 14, 47-61.

Heaton K.W. (1981). Gallstones. In: Trewell H.E, (Ed). Western Diseases: Their emergency and prevention. Cambridge University, UK, pp. 47-59.

Holt S., Brand J., Soveny C. & Hansky J. (1992). Relationship of satiety to postprandial glycemic, insulin and cholecystokinin responses. *Appetite*, 18, 129-141.

Holt S.A. & Brand-Miller J. (1995). Increased insulin responses to ingested foods are associated with lessened satiety. *Appetite*, 24: 43-54.

Hosseini E., Grootaert Ch., Verstraete W. & van de Wiele T. (2011). Propionate as a health-promoting microbial metabolite in the human gut. *Nutrition Reviews*. 69 (5), 245-258.

Howlett J.F., Betteridge V.A., Champ M., Craig A.S., Meheust A. & Julie Miller J.J. (2010). The definition of dietary fiber discussions at the Ninth Vahouny Fiber Symposium: building scientific agreement. *Food & Nutrition Research*, 54: 5750.

Jackson K.G., Taylor G.R., Clohessy A.M. & Williams C.M. (1999). The effect of the daily intake of inulin on fasting lipid insulin and glucose concentrations in middle-aged men and women. *British Journal of Nutrition*, 82: 23-30.

Jenkins D.A. (1978). Dietary fiber and glucose tolerance: importance of viscosity, *British Medical Journal*, 1:1392-1394.

Jonnalagadda S., Harnach L., Liu R.H., McKeown N. Seal C., Luis S. & Fahey G.C. (2011). Putting the whole grain puzzle together: Health benefits associated with whole grains – Summary of American Society for Nutrition 2012 Satellite Symposium. *Journal of Nutrition*, 141(5);1011S-22S.

Krichevsky D. (1995). Epidemiology of fiber, resistant starch and colorectal cancer. *European Journal of Cancer Prevention*, 4, 345-352.

Lairon D., Bertais S., Vincent S., Arnault N., Galan P., Boutron M.C. & Hercberg S. (2003). Dietary fiber intakes and clinical implication in the French Supplementation en Vitamines et Mineraux Antioxidant's (SU.VI. MAX) adult cohort. *Proceeding of the Nutrition Society*, 62: 11-15.

Ludwig DS. (2000). Dietary glycemic index and obesity. *Journal of Nutrition*, 130, 280S-283S.

Meier R. & Gassull M.A. (2004): Consensus recommendations on the effects and benefits of fibre in clinical practice. *Clinical Nutrition*, Suppl 1, 73-80.

Michels K., Fuchs Ch., Giovannucci E., Colditz E., Hunter D., Stampfer M. & Willett W. (2005). Fiber Intake and Incidence of Colorectal Cancer among 76.947 Women and 47.279 Men. *Cancer Epidemiology Biomarkers & Prevention*, 14 (4), 842-849.

Muir J.G. & O'Dea K. (1992). Measurement of resistant starch: factors affecting the amount of starch escaping digestion *in vitro*. *American Journal of Clinical Nutrition*, 56: 123-127.

Niness K.R. (1999). Inulin and Oligofructose: What are they? *American Journal of Clinical Nutrition,* 129 Suppl, 1402S-1406S.

Nordgaard I. Hansen B.S. & Mortensen, P.B. (1995) Digestive processes in the human colon. *Nutrition*, 11, 37-45.

Nyman M. (2002) Fermentation and bulking capacity of indigestible carbohydrates: the case of inulin and oligofructose. *British Journal of Nutrition*, 87, Suppl. 2, S163-S168.

Ohta A., Ohtsuki M., Hosno A., Atachi T., Hara T. & Sakala T. (1998). Dietary fructooligosaccharides prevent osteopenia after gastrectomy in rats. *Journal of Nutrition*, 128, 106-110.

Papathanasopoulos & Camilleri (2010). Dietary fiber supplements: effects in obesity and metabolic syndrome and relationship to gastrointestinal functions. *Gastroenterology*; 138, 65-72.

Park Y., Hunter D.J., Spiegelman D., Bergkvist L., Berrino F., van den Brandt P.A., Buring J.E., Colditz G.A., Freudenheim J.L., Fuchs C.S., Giovannucci E., Goldbohm R.A., Graham S., Harnack L., Hartman A.M., Jacobs D.R. Jr, Kato I., Krogh V., Leitzmann M.F., McCullough M.L., Miller A.B., Pietinen P., Rohan T.E., Schatzkin A., Willett W.C., Wolk A., Zeleniuch-Jacquotte A., Zhang S.M., & Smith-Warner S.A.(2005). Dietaty Fiber Intake and Risk of Colorectal Cancer. A pooled analysis of prospective cohort studies. *JAMA*, 294 (22), 2849-2857.

Pontis H. G. & Del Campillo, E. (1985), Fructans. In: Biochemistry of storage carbohydrates in green plants. Dey, P. M. and Dixon, R. (Eds) London: Academic Press. pp. 205-227.

Pool-Zobel B., van Loo J. Rowland I., Roberfroid M.B. (2002). Experimental evidences on the potential of prebiotics fructans to reduce the risk of colon cancer. *British Journal of Nutrition,* 87 Suppl 2, 273S-281S.

Prosky P., Asp N. G., Schweizer T. F. De Vries, J. W. &Furda, I. (1988). Determination of insoluble, soluble, and total dietary fiber in foods, food products: interlaboratory study. *Journal of AOAC International*, 71,1017-1023.

Prosky L. (1999). Inulin and poligofructose are part of dietary fiber complex. *Journal of AOAC International*, 82, 223-226.

Roberfroid M.B. (1999). Caloric value of inulin and oligofructose. *Journal of Nutrition*, 129, 1436S-1437S.

Roberfroid M.B. (2002). Functional foods: concepts and application to inulin and oligofructose. *British Journal of Nutrition*, 87 Suppl 2, 139S-143S.

Roberts S.B. (2000). High glycemic index foods, hunger, and obesity: Is there a connection? *Nutrition Reviews*, 58, 163-169.

Rolls B.J., Kim S. & Fedoroff I.C. (1990) Effects of drinks sweetened with sucrose or aspartame on hunger, thirst and food intake in men. *Physiology and Behavior*, 48, 19-26.

Sajilata M.G., Singhal R.S., & Kulkami P.R. (2006). Resistant Starch–A Review Comprehensive. *Reviews in Food Science and Food Safety*, 5:1-17 –.

Stubbs J., Mazian N. & Whybrow S. (2001). Carbohydrates, appetite and feeding behavior in humans. *Journal of Nutrition*, 131, 2775S-2781S.

Tahiri M., Tressol J.C., Arnaud J., Bornet F.R.J., Bouteloup-Demage C., Feillet-Coundray C., Brandolini M., Ducros V., Pepin D., Brouns F., Roussel A.M. (2003). Effect of short-chain fructooligosaccharides on intestinal calcium absorption and calcium status in postmenopausal women: a stable-isotope study. *American Journal of Clinical Nutrition*, 77:449-457.

Theander O. & Westerlund, E.A. (1986).Studies on dietary fiber. 3. Improved procedures for analysis of dietary fiber. *Journal Agriculture and Food Chemistry*. 34, 330-336.

Topping D. L., Morell M. K., King R. A. Li ZhongYi, Bird A. R. & Noakes, M. (2003). Resistant starch and health - Himalaya 292, a novel barley cultivar to deliver benefits to consumers. *Starch/Stärke*, 55, 539-545.

Van den Heuvel E.G., Merys T., Van Dokkum W. & Schasfsma, G. (1999). Oligofructose stimulates calcium absorption in adolescents. *American Journal of Clinical Nutrition*, 69, 544-548.

Van Soest P.J. & Wine R.H. (1967). Determination of Plant Cell Wall constituents. *Journal of AOAC International,* 50 (1), 50-55.

Yamashita K., Kawai K., & Itakura M. (1984). Effect of fructo-oligosaccharides on blood glucose and serum lipids in diabetic subjects. *Nutrition Research*, 4, 961-966.

UE , (2008) Union Europea Directiva 2008/100/CE : http://eur-lex.europa.eu

U.S. Food and Drugs Administration (1999). Health Claim Notification for Whole Grain Foods.http://www.fda.gov/Food/LabelingNutrition/LabelClaims/FDAModernizationActFDAMAClaims/ucm073639.htm

Zuleta A. & Araya H. (2009). Hidratos de carbono como ingredientes funcionales, In: Lutz M, León, A, editores. Aspectos nutricionales y saludables de los productos de panificación. Universidad de Valparaíso Editorial, Chile, pp. 52 - 72. ISBN 978-956-214-094-2.

Zuleta. A. & Sambucetti ME (2005). Fructanos: Características Estructurales y Metodología Analítica., Cap. 8, pp. 197-210. In: Carbohidratos en Alimentos Regionales Iberoamericanos. Ed. Franco M. Lajolo y Elizabete Wenzel de Menezes. Editorial de Universidad de Sao Paulo, Brazil.

Index

A

B

C

D

E

F

G

H

I

J

K

L

M

N

O

P

Q

R

S

W

X

Y

Z